PHYSICAL THERAPY
of the GERIATRIC
PATIENT
Second Edition

CLINICS IN PHYSICAL THERAPY
VOLUME 21

PHYSICAL THERAPY of the GERIATRIC PATIENT
Second Edition

Edited by

Osa L. Jackson, PhD, RPT

Associate Professor and Director
Physical Therapy Program
Department of Kinesiological Sciences
School of Health Sciences
Oakland University, Rochester, Michigan
Adjunct Associate Professor
Department of Physical Therapy
School of Health Related Professions
University of Pittsburgh
Pittsburgh, Pennsylvania

CHURCHILL LIVINGSTONE
NEW YORK, EDINBURGH, LONDON, MELBOURNE

Library of Congress Cataloging in Publication Data

Physical therapy of the geriatric patient / edited by Osa L. Jackson.
—2nd ed.
    p. cm.—(Clinics in physical therapy ; v. 21)
    Bibliography: p.
    Includes index.
    ISBN 0-443-08619-2
    1. Physical therapy for the aged. I. Jackson, Osa. II. Series.
RC953.8.P58P48 1989
615.8′2′0846—dc20   89-33721
                                                        CIP

Second Edition © Churchill Livingstone Inc. 1989
First Edition © Churchill Livingstone Inc. 1983

Distributed in the United Kingdom by Churchill Livingstone, Robert
Stevenson House, 1–3 Baxter's Place, Leith Walk, Edinburgh, EH1 3AF,
and by associated companies, branches, and representatives throughout the
world.

Accurate indications, adverse reactions, and dosage schedules for drugs are
provided in this book, but it is possible that they may change. The reader is
urged to review the package information data of the manufacturers of the
medications mentioned.

The Publishers have made every effort to trace the copyright holders for
borrowed material. If they have inadvertently overlooked any, they will be
pleased to make the necessary arrangements at the first opportunity.

Acquisitions Editor: *Linda Panzarella*
Copy Editor: *Kimberly Quinlan*
Production Designer: *Charlie Lebeda*
Production Supervisor: *Christina Hippeli*

Printed in the United States of America

First published in 1989

Contributors

Louis R. Amundsen, RPT, PhD
Director of Graduate Studies, Program in Physical Therapy, Department of Physical Medicine and Rehabilitation, College of Health Sciences, University of Minnesota, Minneapolis, Minnesota

Carl I. Brahce, PhD
Adjunct Professor, Department of Community Health Sciences, Northeastern Ohio Universities College of Medicine, Rootstown, Ohio; Adjunct Professor, Department of Education, Kent State University; Director, Gerontology Center, Kent State University, Kent, Ohio

Dennis J. Chapron, MS
Associate Clinical Professor, School of Pharmacy, University of Connecticut, Storrs, Connecticut; Assistant Director, Pharmacokinetics Laboratory, University of Connecticut Health Center, Farmington, Connecticut

Corinne T. Ellingham, RPT, MS
Assistant Professor, Program in Physical Therapy, Department of Physical Medicine and Rehabilitation, College of Health Sciences, University of Minnesota, Minneapolis, Minnesota

Sue R. Hardy, OTR
Formerly Staff Occupational Therapist, Maryland General Hospital, Baltimore, Maryland

Masayoshi Itoh, MD, MPH
Associate Professor, Department of Clinical Rehabilitation Medicine, New York University School of Medicine; Associate Director, Department of Rehabilitation Medicine, Goldwater Memorial Hospital, New York University Medical Center, New York, New York

Osa L. Jackson, PhD, PT
Associate Professor and Director, Physical Therapy Program, Department of Kinesiological Sciences, School of Health Sciences, Oakland University, Rochester, Michigan; Adjunct Associate Professor, Department of Physical Therapy, School of Health Related Professions, University of Pittsburgh, Pittsburgh, Pennsylvania

Rosalie H. Lang, MA
Consultant to non-profit health, human service, and arts organizations, Orcas Island, Washington

Mathew H. M. Lee, MD, MPH
Professor, Department of Clinical Rehabilitation Medicine; Clinical Professor, Departments of Oral and Maxillofacial Surgery; and Clinical Professor, Departments of Behavioral Sciences and Community Health, New York University School of Medicine and New York University School of Dentistry; Director, Department of Rehabilitation Medicine, Goldwater Memorial Hospital, New York University Medical Center, New York, New York

Nancy L. Mace, MA
Consultant, Office of Technology Assessment, United States Congress, Washington, D.C., and Consultant, Alzheimer's Association, Baltimore, Maryland

David A. Peterson, PhD
Associate Dean, Andrus Gerontology Center, University of Southern California, Los Angeles, California

Barrie Pickles, BPT, MS, MCSP, MCPA
Professor, Departments of Rehabilitation Medicine and Physical and Health Education, Queen's University Faculties of Medicine and Arts and Sciences, Kingston, Ontario, Canada

Peter V. Rabins, MD, MPH
Associate Professor, Department of Psychiatry, and Director, T. Rowe and Eleanor Price Teaching Service, Johns Hopkins University School of Medicine, Baltimore, Maryland

Kenneth Solomon, MD
Associate Clinical Professor of Geriatric Psychiatry, Department of Psychiatry, University of Maryland School of Medicine; Chief, Geriatric Psychiatry Inpatient Unit, Sheppard and Enoch Pratt Hospital, Baltimore, Maryland

Preface

Rehabilitation and physical therapy techniques were developed at a time when the patient over the age of 70 was not only uncommon, but also usually not considered a candidate for rehabilitation or physical therapy. Today, the majority of patients seen in hospitals are over the age of 55; the average age of nursing home patients is 80 or higher; and the number of persons over the age of 65 is projected to continue to increase for at least the next 25 years. We are now compelled to increase the functional level of these older people in our rehabilitation programs, and in *Physical Therapy of the Geriatric Patient*, second edition, we hope to show our students and colleagues effective means through which the older person can gain functional independence.

At the age of 60 and above, a person embarks on a stage in life that presents enormous challenges for adaptation. At this stage, deaths of loved ones and role changes are normal events that require support in the best of circumstances. However, when a person over 60 becomes ill, that person needs an even greater understanding from the health care team. The health care professional who recognizes and acknowledges that an older patient is capable of responding to physical therapy at a level above the obvious potential will enjoy working with the patient and the success that results. This effective response is made possible through the emotional, cognitive, physical, social, and environmental resources that are available to the patient, and through the basic concepts and principles of geriatric rehabilitation mastered and communicated effectively by the health care team.

In this edition we present those patient resources and those basic concepts and principles, as well as presenting ways of effective interaction, as we introduce the reader to the basic applied science of normal aging, the medical and functional problems common in the elderly, and the implications for therapeutic intervention. We have sought to present the unique manifestations of physical, psychological, sociologic, and environmental adaptation commonly seen in patients of advanced age. While we have tried to be comprehensive, we have not attempted to be a forum for original research.

Chapter 1 examines the demographics of the aged population and the degenerative medical problems common in these patients. Also discussed are the implications of the changing demographics for the structure and process of rehabilitation for the elderly.

Chapter 2 assumes the reader has a working knowledge of normal physiology, and from that point of view presents a brief review of those aspects (connective tissue, bone, muscle, nerve, hormone) that are commonly altered with advanced age. It then describes the most relevant physiologic changes seen in advanced aging and the implications of these changes for clinical intervention.

Chapters 3, 4, and 5 present an overview of normal cognitive function versus altered function in the elderly. Learning styles of the older adult are compared with those of younger persons in learning new psychomotor and cognitive skills, and the rationale for the specific modifications necessary in the clinical assessment of aging patients with normal and common abnormal psychological changes is given. The authors discuss the most common psychological dysfunctions that interfere with positive rehabilitation (depression, Alzheimer's disease, pseudodementia), and the modes of supportive intervention and environmental manipulation that will promote the most successful rehabilitation in these patients.

Medicinal metabolism in the geriatric patient is discussed in Chapter 6. The author describes the common physiologic side effects of drugs that may present an obstacle to successful rehabilitation, as well as ways to differentiate those symptoms that can be corrected or minimized by an adjustment of dosage, route, or timing.

The vulnerability of emotional resources in the face of acute or prolonged illness is discussed in Chapter 7. The common patterns of interaction between patient, family, meaningful others, and acquaintances are discussed, and descriptions are given of family orientation and education programs that will help promote an environment for healing in both the patient and those around him or her.

Chapter 8 discusses the potential of the aging patient in an exercise training program to improve cardiopulmonary function, and the modifications necessary to ensure the highest rate of success in older patients.

In Chapter 9 we bring the theory into practice by examining the normative functional changes seen in the elderly who are now at ages 65 to 74, 75 to 84, and over 85, and the most common functional problems noted in each age category. We discuss the relationship of functional status in each age group with the ability to determine the elderly who are at risk of institutionalization, and the evaluation of major acute and chronic problems. Two assessment approaches are presented: one for use by the rehabilitation team to organize care of the elderly, and the other for the detailed assessment of functional skills.

I want to thank William McGrane of the Self-Esteem Institute in Cincinnati, Ohio, for his pioneering work in therapeutic language derived from the psycholinguistics of interaction. In the hands of the therapist, this new tool provides the older patient with clear, supportive communication that encourages self-determination and motivation. It is this communication concept that has provided the basis for the presentation of material in this second edition.

I am deeply grateful to Dr. Otto Payton for giving me the opportunity to present this text in its second edition and to the contributing authors who gave of their precious time to write insightful and practical chapters. I am also grateful to Dr. Moshe Feldenkrais, who through his understanding of the human spirit and neurophysiology, has helped me to organize my thinking about the rehabilitation and physical therapy modalities that are needed if we are to be truly supportive of each individual in his or her efforts to attain maximum independence and satisfaction with life.

We hope that this text will help the student and the clinician to examine current rehabilitation and physical therapy practices, to modify these practices toward more successful geriatric rehabilitation, and to strive toward the goal of *independent living* for these geriatric patients.

Osa L. Jackson, Ph.D., P.T.

Contents

1 | Rehabilitation for the Aged

Masayoshi Itoh
Mathew H. M. Lee

Improvements in medical surgical technology and public health have dramatically increased life expectancy. In 1900 only 4 percent of the United States population was age 65 or over, but by 1980 this figure had increased to 11 percent. It is projected that by the year 2030 more than 50 million people, or 17 percent of the total United States population, will be in this age group.[1]

For the most part, the aged are men and women who worked and sacrificed all their lives to maintain our society, to improve our standard of living, and to assure the future of our children. The elderly in Eastern cultures may enjoy respect for their wisdom and recognition for their contributions to society, whereas in the United States, the view of the elderly is unclear and seems dependent on individual circumstances as to how much they are either respected or recognized.

In recent years our youth have been surrounded by subliminal messages suggesting that there is something so wrong or distasteful about aging that it either should not be seen or should be regarded as a joke. Movies present children, teenagers, and young adults in the leading roles, but since John Wayne died, we seldom see an elderly hero in films. Television has portrayed the elderly as fatuous and insane, while mimicking their physical and functional limitations. In neither medium are the elderly portrayed in such a way as to promote appreciation and respect. Advertisements consistently stress youth and the necessity for superficial youthfulness. The clothing, food, and home products industries rarely use a middle-aged or elderly model in the promotion of their wares. Acceptable elderly role models are scarce in the media. Euphemisms such as "senior citizen" and "golden ager" are merely compensatory; they do not change many of the negative attitudes now held by the young population.

Those who engage in clinical medicine, particularly rehabilitation, are finding an ever-increasing elderly population who become ill and disabled. So-called geriatric rehabilitation is becoming a large part of the daily practice in the field of rehabilitation. If one is to provide meaningful and supportive rehabilitation services to the aged, stereotyped concepts must be abandoned. Every effort must be made to understand value systems, life-styles, and the individual problems of each elderly person.

One of the pitfalls in the scientific discussion is the loose use of a term or terms. Rusk's[2] definition of rehabilitation, "the ultimate restoration of a disabled person to his maximum capacity—physical, emotional, and vocational," seems to be comprehensive enough and has been universally accepted. It is interesting, however, to examine this definition. There are two key phrases, "ultimate restoration" and "maximum capacity." If the emphasis is placed on *restoration,* then the goal of the rehabilitation is to bring the functional capacity to the premorbid level. If the patient was not functioning at maximum capacity premorbidly, then successful rehabilitation services may achieve a goal higher than restoration. Rehabilitation may make a person as good as before or better than before. If the patient is adult or aged, the former goal may be applicable. If the patient is a child, adolescent, or young adult, the latter may be more appropriate.

In the field of gerontology and geriatrics, the most ill-defined word is "aged" or "elderly." While evaluating a healthy 50-year-old male traumatic above-knee amputee, a very young resident physician from a developing nation stated, "This patient is too old to have an above-knee prosthesis." His statement astonished as well as amused us. Perception of "old" depend on each person's cultural and social background. To test this theory, the question "What is your definition of an old person?" was asked of laypersons. Many responded, "A person 65 years of age or older." Until recently the mandatory retirement age was 65, and after the 65th birthday one can receive Social Security benefits. Responders based their answers on the Social Security system rather than on any theory of what constitutes "old." One wonders, now that the mandatory retirement age is 70, what the concept of "old person" will become.

From the womb to death in old age, there are certain benchmarks that divide the epochs of the life of a human being (Fig. 1-1). Such benchmarks as newborn, infant, child, and adolescent cause very little disagreement. Aging is a continuous and cumulative process taking place in humans from conception to death. It is generally agreed that the first two decades of human life is the phase of the productive aging process and that the degenerative aging process commences in the third decade of life. Puberty is generally accepted as the division between childhood and adolescence, but few if any would agree that the climacteric is the division between middle age and old age. There seems to be no universally accepted benchmarks after adolescence.

Certain morphologic and histopathologic degenerative changes that alter one's functional status are commonly found among those who are advanced in age. These degenerative changes are insidious, progressive, and irreversible

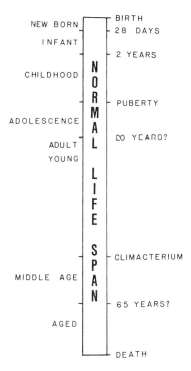

Fig. 1-1. Benchmarks of a normal life span.

and involve multiple organ systems. When many such changes can be detected objectively or subjectively, the individual may be called "aged." If biological or chronological age is used as a basis for defining "old" or "aged," then it is necessary to make qualifying exceptions and explanations. Many well-known statesmen, scientists, artists, and musicians functioned superbly and were completely capable of pursuing high levels of achievement well into the sixth, seventh, or eighth decade of life or beyond.

Once in a great while, the description of a patient in the medical records reads, "This is a 70-year-old white male appearing younger than his age," or even "This is a 70-year-young white male." On the other hand, there are many persons in younger age groups, particularly those who have undergone prolonged physical, emotional, or socioeconomic stress, who exhibit very advanced aging processes. However, such deviations are seldom noted in medical records, perhaps because of stereotypic perceptions of aging in the minds of medical and paramedical professionals.

Another aspect of defining the aged is self-perception. Mortimer Collins said, "A man is as old as he's feeling, a woman as old as she looks." Perhaps the most significant factor that makes a person feel old is the realization that one has some of the characteristics of the aged. Often this comes as a shock even to the older person. The realization may stem from something big or something small. Having to use a cane or wear orthopedic shoes can be just as devastating as recognizing a severe disability. It is vitally important for those who provide care to the elderly to comprehend this psychologically vulnerable state in a patient.

John Godfrey Saxe wrote in his *I Am Growing Old:*

I'm growing fonder of my staff;
I'm growing dimmer in the eyes;
I'm growing fainter in my laugh;
I'm growing deeper in my sighs;
I'm growing careless of my dress;
I'm growing frugal of my gold;
I'm growing wise; I'm growing—yes,—
I'm growing old!

Rollin John Wells in his poem *Growing Old* stated:

A little more tired at close of day,
A little less anxious to have our way;
A little less ready to scold and blame;
A little more care of a brother's name;
And so we are nearing the journey's end,
When time and eternity meet and blend.

These writings vividly describe persons who recognize the changes that imply that death is very near based on changes in their own physical and mental functions. Advanced old age and predeath changes are two distinctly different physiological/psychological experiences as described by Kleemeier. The average person today and especially the health-care provider needs to examine the important differences in these two human experiences.

HEALTH STATUS OF THE AGED

Publilius Syrus, now a relatively obscure writer but in his day a popular writer of maxims in the Roman Empire, first century B.C., said, "Good health and good sense are two of life's greatest blessings." A Greek poet, Simonides of Ceos, in the sixth century B.C. noted in his *Sextus Empiricus:* "There is no joy in beautiful wisdom, unless one have holy health." The Scottish essayist and philosopher Thomas Carlyle stated in 1838: "Ill-health of body or of mind, is defeat. . . . Health alone is victory. Let all men, if they can manage it, contrive to be healthy." Health and ill health have been a great concern of the human race for centuries. Numerous writings related to this subject can be found throughout the literature of many cultures.

The most quoted and widely accepted concept of health is the definition by the World Health Organization (WHO):[3] "A state of complete physical, mental, and social well being and not merely the absence of disease or infirmity." Although no one disputes this definition of health, one may wonder if such a condition exists. The existence of a state of complete physical well-being is conceivable; the term *mental* implies in this context not only mental but also emotional and psychological. Today, the average intelligent person is concerned about local, national, and international politics; war and peace; future environmental safety; violence and crime, and so on. Thus, in our contemporary society the state of a complete feeling of mental well-being may need to be worked for consciously in order to be achievable. Social well-being includes economic and vocational components. In view of current national and international economic conditions, there are ongoing changes resulting in economic problems and unemployment. Thus, presently, attainment of perfect health as defined by WHO can be equated to a search for the fountain of youth or immortality.

Therefore it seems to be more appropriate in this chapter to discuss the different aspects of physical health. It is presumed however, that there is a direct interplay between physical health and emotional well being—that is, the degree to which people have a sense of control over their lives and a joyful acceptance of the gift of each day with the opportunities that present themselves.

Rogers[4] developed a conceptual model of human health. This model recognizes five levels or states of health, *Optimum Health* being one extreme and *Death* being the other (Fig. 1-2). Assuming the total sum of health to be a constant, Optimum Health represents complete presence of health and Death represents total absence of health. Optimum Health is the physical health that WHO defined.

However, there is a state that is not Optimum Health but is a state with "absence of disease or infirmity." This particular state is called *Suboptimum Health*. The majority of the aged are in this state of health owing to arteriosclerotic, osteoarthritic, or osteoporotic changes that accompany aging, even though they may be asymptomatic.

The state of *Overt Illness* or *Disability* is usually recognizable. However, illness that has an insidious onset, such as multiple sclerosis, or Parkinson's disease, may be difficult to detect until the overt symptoms appear.

Despite the increase in knowledge and understanding of disease processes and the improvement of diagnostic and therapeutic techniques, a disease may progress to a point that threatens life. This state is called *Approaching Death*. Cardiac pacemakers, cardiac bypass surgery, organ transplantation, hemodialysis, and such techniques may allow those who were in this state of health to return to a relatively normal life in the state of Suboptimum Health. Others in the Approaching Death state can be maintained at this level for weeks, months, or even years if all necessary life-support systems are artificially provided. But these efforts to prolong life or postpone death often become the subject of medicolegal, religious, or ethical controversy. Finally, every man and woman reaches the state of Death. Death by definition is absolute and irreversible. But with effective cardiopulmonary resuscitation, many people previously considered to be dead are returned to the state of Approaching Death.

Once it was thought that a human life begins at birth and terminates at

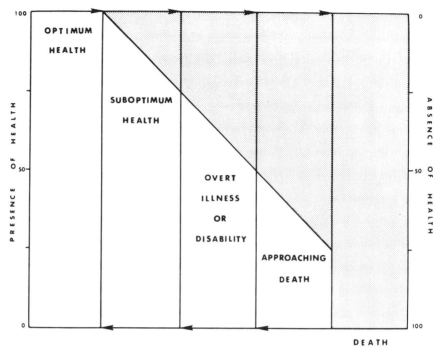

Fig. 1-2.   Health status scale. (Modified from Rogers,[4] with permission.)

death. In recent years there have been fierce debates over the time a human life starts. It is universally agreed that some form of life starts at the time of conception, and two cells, ovum and sperm, eventually become a human being. A dewdrop on a leaf on a high mountain cannot be called an ocean, although this dewdrop may eventually become a part of an ocean. By the same reasoning, not by any stretch of the imagination can these two cells be called a human being. There seems to be little disagreement in the medical community that a human life starts when the oxygen supply to the body enters through the lungs and ceases to pass through the umbilical cord. The basis of the "when life begins" controversy is perhaps more of an emotional, religious, or legal conflict than a scientific one.

Similarly, there have been disagreements as to the point at which a human being is considered dead. Customarily, death is pronounced when all vital functions cease or no vital signs can be detected. However, with the development of artificial life-support systems, we are able artificially to maintain cardiopulmonary functions, nutritional requirements, and electrolyte and fluid balance. To refine the definition of death, the concept of brain death was introduced. If the electroencephalogram, which is a record of brain activity, shows a flat line, brain death is pronounced, even though the electrocardiogram can register cardiac activity because of the use of life-support equipment. In many states, after confirmation of brain death by two physicians and if the family consents, it is legal to remove body organs for organ transplantation. On the other hand, under the same circumstances, if medical practitioners turn off the artificial life-support systems, they may face criminal prosecution. One thus recognizes that there is no longer one simple definition of death in contemporary medical practice. There is great need for a reappraisal of the definition of death, but one can assume that as science discovers additional means to nullify death other disagreements or problems will arise.

In the Rogers' Health Status model,[4] no human condition remains static at any level of health for a prolonged period. It constantly changes in either direction, down to Approaching Death or up to Optimum Health. The changes of the health status toward Death is a natural process similar to the skier being pulled down the mountain slope by gravity. On the other hand, raising of the health status toward Optimum Health may require a conscious effort. The extent of that effort depends on the person's health classification. If a human is in Suboptimum Health, simple rest may suffice, but for one in the state of Approaching Death rigorous and sometimes heroic medical and/or surgical intervention may be required, similar to the skier at the bottom of the mountain who uses a ski lift to return to the peak, representative of Optimum Health.

The Rogers' Health Status Scale was devised to apply to the general population and not to a particular subgroup of the population, such as the aged. However, the Rogers model, demonstrating fluidity in human health status, is applicable to the aged. As has been stated, degenerative aging processes begin in the third decade of human life. These processes are natural, inevitable, progressive, cumulative, and irreversible. Such cumulative effects may become clinically more evident in the sixth decade of life. Obviously, these aging degenerative changes do not affect all organ systems equally. Such changes may be discovered as incidental findings in a clinical investigation of a totally unrelated physical problem. Nevertheless, it is reasonable to assume that the health status of those who reach the sixth and subsequent decades of life are at best in Suboptimum Health. Currently, medical science has no known method to restore the aged to the level of Optimum Health. Thus the scope of the health status for the aged is more limited and narrower than that of the younger population.

SUSCEPTIBILITY OF THE AGED

In the early twentieth century, Stallybrass[5] defined epidemiology as "the science which considers infectious diseases—their course, propagation, and prevention." Welch[6] defined epidemiology as "a study of the natural history of disease," and Lilienfeld[7] described it as "the distribution of a disease or condition in a population and of the factors that influence this distribution." Sartwell and Last[8] defined it simply as "the study of the distribution and dynamics of disease in populations."

As the evolution of definitions of epidemiology indicates, the focus of this branch of medicine now encompasses communicable diseases and all types of diseases as well as physical and mental disabilities.[9] Clinical medicine, and geriatrics in particular, has dealt with each disease entity of the aged from etiology to treatment. Epidemiologic investigations into the problems of the aged also probe to find the developmental processes of a specific condition, disease, or disability. This is the first step toward a scientific approach to limitation and prevention. Such epidemiologic investigation and analyses employ the same conceptual approach and methodology that is always used to study communicable diseases.

The first consideration in epidemiology is the host and the host's susceptibility. The word "susceptibility" was derived from the Latin word *suscipere,* meaning to receive or undertake. In general use susceptible means "easily affected emotionally" or "having a sensitive nature or feelings." *Dorland's Medical Dictionary* defines susceptible as "not having immunity to an infectious disease and thus at risk of infection." Immunity is generally regarded as the capacity of a person, when exposed to infection, to remain free of illness or infection.[8] For example, all human races are susceptible to *Borreliota variolae,* which causes smallpox, unless they have been vaccinated recently. A human who is vaccinated loses susceptibility and gains immunity to variola. Immunity is security against a particular disease or poison. Specifically, it is the power a person sometimes possesses naturally or acquires to resist and/or overcome an infection to which most people are susceptible.

Susceptibility and immunity are two opposite host reactions to a disease. Immunity and susceptibility, however, seldom are considered as absolute states. When one is discussing the presence or absence of susceptibility, it is almost the same as discussing the absence or presence of immunity (Fig. 1-3).

If a given population is highly susceptible to a disease or condition, that particular group of people is considered to be a high-risk population. It is commonly known that a majority of the aged are least susceptible to the common childhood diseases such as rubella, varicella, and pertussis. This is because most of the aged had these diseases in their childhood and developed active immunity. Statistics show that the aged are less susceptible to highway traffic accidents than adolescents or young adults but more susceptible to automobile accidents as pedestrians. The former is probably due in part to their maturity—they avoid speeding and alcoholic consumption or drug abuse. Thus in this case the aged as drivers are a lower risk population. Pedestrian accidents may be explained by such factors as visual and/or auditory disabilities, kinesthetic disturbance, incoordination, slowed reflex time, and medication side effects causing a variety of symptoms including those just listed. The visual disability in this case is not hyperopia but possibly a condition such as senile immature cataract. Central or conduction deafness is the common hearing problem of the aged. Kinetic abnormalities, incoordination, and retarded reaction time may be the result of neurovascular degeneration. A study in Gothenburg, Sweden, indicated that the incidence of fatal pedestrian accidents was about four times higher in an elderly group, 65 years or older, than in a group aged 5 to 14 years.[10] Another study[11] showed no women and only 20 percent of healthy men aged 80 years were able to walk at a speed of

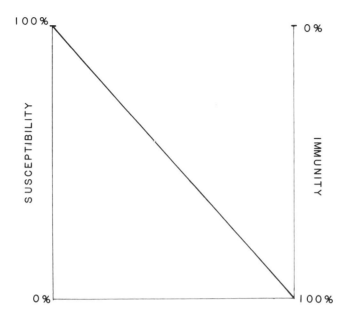

Fig. 1-3.   Relationship between susceptibility and immunity.

1.4 m/sec, which is necessary to cross the street at intersections regulated by traffic lights in the city of Gothenburg. Aged pedestrians therefore are a high-risk population because their age-related functional abilities make them most susceptible to accidents while walking. It is likely that aged persons subject to these disabilities do little if any driving.

It has been stated that the health status of the aged is at best Suboptimum Health owing to the presence of degenerative aging processes. Each degenerative change may cause a specific disease condition. For example, arteriosclerosis, one of the most common degenerative aging changes, may eventually result in arteriosclerotic heart disease or myocardial infarction. On the other hand, cerebral arteriosclerosis may contribute to the development of parkinsonism or senile dementia. However, these conditions can hardly be called symptoms of arteriosclerosis, but those who have arteriosclerosis are indeed increasingly susceptible to such diseases.

A multiplicity of degenerative changes associated with aging may increase the susceptibility of the aged to a variety of diseases, conditions, and functional changes. One very common traumatic condition among the aged is fracture of the neck of the femur. There are different theories on whether hip fracture is the result of a fall or the cause of a fall.[12] For this discussion we shall assume that hip fracture is the result of a fall.

Visual disability, kinetic abnormalities, and retarded reaction time have been described previously. Other symptoms, such as syncopic episodes and vertigo, are related to neurovascular degeneration and may also cause a falling accident. Because it is not uncommon for the aged to be taking hypotensive, hypoglycemic, or psychotropic medication, it should be noted that these symptoms may be iatrogenic.

Osteoporosis is another well-known degenerative aging process that makes bones brittle. Bones of children are far more resilient than those of the aged. In a fall children may suffer from greenstick fracture of the forearm. The aged in a similar accident may sustain a Colles' fracture, which has almost become the hallmark of the old. Hip fracture is found most often among aged women, and osteoporotic changes are known to be accelerated by postmenopausal hormone imbalance. Osteoporotic processes are also known to take place when there is a lack or absence of stress to bones in all age groups. Weight bearing and isometric muscle contraction are main sources of such stress. Whatever the rationale may be, the aged tend to lead a sedentary life. This sedentariness, often self-imposed, and lack of physical exercise may also contribute to the progression of osteoporosis.

Many environmental factors may be viewed as causative elements for falling accidents. In a given household there may be three generations exposed to the same environment. The grandparents would be less exposed to any hazardous physical conditions in this house, owing to their sedentariness, than the grandchildren, who are physically very active. Nevertheless, the facts show that they (grandmother more than grandfather) are more likely to fall and fracture a hip. This situation indicates that there is also a greater susceptibility to hip fracture among aged females than there is in the younger population.

It is reasonable to assume that the aged are susceptible to certain diseases and conditions and immune to others. This group's specific susceptibility has its origin in degenerative aging changes. While these changes singly can increase susceptibility, in some cases a combination of them may result in a drastic increase in susceptibility. This epidemiologic analysis illustrates the complexity of susceptibility among the aged and is basic to understanding the natural history of disabilities as commonly found in advanced age groups.

DISABILITIES AMONG THE AGED

Edentulous, stooped, with poor vision, hard of hearing, walking with a shuffling gait—a common concept of an old man. Old age is closely associated with disability in the minds of the general public. Various degenerative aging processes can be responsible for the development of disabilities such as hemiplegia, amputation of lower extremities owing to vascular insufficiency, hearing loss, senile cataract, organic brain syndrome, or senile dementia. These disabilities are direct results of disease processes and are often called primary disabilities.

In the daily practice of rehabilitation the major effort is not limited to treatment of these primary disabilities but also includes treatment to prevent the development of secondary disabilities. Secondary disability is defined as disability that does not exist at the onset of primary disability but develops subsequently.[9] Examples of secondary disability include flexion contractures of joints, subluxation of the shoulder joint in hemiplegics, decubitus ulcer, and disuse atrophy of muscles. Development of the secondary disability is closely related to a long-lasting primary disability, resulting in spasticity, flaccidity, imbalanced power in antagonists, hypoesthesia or anesthesia of skin, pain, disuse, or immobilization.

The onset of the primary disability is, in general, acute or sudden, whereas development of secondary disability is often insidious. Flexion contracture of joints in hemiplegics and rheumatoid arthritics may develop over a period of weeks and months. It is not unusual to find an elderly patient with rheumatoid arthritis contracted almost into the fetal position. Such deformities are vivid illustrations of the damage done by long-term illness, pain, lack of proper exercise, neglect, and perhaps self-resignation.

A decubitus ulcer, on the other hand, may develop in a relatively short period. Whereas contracture of a joint causes kinetic functional deficiencies, a decubitus ulcer could result in life-threatening consequences. A person with an extensive ulcer loses a large amount of body fluid and consequently dehydration, electrolyte imbalance, and hypoproteinemia can develop. Nutrition for the elderly is often poor. Subcutaneous fat tissues are depleted, and bony prominences protrude directly under the skin. Diminished activity in sebaceous glands makes the skin of the aged less elastic and drier. These common characteristics are the reason that the elderly with primary disability develop an extremely high susceptibility to decubitus ulcer. From the onset the nutritional condition is precarious; appearance of the ulcer upsets nutritional balance further and creates a vicious cycle to the point of cachexia. At this stage there are often multiple decubiti. Another complication of decubitus ulcer is infection, often with gram-negative organisms. Such infection not only destroys surrounding soft tissue but also causes osteomyelitis. Septicemia due to an infected decubitus ulcer is not uncommon.

Certainly in any age group, a primary disability may alter one's life-style. The sequelae of secondary disability can put an end to one's life-style and to one's life. Susceptibility to secondary disability in the aged, like primary disability, is a consequence of degenerative aging changes.

Rusk's[2] definition of rehabilitation refers to restoration of the total human being. To accomplish this goal, the individual's ability as well as disability must be assessed thoroughly by a group of medical and allied health professionals. Their findings are most often presented in a descriptive and narrative form. To simplify such presentations, methods of rating functional capacity have been devised. Classic examples are the Cardiac Function Classification by the American Heart Association and the Manual Muscle Power Rating by the National Foundation of Infantile Paralysis. These use an ordinal scale with letters or numbers or a combination of the two to indicate the ratings. Whether a letter or number is used, such as F or 3 in muscle-power grading, is immaterial as long as each gradation is clearly defined so that the ratings are reproducible. Nominal scales are more descriptive; however, unless the definitions are exceptionally clear they are often confusing. Nominal scales are frequently used when rating Activities of Daily Living (ADL)—for example, partial independence or minimum assistance.

There are many disability assessment methods, from rather simple ones to lengthy ones, that examine not only physical but psychosocial and vocational factors.[13–17] When a numerical scoring system is used, certain significant factors are weighted. Workmen's compensation uses a weighted percentage system, 100 percent being total disability. Most of these methods focus on the general population; there are very few disability rating systems specifically designed for the aged population.

The PULSES Physical Profile by Moskowitz and McCann[18] is perhaps the earliest method in the literature for evaluation of disabilities in the aged. Each of the six letters in PULSES represents a particular category of human function, and each category is rated on a scale of 1 to 4; normal function according to age is indicated by 1 and poorest function by 4 (Table 1-1).

Table 1-1. PULSES Patient Profile

P. *Physical condition,* including diseases of the vicera (cardiovascular, pulmonary, gastrointestinal, urologic, and endocrine) and cerebral disorders not enumerated in the lettered categories below.
1. No gross abnormalities considering the age of the individual
2. Minor abnormalities not requiring frequent medical or nursing supervision
3. Moderately severe abnormalities requiring frequent medical or nursing supervision yet still permitting ambulation
4. Severe abnormalities requiring constant medical or nursing supervision confining individual to bed or wheelchair

U. *Upper extremities,* including shoulder girdle and cervical and upper dorsal spine
1. No gross abnormalities considering the age of the individual
2. Minor abnormalities, with fairly good range of motion and function
3. Moderately severe abnormalities but permitting performance of daily needs to a limited extent
4. Severe abnormalities requiring constant nursing care

L. *Lower extremities,* including the pelvis and lower dorsal and lumbosacral spine
1. No gross abnormalities, with fairly good range of motion and function
2. Minor abnormalities, with fairly good range of motion and function
3. Moderately severe abnormalities permitting limited ambulation
4. Severe abnormalities confining the individual to bed or wheelchair

S. *Sensory components* relating to speech, vision, and hearing
1. No gross abnormalities considering the age of the individual
2. Minor deviations insufficient to cause any appreciable functional impairment
3. Moderate deviations sufficient to cause appreciable functional impairment
4. Severe deviations causing complete loss of hearing, vision, or speech

E. *Excretory function,* i.e., bowel and bladder control
1. Complete control
2. Occasional stress incontinence or nocturia
3. Periodic bowel and bladder incontinence or retention alternating with control
4. Total incontinence, either bowel or bladder

S. *Status*—mental and emotional
1. No deviations considering the age of the individual
2. Minor deviations in mood, temperament, and personality not impairing environmental adjustment
3. Moderately severe variations requiring some supervision
4. Severe variations requiring complete supervision

(From Moskowitz and McCann,[18] with permission.)

Experience in the Skilled Nursing Facility of Goldwater Memorial Hospital over the past 20 years reveals the extremely high reproducibility of PULSES scores. An attending physician in this facility scores a PULSES profile on each admission and annual physical examination. Comparison of two or more PULSES profiles of a patient clearly illustrates progress or decline over the years. Furthermore, individual PULSES records are adaptable to wall charts or card files to provide a comprehensive record of a group's scores. The Moskowitz[18] and the Goldwater groups have independently developed color-coding systems.

Another approach to assessment of disability in elderly people is to measure the amount of assistance required. Long-Term Care Placement Form–Medical Assessment Abstract (DMS-1) by the New York State Department of Health is an example (Fig. 1-4). Their form DMS-9 (Fig. 1-5) shows the weighted scores of each entry. A total score indicates the amount of nursing care needed. These forms are an administrative tool that determines a patient's eligibility for admission to a long-term care facility and are not designed primarily for disability/functional assessment. However, an experienced reviewer of DMS-1 can visualize the state of the total score. The shortcoming of this form is its ambiguous terminology, which tends to decrease its reproducibility. Studies show that DMS-1 is a reliable method for its original intended purpose.[19,20] In 1986, New York State replaced DMS-1 with the Resource Utilization Groups (RUGs). The purposes of the RUGs are determination of the reimbursement rate for each residential health care facility and of the level of care required for each patient, that is, skilled nursing or health-related facility. Although the RUGs serves its purposes, as a disability assessment scale it is inferior to the DMS-1.

It is likely that more disability assessment methods will be devised for the growing elderly population. Although most of the disability evaluation methods, including PULSES, attempt to express physical and mental disability directly, measurement of other parameters such as emotional support, sense of control, and nursing care needs can also illustrate the scope of physical and mental limitations.

PAIN IN THE AGED

Although almost all people are subject to pain, somehow nagging muscle aches and joint pains are often referred to commonly as being caused by old age. There are no statistical data or research substantiating this belief.

Pain is one of the most difficult pathophysiologic phenomena to define. Pain is human perception or recognition of a noxious stimulus in a part of the body. Crue's definition of pain, "anything the patient said it is,"[21] illustrates the mysterious nature of pain. The mystery is due to our insufficient knowledge and understanding of neurophysiology and neurochemistry. There is a disagreement among experts on transmission and perception of noxious stimulus, and various hypotheses have been advanced. Melzak's gate theory[22] is

NEW YORK STATE DEPARTMENT OF HEALTH
LONG TERM CARE PLACEMENT FORM
MEDICAL ASSESSMENT ABSTRACT
PREDICTOR SCORE

CURRENT PAT. LOCATION
☐ HOSP. ☐ DCF
☐ SNF ☐ HOME CARE
☐ HRF ☐ OTHER
SPECIFY ______

REASON FOR PREPARING FORM
☐ DISCHARGE/TRANSFER TO ______
☐ ADMISSION FROM ______
☐ REVIEW FOR PERIOD FROM ______ TO ______
☐ MEDICAID REVIEW ☐ DEATH
☐ OTHER, SPECIFY ______

PATIENT NAME LAST FIRST M.I. | STREET CITY STATE ZIP | SEX ☐ MALE ☐ FEMALE

PATIENT NUMBERS
S.S. NO. ______
MEDICARE NO. ______
MEDICAID NO. ______
SOC. SERVICE DIST. ______
MEDICAL RECORD NO. ______
ROOM NO. ______

PATIENT DATES
DATE OF BIRTH ______ AGE ______
DATE LATEST HOSP. STAY –
FROM ______
TO ______
DATE THIS ADMISSION ______
RESPONSIBLE PHYSICIAN ______

PROVIDER INFO
NAME ______
ADDRESS ______
MEDICAID NO. ______
MEDICARE NO. ______
DOES PATIENT HAVE PRIVATE INSURANCE?
☐ NO ☐ YES ______

MEDICAL COVERAGE: PATIENT'S CONDITION AND TREATMENT REQUIRING SKILLED SUPERVISION (ALL ITEMS MUST BE COMPLETED)

1. A. DIAGNOSES OCCASIONING CURRENT USE OF SERVICES:
PRIMARY ______
OTHER ______
OTHER ______
OTHER ______
B. NATURE OF SURGERY ______ DATE ______
C. IF PATIENT HAD CVA/MI SPECIFY ______ DATE ______
D. ALLERGIES OR SENSITIVITIES, SPECIFY ______

2. LIST SIGNIFICANT MEDS/INJECTIONS.
(FOR PARENTERAL MEDS ALSO CHECK ITEM 3 A)

MED	DOSE	FREQUENCY	ROUTE

1. A. NURSING CARE & THERAPY (SPECIFY DETAILS IN 3D, 3E OR ATTACHMENT)	FREQUENCY			SELF CARE		CAN BE TRAINED	
	NONE	DAY SHIFT	NIGHT/EVE SHIFT	YES	NO	YES	NO
PARENTERAL MEDS							
INHALATION TREATMENT							
OXYGEN							
SUCTIONING							
ASEPTIC DRESSING							
LESION IRRIGATION							
CATH/TUBE IRRIGATION							
OSTOMY CARE							
PARENTERAL FLUIDS							
TUBE FEEDINGS							
BOWEL/BLADDER REHAB.							
BEDSORE TREATMENT							
OTHER (DESCRIBE)							

B. INCONTINENT
URINE OFTEN* ☐ SELDOM** ☐ NEVER ☐ FOLEY ☐
STOOL OFTEN* ☐ SELDOM** ☐ NEVER ☐

C. DOES PATIENT NEED SPECIAL DIET? NO ☐ YES ☐
IF YES, DESCRIBE ______

*MORE THAN ONCE A WEEK **ONCE A WEEK OR LESS

3. D. Is the patient's condition unstable so that an R.N. must detect/evaluate need for modifications of treatment/care on a daily basis?
NO ☐ YES ☐
If yes, describe instability and specific need for nursing supervision, vital signs ranges, lab values, symptoms, etc.

E. Is there high probability that complications would arise in caring for the patient without skilled nursing supervision of the treatment program on a daily basis?
NO ☐ YES ☐
If yes, describe (a) patient's condition requiring skilled nursing supervision (b) the aggregate of services to be planned and managed in the treatment program. Indicate services needed and potential dangers of complicating clinical factors.

F. Circle the minimum number of days/week of complex skilled nursing supervision:

REQUIRES
0 1 2 3 4 5 6 7

RECEIVES
0 1 2 3 4 5 6 7

DMS–1 (1/77)

Fig. 1-4. New York State Department of Health, Long-Term Care Placement Form. Medical Assessment Abstract (DMS-1).

PATIENT NAME	LAST	FIRST	M.I.		PATIENT S.S. NO.	MEDICAL RECORD NO.	ROOM NO.

4. FUNCTION STATUS	SELF CARE	SOME HELP	TOTAL HELP	CAN NOT	REHAB* Poten.
WALKS WITH OR W/O AIDS					
TRANSFERRING					
WHEELING					
EATING/FEEDING					
TOILETING					
BATHING					
DRESSING					

7. SHORT TERM REHAB. THERAPY PLAN
(TO BE COMPLETED BY THERAPIST)

A. DESCRIBE CONDITION (NOT DX) NEEDING INTERVENTION   SHORT TERM PLAN OF TREATMENT AND EVALUATION & PROGRESS IN LAST 2 WEEKS   ACHIEVEMENT DATE

5. MENTAL STATUS	NEVER	SOME TIMES	ALWAYS		REHAB* Poten.
ALERT					
IMPAIRED JUDGMENT					
AGITATED (NIGHTTIME)					
HALLUCINATES					
SEVERE DEPRESSION **					
ASSAULTIVE					
ABUSIVE					
RESTRAINT ORDER					
REGRESSIVE BEHAVIOR					
WANDERS					
OTHER (SPECIFY)					

6. IMPAIRMENTS	NONE	PARTIAL	TOTAL		REHAB* Poten.
SIGHT					
HEARING					
SPEECH					
COMMUNICATIONS					
OTHER (CONTRACTURES, ETC.)					
SPECIFY					

B. CIRCLE MINIMUM NUMBER OF DAYS/WEEK OF SKILLED THERAPY FROM EACH OF THE FOLLOWING:

REQUIRES		RECEIVES
0 1 2 3 4 5 6 7	PT	0 1 2 3 4 5 6 7
0 1 2 3 4 5 6 7	OT	0 1 2 3 4 5 6 7
0 1 2 3 4 5 6 7	SPEECH	0 1 2 3 4 5 6 7

8. DO THE WRITTEN ORDERS OF THE ATTENDING PHYSICIAN AND PLAN OF CARE DOCUMENT THAT THE ABOVE NURSING AND THERAPY ARE NECESSARY?   NO ☐ YES ☐

9. A. SHOULD THE PATIENT BE CONSIDERED FOR ANOTHER LEVEL OF CARE: NO ☐ YES ☐   IF YES: WHEN? _____ WHAT LEVEL? _____

   B. AS A PRACTICAL MATTER, COULD PATIENT BE CARED FOR AS AN OUTPATIENT?   NO ☐ YES ☐

   C. AS A PRACTICAL MATTER, COULD PATIENT BE CARED FOR UNDER HOME CARE?   NO ☐ YES ☐
     IF YES TO ANY OF ABOVE, ATTACH A DISCHARGE PLAN.

10. SHOULD THE PATIENT/RESIDENT BE MEDICALLY QUALIFIED FOR SNF CARE?   COVERED ☐ QUESTIONABLE ☐ NON-COVERED ☐ ***

11. ADDITIONAL COMMENTS ON PATIENT CARE PLAN/REHAB. POTENTIAL _____
_____
_____

12. I CERTIFY, TO THE BEST OF MY INFORMATION AND BELIEF, THAT THE INFORMATION ON THIS FORM IS A TRUE ABSTRACT OF THE PATIENT'S CONDITION AND MEDICAL RECORD.

_____ (SIGNATURE OF DESIGNATED RN AND TITLE)   DATE ASSESS. COMPLETED

TO BE COMPLETED BY U.R. AGENT OR REPRESENTATIVE UPON CONTINUED STAY REVIEW

13. ADDITIONAL INFORMATION BY U.R. REPRESENTATIVE   15. U.R. REPRESENTATIVE PLACEMENT _____

SIGNATURE _____ DATE _____

16. U.R. PHYSICIAN: PLACEMENT _____

SIGNATURE _____ DATE _____

14. NEXT SCHEDULED REVIEW DATE _____

*CHECK THE BOX CORRESPONDING TO APPROPRIATE CRITERION IF THERE IS A LIKELIHOOD THAT THE PATIENT WILL RESPOND UNDER A COORDINATED PLAN OF RESTORATIVE TREATMENT. (INDICATE PLAN IN ITEM 3 E OR 11).

**IF PATIENT HAS SEVERE DEPRESSION, PSYCHIATRIC CONSULTATION SHOULD BE OBTAINED.

***IF CHECKED "NON-COVERED", SNF PLACEMENT CANNOT BE APPROVED BY MEDICAID.

A. ITEMS 1, 2, 3, 4, 5, 6 SHOULD BE COMPLETED BY NURSE
B. ITEM 7 SHOULD BE COMPLETED BY THERAPIST.
C. ITEMS 8, 9, 10, 11, 12 TO BE COMPLETED IN CONSULTATION WITH THE HEALTH TEAM.

DMS 1 (1/77)

Fig. 1-4. (*continued*)

New York State Health Department Numerical Standards Master Sheet
Numerical Standards for Application for the Long Term Care Placement Form
Medical Assessment Abstract
(DMS-1)

3.

a. Nursing Care and Therapy (Specify details in 3d,3e or attachment)

	Frequency			Self Care		Can Be Trained	
	None	Day Shift	Night/Eve. Shift	Yes	No	Yes	No
Parenteral Meds	0	25	60	-15	0	0	0
Inhalation Treatment	0	38	37	-20	0	0	0
Oxygen	0	49	49	-4	0	0	0
Suctioning	0	50	50	-1	0	0	0
Aseptic Dressing	0	42	48	0	0 +1	0	0
Lesion Irrigation	0	49	49	-20	0	0	0
Cath/Tube Irrigation	0	35	60	-1	0 +4	0	0
Ostomy Care							
Parenteral Fluids	0	50	50				
Tube Feedings	0	50	50				
Bowel/Bladder Rehab.	0	48	48				
Bedsore Treatment	0	50	50				
Other (Describe)	0	0	0				

b. Incontinent

Urine: Often* [ ] 20 Seldom** [ ] 10 Never [ ] 0
 Foley [ ] 15

Stool: Often* [ ] 40 Seldom** [ ] 20 Never [ ] 0

c. Does patient need a special diet? No [ ] Yes [ ]

If yes, describe: _____

DMS-9 (2/77)

4. FUNCTION STATUS

FUNCTION STATUS	Self Care	Some Help	Total Help	Can Not
Walks with or w/o aids	0	35	70	105
Transferring	0	6	12	18
Wheeling	0	1	2	3
Eating/Feeding	0	25	50	
Toileting	0	7	14	
Bathing	0	17	24	
Dressing	0	40	80	

5. MENTAL STATUS

MENTAL STATUS	Never	Sometimes	Always
Alert	40	20	0
Impaired Judgment	0	15	30
Agitated (nighttime)	0	10	20
Hallucinates	0	1	*
Severe depression			*
Assaultive	0	40	80
Abusive	0	25	50
Restraint Order	0	40	80
Regressive Behavior	0	30	60
Wanders			
Other (Specify)			

6. IMPAIRMENTS

IMPAIRMENTS	None	Partial	Total
Sight	0	1	2
Hearing	0	1	2
Speech	0	10	20
Communications			
Other (Contractures, etc.)			

7.

Short Term Rehab. Therapy Plan (To be completed by therapist)

a.

Describe Condition (not Dx) Needing Intervention	Short Term Plan of Treatment & Eval. and progress in last 2 weeks.	Achievement Date

b. Circle Minimum number of days/week of skilled therapy from each of the following:

REQUIRES		RECEIVES
0 1 2 3 4 5 6 7	PT	0 1 2 3 4 5 6 7
0 1 2 3 4 5 6 7	OT	0 1 2 3 4 5 6 7
0 1 2 3 4 5 6 7	Speech	0 1 2 3 4 5 6 7

✦ 37 for skilled rehab/therapy (received & required both≥0)

Fig. 1-5. New York State Department of Health Numerical Standard Sheet (DMS-9).

representative of the school of peripheralists. To account for various unexplainable symptoms such as hemiplegic pain or thalamic pain, the school of centralists has advanced a theory of central pain. There is also a difference of opinion as to whether phantom pain should be considered as peripheral or central pain. In addition, the newly discovered brain peptides, such as β-endorphin, and their relation to pain are being studied, but information is still inconclusive.

Pain may be classified as acute, chronic, or malignant. Acute pain is characterized as severe, its onset often sudden, with corresponding objective symptoms; owing to the existence of definitive treatment methods, it has a predictable duration and good prognosis. Pain due to trauma such as fracture, laceration, sprain, or acute abdominal infection is an example of acute pain.

Chronic pain may vary from mild to severe. It may follow acute pain, it may begin suddenly or gradually, and it often is recurrent. Corresponding objective symptoms may or may not be present. There is often no effective treatment method, its duration is unpredictable, and its prognosis is guarded. Although acute pain is generally considered to be peripheral pain, some hold that chronic pain may be central pain.[23]

Malignant pain has many of the characteristics of acute pain, but it lacks definitive treatment methods and its prognosis is extremely poor. Malignant pain is caused by malignant tumors in their terminal stage. Obviously this classification is based on methods of clinical management rather than any other consideration.

It seems more reasonable to group pain into two categories, acute and chronic. Chronic pain may be subgrouped into an acute-chronic model and a recurrent-chronic model (Figs. 1-6 to 1-8). In the acute-chronic model the precise point when pain changes clinically from acute to chronic is unknown.[24]

Treatment of the cause is the choice for management of acute pain. A liberal use of narcotic analgesics to free the patient from discomfort is the acceptable approach to malignant pain, and in such cases the possibility of addiction should not prevent the use of narcotics.

On the other hand, the chronic pain that is frequently observed in the aged is most difficult to control and is a challenging task for clinicians. Chronic pain, particularly the recurrent type, may or may not be accompanied by objective findings. Even if such findings can be treated surgically, such as a herniated disk, there is no guarantee that pain will be totally eliminated after the surgery. Pain is a somatic and subjective symptom, and chronic pain may not always correspond to any objective physical findings. The degree and extent of pathologic or abnormal findings are not necessarily indicators of severity and chronicity in pain.

It has been well recognized that emotional and socioeconomic factors play an important role in the causation of chronic pain. Whereas tension and anxiety are normal emotional reactions to the presence of severe acute pain, various complex psychological factors may contribute to chronic pain. Chronic situational depression is often due to a realization of aging, loneliness, or unmet physical and/or socioeconomic needs; it is frequently found to be the contributing emotional factor.

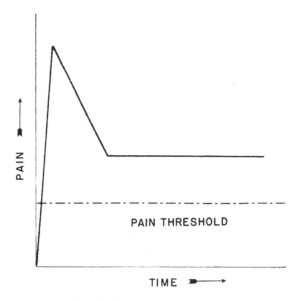

Fig. 1-6.   Acute pain model.

As with other somatic complaints, careful evaluation of the physical condition is the best basis for developing a management plan for chronic pain. Even if a definite pathology, such as osteoarthritic change, is found, the investigation for the source of chronic pain needs to include the psychosocial state of the patient. Such comprehensive assessment is fundamental to establishing a rational and meaningful patient-care plan.

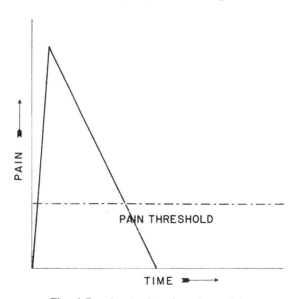

Fig. 1-7.   Acute-chronic pain model.

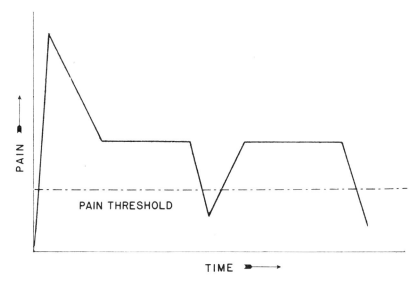

Fig. 1-8.   Recurrent chronic pain model.

The constant presence of pain, even intermittent nagging pain, interferes with normal ADL. Self-imposed immobilization will result in joint contractures, causing severe disability. A feeling of isolation and the development of deformities would aggravate a precarious emotional balance. Therefore, every effort should be made to eliminate the pain or to make it more tolerable.

In the management of chronic pain a surgical approach is usually not the first choice of treatment. Various nonnarcotic analgesics can be prescribed, but the aged are more susceptible to the cumulative effects as well as side effects (see Ch. 6). Some patients may be under a medication regimen for an illness totally unrelated to the condition causing the pain. In such cases possible drug interaction between other medications and analgesics must be carefully considered. When a psychological state such as chronic situational depression is an outstanding component of chronic pain, antidepressants may be prescribed. There are also a variety of physical therapy modalities that are effective in lessening discomfort. In addition, it is important to remember that psychological and social counseling are also helpful.

GERIATRIC REHABILITATION

Advancement in medical knowledge and technology since the turn of the century is unprecedented in human history. The first half of the twentieth century was marked by great contributions to the understanding of disease; the latter half of this century has been a period of superspecialization in the field of clinical medicine. For the past two decades the terms *geriatric rehabilitation* and *pediatric rehabilitation* have been used. Does this mean the users of these terms advocate a subspecialty in rehabilitation medicine? Probably not. It is more than likely done to emphasize certain characteristic approaches to rehabilitative care specially designed for the two age groups. In this chapter the term geriatric rehabilitation is used to signify certain other conceptual and practicable aspects of rehabilitation for the aged.

As mentioned previously, the goal of rehabilitation for the aged is restoration of physical function to the premorbid level. The aged population's high susceptibility to certain primary and secondary disabilities and a health status that is at best suboptimum have also been discussed. The images of the aged drawn from these discussions indicate the distinctly different characteristics of their disabilities and rehabilitation.

Prior to development of the treatment strategy, an assessment of the premorbid life-style, functional level, and health status is mandatory in geriatric rehabilitation. In general, the younger population maintains a certain life-style according to occupations and social obligation. They maintain Optimum Health most of the time and are able to perform not only all ADL but can participate in rigorous recreational activities as well.

On the other hand, it is difficult to generalize about the aged population. One person may follow a very sedentary life pattern, whereas another may enjoy a life-style as active as someone a decade younger. Some may be assisted by relatives and friends in ADL, whereas many others are functioning physically and mentally at their optimum level. Although it is true that various degenerative aging processes are present, not every elderly person is ill and infirm. In these respects more exceptions will be found among the aged than among the younger population.

The primary goal of geriatric rehabilitation is so limited that the health-care team must have a clear understanding of the function level to be achieved through the rehabilitation process. A careful assessment will provide a clearer picture of the patient and indicate what may be achieved by the individual. This will help the patient establish realistic goals. In addition, a thorough evaluation of the physical condition is mandatory prior to initiation of physical restoration because such evaluation will reveal the extent of the aging process. This evaluation includes not only routine physical examination but cardiopulmonary functions, peripheral blood circulation, degree of osteoporosis if so indicated, as well as mental condition. Findings from these assessments would suggest the patient's endurance, indications or contraindications for certain treatment regimens, the pace of the rehabilitation process, and possibly prognosis of final functional ability and can be interrelated to the patient's motivation.

After the acute onset of the primary disability, a patient often requires relatively protracted bed rest until he or she is ready for rehabilitation. Such prolonged inactivity will decondition anyone, including young people. The degree and speed of deconditioning is more severe in elderly people, even if they led active lives premorbidly. Thus regardless of disability the most important step in beginning a rehabilitation process is to motivate the patient to desire general conditioning activities (including ADL) to build up endurance. If this conditioning process is omitted, cardiovascular or respiratory disturbance may ensue. Once such complications develop, not only will the rehabilitation process be interrupted and delayed but the patient may become fearful of the process and withdraw into depression. This physical conditioning period is also an excellent time to prepare the patient for resuming as normal a life as is possible in the future.

Sometimes the process of geriatric rehabilitation can be agonizingly slow. The reasons for this slow progression are many; some are psychological and others are physical. Shyness, resentment, shame, anger, and depression interfere with the performance of even simple physical exercise. Members of the rehabilitation team must be able to appreciate these feelings and play supportive roles. Physically, elderly patients may have neuromuscular inco-ordination, delayed reaction time, diminished vision and hearing. Their muscle power may not be strong enough to perform a demanded task. Physically elderly patients may have good days and bad days. One day they may be very energetic and perform extremely well; on another day they may not be able physically to muster the required energy to perform the task. This does not indicate regression. Elderly patients merely lack the "reserves" of youth and can no longer "push" themselves to function beyond a certain pace. Furthermore, they may have difficulty concentrating and may simply forget what was taught the day before (possibly stress induced).

The key word for therapists is "patience," and they must be able to understand these subtle mental and physical characteristics of the disabled elderly person. Words of empathetic encouragement by a therapist are more effective than scolding. Repetition of the same physical action, though necessary at times, can be dull and boring. The patient may begin to feel that repetition is necessary due to some deficiency within himself or herself. The therapist must interpret the reasons for repetitive exercise if it is used. Sincere praise by the therapist, even for slight progress, can promote self-confidence, fortitude, and motivation. Self-confidence is believing that a task can be done; fortitude is strength, courage, and endurance to do it; and motivation is the desire to do it.

The fear of falling is another very common phenomenon among the aged. Sometimes this fear is so strong that a patient is petrified and refuses to get out of a wheelchair. An analysis of this fear indicates that the source of fear is the fall itself rather than the consequences, such as fractures. This fear is particularly common among women who did not participate in some sort of sport when younger. One approach for this type of patient is to provide maximum physical support, such as direct physical contact or contact guarding by a therapist while a second therapist stands next to the patient. The patient is more confident knowing that two therapists will be able to prevent a fall. Once sufficient confidence is established, these supportive measures may be gradually withdrawn.

Another, more complex method is to condition the patient. This has been done with actors and athletes for many years. It involves training the patient to fall without injury by practice-falling onto a mattress. However, the patient must be constantly supervised and the therapist must be specifically trained in falling techniques in order to teach them.

Regardless of patient age, every opportunity should be given the patient to gain maximum restoration of function. For example, it is often said that a patient "is too old to use an above-knee prosthesis." Age per se is not a contraindication for most therapeutic interventions. There must be some irrefutable reason, such as cardiac or respiratory deficiency, extreme weakness, flexion contractures in the lower extremities, poor muscle coordination, or lack of trainability due to poor memory, to deny the patient a prosthesis. It is both a fallacy and a misconception to believe that rehabilitation potential is equated directly with patient age.

PREVENTIVE REHABILITATION

Efforts to restore health from Overt Illness or Approaching Death to Optimum Health are usually called therapeutic medicine. In a broad sense the goal of therapeutic medicine is restoration of health to the premorbid level. Considering the definition of rehabilitation, one might call therapeutic medicine an "act of rehabilitation."[25] As previously discussed, rehabilitation for children and adolescents may restore physical, intellectual, and/or vocational function to a state better than the premorbid level, but this exception cannot be applied to therapeutic medicine.

The restorative and curative aspects of clinical medicine can be illustrated in acute and episodic illnesses such as acute appendicitis, upper respiratory infection, or acute gastroenteritis. However, when clinical medicine is applied to a chronic disease, these same aspects become less distinct. For example, a given patient with arteriosclerotic heart disease goes into acute cardiac decompensation. Control of acute congestive heart failure usually is not very difficult, and within a few days cardiac function would be restored. This patient will most likely be on a maintenance dose of cardiac medication for a long period. At this point therapeutic medicine becomes preventive medicine because administration of a maintenance medicine prevents a recurrence of congestive heart failure. Here it is easy to see how the distinction between therapeutic and preventive medicine becomes less prominent. A similar meld exists for therapeutic rehabilitation and preventive rehabilitation.

A cursory observation of the activity of physical therapists, occupational therapists, and nurses gives the impression that they are engaged in restoration of disabilities. However, a close analysis reveals that a major part of their effort is to prevent secondary disabilities such as joint contractures, disuse atrophy, osteoporosis, or decubitus ulcer. If these preventive activities were not mandatory, the rehabilitation process would be much simpler and faster. To stress this aspect of rehabilitation, the term *preventive rehabilitation* was introduced.[25-27]

Contemporary therapeutic rehabilitation concentrates on the treatment of primary disability and the prevention or treatment of secondary disability. Once primary disability develops in a person, rehabilitation processes cannot always achieve a complete restoration. Even if full restoration is accomplished, it costs the patient as well as the community time, energy, resources, and emotional anguish. Preventive rehabilitation focuses on prevention or eradication of both primary and secondary disabilities (Table 1-2). Some may argue that this is preventive medicine and should not be a part of rehabilitation, which is a therapeutic specialty; however, it should be noted that today there are many components of preventive medicine in every clinical specialty.

The aged population is susceptible to various disabling diseases and conditions. Residual disabilities often interfere with their normal daily functions, and they may need assistance at home or care in an institution. Thus preventive rehabilitation is most meaningful for the elderly population.

Various public-health measures, discoveries, and innovations in preventive medicine are practiced in the United States and worldwide in order to prevent numerous infectious diseases and decrease potentially disabling diseases and conditions. Some of these preventive measures are more effective than others. For example, a well-planned and properly executed vaccination program can eliminate poliomyelitis in a given geographic area; on the other hand, well-publicized high-school driver-education programs have not had the expected impact on highway fatalities.[28] A major focus of preventive medicine has been the population of childhood, adolescence, young adult, and middle-age adult. It appears that the aged are somewhat neglected in this area.

Certain preventive rehabilitation measures for the aged should start before a person has become ''aged'' (e.g., in their thirties and forties). Hypertension is one of the most common causes of cerebrovascular accident; however, in recent decades the incidence of cerebrovascular accident due to hypertension has drastically decreased because of advancement in drug therapy and other means of controlling hypertension. Early detection and proper control of diabetes mellitus may prevent diabetic retinopathy, peripheral neuropathy, or peripheral vascular insufficiency. If these are combined with meticulous foot care, lower extremity amputation due to diabetic gangrene may be prevented in the advanced age group. Physicians who treat patients with these diseases need to stress both the importance of controlling these diseases and the preventive aspects of the treatment regimen. Unless patients and their families understand both therapeutic and preventive aspects of the prescribed treatment, they may not adhere to the regimen as strictly as they should.

In considering other aspects of preventive rehabilitation medicine for the aged it is necessary to assess susceptibility to certain diseases or trauma. For example, fracture of the neck of the femur is found almost exclusively in the

Table 1-2. Components of Rehabilitation

Disability	Rehabilitation	
	Therapeutic	Preventive
Primary	Treatment	Prevention Eradication
Secondary	Prevention Treatment	Prevention Eradication

aged population, particularly in females. The physical characteristics of this population require a conscious effort to enhance relaxation (i.e., flexibility exercises in order to maintain the ability to allow passive range of motion to each joint). Patients need to be highly motivated to work to enhance their coordination; therapeutic improvement is not always possible. Therefore, the easiest preventive measures are environmental. Neatness in the home, improved lighting, and handrails on steps and stairways are examples of environmental protection. An elderly woman with shuffling gait needs to be encouraged to wear shoes instead of house slippers, and throw rugs should never be used in a household where elderly people live.

Primary health-care personnel who treat the aged, such as physicians, hospital nurses, visiting nurses, physical therapists, and occupational therapist, need to recognize the danger of falling accidents among the elderly. Dizziness or transient cerebral ischemic attack is one of the most common causes of a fall, aside from environmental obstacles. Some such attacks are drug-induced, whereas others may be due to vascular spasm. Therefore, health-care personnel should give instructions to the aged and those who help them as to what they should do in case of a dizzy spell.

Hip fracture is a common injury among hemiplegics who have successfully completed rehabilitation. The fracture occurs almost invariably on the side of paralysis, probably because of muscle weakness or incoordination. As part of a prosthesis-rehabilitation program a lower extremity amputee is routinely trained in the technique of falling. If all hemiplegics are trained how to fall by a physical therapist during their rehabilitation, the incidence of hip fracture among hemiplegics may decrease.

The foregoing examples of preventive rehabilitation illustrate that some measures are designed primarily for prevention of primary disability and that others are indirectly preventive. Many existing means of preventive rehabilitation and the need for new approaches and preventions can be identified by continued analysis of the susceptibility of the aged to primary disability, medical care practices, and community action and services carried out on behalf of the elderly. Levy and Moskowitz[29] state, "A focus on prevention means educating the public and the health professional alike on how to obtain information on risk factors or ways to change life-styles and habits or means to promote behavioral changes."

The concept of preventive rehabilitation is rational, and obviously its potentials are unlimited. The question is, Who logically should be responsible for this health-related issue of the elderly? The members of the rehabilitation team have a wealth of knowledge on the natural history and treatment of primary and secondary disabilities. The team practices comprehensive care for the total human being. Its practice is not confined to physical therapy, occupational therapy, hospital patient room, private office, or clinic, but includes years of consistent action at the community, state, and federal levels. This concerted effort has in the past resulted in many changes that have improved the quality of life for those who are handicapped and those who are not. Those who engage in rehabilitation are the best equipped to undertake this new frontier of geriatric rehabilitation.

REFERENCES

1. Butler RN: Introduction. In Haynes SG, Feibleib M (eds): Second Conference on the Epidemiology of Aging. NIH Publication No. 80-968. US Department of Health and Human Services, Washington, DC, 1980.
2. Rusk HA, Hilleboe HE: Rehabilitation. In Hilleboe HE, Larimore GW (eds): Preventive Medicine. WB Saunders, Philadelphia, 1965
3. World Health Organization: Constitution of the World Health Organization. World Health Organization, Geneva, 1964
4. Rogers ES: Human Ecology and Health. Introduction for Administrators. Macmillan, New York, 1960
5. Smillie WG: Epidemiology. In: Preventive Medicine and Public Health. Macmillan, New York, 1952
6. Welch WH: Institute of hygiene. In Rockefeller Foundation Annual Report. Rockefeller Foundation, New York, 1916
7. Lilienfeld BE: Epidemiologic methods and inferences. In Hilleboe HE, Larimore GW (eds): Preventive Medicine. WB Saunders, Philadelphia, 1965
8. Sartwell PE, Last JM: Epidemiology. In Last JM (ed): Public Health and Preventive Medicine. Appleton-Century-Crofts, East Norwalk, CT, 1980
9. Itoh M, Lee M: The epidemiology of disability. In Krusen FH, Kottke FJ, Ellwood PM (eds): Handbook of Physical Medicine and Rehabilitation. WB Saunders, Philadelphia, 1971
10. World Health Organization Regional Office for Europe, Wilson J (ed): The Age Factor in Disability Prevention: The Global Challenge. Oxford University Press, Oxford, 1983
11. Dahlsted S: Slow pedestrians—walking speeds and walking habits of old-aged people. Report R2. Swedish Council for Building Research, Stockholm, 1978
12. Itoh M, Dasco MM: Rehabilitation of patients with hip fracture. A clinical study of 126 cases. Postgrad Med 28:134, 1960
13. Knapp ME: Disability evaluation, 1. Postgrad Med 46:184, 1969
14. Knapp ME: Disability evaluation, 2. Postgrad Med 46:201, 1969
15. World Health Organization: Classification of disability resulting from leprosy, for use in control program. Bull WHO 40:609, 1969
16. Sokolow J, Silson J, Taylor EJ, et al: A method for the functional evaluation of disability. Arch Phys Med Rehabil 40:421, 1959
17. Pool DA, Brown RA: A functional rating scale for research in physical therapy. Tex Rep Biol Med 26:133, 1968
18. Moskowitz E, McCann CB: Classification of disability in chronically ill and aging. J Chronic Dis 5:342, 1957
19. Foley WJ, Schneider DP: A comparison of the level of care predictions of six long-term care patient assessment systems. Am J Public Health 70:1152, 1980
20. Harris JF, Orr M, Allaway NC: Long-term care criteria and standards agreement with professional placement determination. Am J Public Health 72:602, 1982
21. Crue BL, Felsoory A, Agnew D, et al: The team concept in the management of pain in patients with cancer. Bull Los Angeles Neurol Soc 44:70, 1979

22. Melzak R: The gate-control theory of pain. In Melzak R (ed): The Puzzle of Pain. Basic Books, New York, 1973
23. Crue BL: A physiological view of the psychology of pain. Bull Los Angeles Neurol Soc 44:1, 1979
24. Itoh M, Lee MH: Epidemiology of pain. Bull Los Angeles Neurol Soc 44:14, 1979
25. Itoh M, Lee M: The future role of rehabilitation in community health. Med Clin North Am 53:719, 1969
26. Itoh M: Preventive rehabilitation for leprosy—a new approach to an old problem. Rehabil Rev 19:13, 1968
27. Karat S: Preventive rehabilitation in leprosy. Leprosy Rev 39:39, 1968
28. Robertson LS, Zador PL: Driver education and fatal crash involvement of teenaged drivers. Am J Public Health 68:959, 1978
29. Levy RI, Moskowitz J: Cardiovascular research: decades of progress, a decade of promise. Science 217:121, 1982

2 | Biological Aspects of Aging

Barrie Pickles

This chapter summarizes the major biological changes that occur during normal aging in those tissues of the body of particular significance to the physical therapist. The effect of these aging changes on function are outlined, and suggestions for dealing with these clinically relevant changes are presented.

FIBROUS CONNECTIVE TISSUE

All connective tissue cells have a common ancestry—all develop from the same primitive type of mesenchymal cell. As the result of this common ancestry, different types of connective tissue cells have many features in common. All connective tissue cells secrete collagen, elastin, glycoproteins, hyaluronic acid, and contractile proteins. In different tissues the proportion of these substances varies; in white fibrous tissue the predominant secretion is collagen, in yellow elastic tissue elastin is particularly prevalent, and in cartilage glycoprotein secretion is especially pronounced. Under different environmental conditions within the body, the pattern of secretions by connective tissue cells will be altered. The production and functional significance of each of these secretions is summarized next, and the effects of aging on each are considered.

Collagen

Some ribosomes within the connective tissue cells produce a secretion of procollagen, a protein material.[1] Molecules of procollagen are then extruded from the cell into the surrounding tissue fluids. Once they have left the cell the individual procollagen molecules stick together in an end-to-end fashion to form a strand of tropocollagen. One part of each tropocollagen strand is positively charged; another area possesses a negative charge. A number of tropocollagen strands come together in a staggered fashion as the result of electrical attraction between the positively and negatively charged portions of adjacently lying strands. Later, chemical bonds also develop between adjacent tropocollagen strands, causing the strands to become tightly wound in a spiral fashion to form a mature collagen fiber.[2,3]

Tropocollagen is quite soluble in cold water, but as the conversion of tropocollagen into collagen takes place, and as maturation of the collagen fiber progresses, the fiber becomes less soluble. The greater the number of chemical bonds that develop between the strands, the less soluble the material becomes. The development of other chemical bonds results in shortening or contracture of the maturing collagen mass.

Collagen fibers grow in diameter by the surface aggregation of additional tropocollagen strands. As this occurs the center of the fiber is compressed and becomes more dense. The mature fiber is characterized by a central portion of intermolecularly cross-linked insoluble collagen surrounded by less completely cross-linked material.[4]

The eventual diameter of the fibers depends on the chemical composition of the matrix in which they are embedded, but even when the fibers have reached their ultimate size, further cross-linkages continue to be added.[5]

The diameter of collagen fibers in a given location within the body is usually greater in old persons than in younger persons. The increased diameter of these fibers is possibly a reflection of the chemical changes in the matrix in older persons and the addition of more tropocollagen to the surface of the collagen fiber. When the oxygen concentration in the matrix is moderately low, the secretion and maturation of collagen continues to take place, even when secretion of other materials has ceased. In general, therefore, the tensile strength of connective tissue in a given location in older persons is greater than in younger adults.

No evidence suggests that a connective tissue cell's ability to produce collagen is reduced as part of the normal aging process, although the ability to divide and replicate is lower in cells taken from older persons than in cells taken from younger persons.[6]

In two situations, however, there will be a reduction in the tensile strength of collagen. In many older persons a vitamin C lack (scurvy) exists, which reduces the amount of procollagen the cell can secrete. Vitamin C is required to convert the amino acid proline into hydroxyproline, a component of the procollagen molecule.[7] Many older persons also suffer from chronic stress, which appears to have an inhibitory effect on both the production and maturation of collagen.[8]

Elastin

A different group of ribosomes within the connective tissue cells of children and young adults secrete elastin. When elastin molecules are brought together in the extracellular fluid after being ejected from the cell body they link up with each other, not only in an end-to-end fashion but also in a branching arrangement, thus creating a latticetype network of elastin material. As its name implies, elastin possesses the power to recoil to its original length after it has been stretched and the stretching force has been removed.

The amount of elastin in the skin, in the bronchial tree, and in the walls of larger arteries is reduced progressively throughout life.[9] If overstretching of part of an elastin network occurs in adults and elastin fibers are torn, healing by scar tissue (collagen) will follow. The elastin properties of these tissues (skin, the bronchial tree, arterial walls) will therefore be progressively reduced during life.

Glycoproteins

Glycoproteins are substances formed when polysaccharide carbohydrates link with protein molecules. A variety of glycoprotein substances are manufactured by connective tissue cells; they form a group of relatively small molecules of soluble protein material. The presence of glycoprotein materials in the extracellular fluid produces an osmotic force that is important in maintaining the fluid content of the tissues. The higher their concentration in the extracellular fluid, the greater will be the amount of fluid retained within the tissue by osmotic attraction forces. Both the production and liberation of glycoproteins are considerably reduced in old age; consequently, it becomes progressively more difficult for the tissues to retain their original fluid content, and so a progressive dehydration occurs in the tissues of older persons.

The nature of glycoproteins varies among different tissues and may alter in a particular location as part of the aging process.[10] There appears to be a definite relationship between the type of glycoprotein present and the average thickness of the collagen fibers in an area. In the elderly, where dermatin sulfate is the predominant glycoprotein secretion in the skin, the collagen fibers that are formed have a larger diameter than those found in the same location in younger persons, in whose tissues chondroitin sulfate is the most predominant glycoprotein. In the skin of elderly persons, the increased average diameter of the collagen fibers may be largely accounted for by an increase in the dermatin sulfate secretion; the accompanying dehydration of the skin indicates that although the secretion of dermatin sulfate has increased, the total glycoprotein secretion is reduced.

The secretion of collagen and glycoproteins is independent of each other. Strains of fibroblasts have been grown that produce only glycoprotein, but no cells have been found that secrete only collagen.

Hyaluronic Acid

Some ribosomes in the connective tissue cells produce hyaluronic acid, which helps to regulate the viscosity of the tissues. Friction between different cellular components during movement or as the result of biochemical activity will be reduced to a minimum if adequate amounts of hyaluronic acid are produced. In older persons the secretion of hyaluronic acid by the connective tissue cells is reduced; the viscosity of the connective tissues is altered, and movements become progressively more difficult.[11]

Contractile Proteins

Contractile proteins are secreted to some degree by all types of connective tissue cells.[12] The presence of contractile proteins in these cells gives them the power of motility—the ability to push out a pseudopodium to ingest a particle of tissue debris, the power of some cells to move bodily within the tissue spaces, and the capacity to force a way through the wall of a capillary or lymphatic channel. The presence of contractile proteins within a cell is by no means restricted to muscle fibers; indeed, muscle fibers betray their mesenchymal origin by the presence of contractile protein within their substance. The reduced motility of connective tissue cells in older people may be explained in terms of reduced secretion and organization of contractile proteins within these cells.

Clinical Problems of Aging in Fibrous Connective Tissue

Fibrinous Adhesions

During life a small but regular exudation of molecules of the soluble plasma protein fibrinogen occurs through the capillary walls into the neighboring tissue spaces, where they will be converted into sticky strands of insoluble fibrin. These stands adhere to nearby structures in a random fashion and tend to restrict movement of these structures. In young persons and in active adults these fibrinous strands are broken down during the performance of normal everyday activities, and the resulting debris is removed by scavenging macrophages of the reticuloendothelial system.

In the elderly, although the exudation of fibrinogen into the tissue spaces may be less than in younger persons, the overall accumulation of fibrinogen in the tissues tends to be greater, owing to a combination of reduced levels of physical activity and reduced effectiveness of scavenging by the macrophages. If adequate activity is not maintained, complete breakdown of fibrin may not occur. Increased amounts of sticky fibrin will accumulate in the tissue spaces and produce adhesions, which will restrict movement between adjacent structures. Fibrinous adhesions also form in a localized area following damage to the tissues.

In many cases the maintenance or restoration of regular normal activity is sufficient to cause breakdown of these fibrinous adhesions. If the mass has become consolidated, it may be necessary for stretching to be applied using passive movements or manipulation to cause the breakdown.

Collagenous Contractures

As secondary chemical bonds develop between adjacent tropocollagen strands during the maturation process to pack the strands more tightly together, other bonds are produced that cause shortening and distortion of the collagen fibers. Shortening of the collagen fibers through this mechanism may result in the development of contractures. As more collagen fibers in a mass of connective tissue are shortened in this way, a progressive restriction of movement is observed.

When connective tissue is stretched, it demonstrates viscoelastic properties; that is, part of the deformation remains after the load is removed (the viscous or plastic component), whereas part of the elongation produced is reversed after the load is removed (the elastic component).[13] In older persons the elastic component is progressively reduced. Collagen fibers are tough and inelastic, and most of the linking chemical bonds are too strong to be broken down by mechanical stretching forces along. Indeed, the use of strong, rapid mechanical stretching is more likely to produce rupturing of the tropocollagen strands than a breakdown of the secondary chemical bonds.[14] If the mechanical stretch is applied more gradually, and maintained for lengthy periods, as is the case when serial corrective casting methods are used, a permanent plastictype elongation is produced, as the result of breakdown of the secondary linking bonds.

Some of these secondary bonds, however, are temperature sensitive. At 42.5° C and above these bonds become unstable and may then be readily broken. To break down these bonds and prevent their immediate reformation three conditions have to be met:

1. The collagen must be heated to 42.5° C or above.
2. A continuous stretching force must be applied while tissues are being heated.
3. The stretching force must be maintained for at least the first 30 minutes of the cooling period.[15]

Ultrasound may be used to raise the temperature of the collagen to the required level, using a continuous beam with a frequency of 1 MHz at an intensity of 1.0 W/cm^2 for a period of 10 minutes.[16]

In practice, any soft-tissue contracture should be regarded as a mixture of fibrinous adhesions and collagenous shortening. In newly developed contractures the proportion of the total problem attributable to the presence of fibrinous adhesions is high, whereas in more chronic contractures collagenous shortening will predominate. If attempts at normal activity are insisted on, some improvement will follow the breakdown of fibrin strands. When collagenous shortening is present and interlinking chemical bonds have become established between adjacent collagenous structures, only breaking down these bonds through the use of combined heating and stretching or the use of serial corrective casts, forced manipulation, or correction of the deformity by surgery will lead to improvement.

Myofibroblast Production

In normal fibroblasts the secretion of contractile protein is small. Under certain conditions, as the result of a combination of stimuli that are not completely understood, the production of actin and myosin may be increased to a significant degree. Connective tissue cells that produce unusually large amounts of contractile protein are termed *myofibroblasts*.[17]

The response of connective tissue cells to damage or irritation normally occurs in two stages. In the first stage some cell multiplication occurs, followed by a second phase during which the increased number of cells become actively secretory. If considerable hyperplasia has occurred before the secretory phase begins, and if the production of actomysin is unusually large, the contractile force exerted by the developing mass may be sufficient to progressively restrict the normal range of movements in the affected area.

In some older persons this process occurs in the fibroblasts in the rotator cuff at the shoulder to give rise to a particular form of "frozen shoulder," in which the restriction of movement becomes progressively worse over a period of about 6 months, remains at its severest level for the next 6 months regardless of the treatment given, and takes a further 6 months to clear. Myofibroblasts may also develop in the palmar fascia of patients with Dupuytren's contracture, although in this case the shortening is permanent, rather than showing a spontaneous improvement after a period of time.

CARTILAGE
Normal Development and Function

Cartilage tissue is formed when primitive mesenchymal cells are subjected to compression forces in an environment of low oxygen concentration. Under these conditions the predominant secretions of the chondroblast will be a glycoprotein chondroitin sulfate and hyaluronic acid with some collagen also being produced to a lesser degree.

The initial secretion of the mesenchymal cells is procollagen. The conversion of procollagen into tropocollagen, and the subsequent consolidation into collagen occurs in the same manner as that described earlier. The collagen fibers in hyaline cartilage are thinner and less evident than in many other tissues. In a mass of articular cartilage the collagen fibers are arranged in an arcade fashion, with one or both ends of the fiber firmly embedded in the deepest portion of the cartilage or even in the subchondrial bone. The loop of this collagenous arcade runs parallel to the joint surface.

Once the collagenous base has been developed, the chondroblasts secrete chondroitin sulfate and hyaluronic acid—both glycoproteins—into the extra-cellular spaces. Chondroitin sulfate forms the largest component of the cartilagenous matrix and gives this matrix its characteristic opalescent appear-ance, its ability to retain fluids, and its strong resistance against deformation. The hyaluronic acid provides lubrication for the joint.[18]

Cartilage differs from other tissues in that it has no direct blood supply. Nutrients are supplied to the cartilage cells, the chondroblasts, from blood flowing in the adjacent bones and from the synovial fluid in the joint cavity. The glycoprotein materials within the matrix exert a strong osmotic force that attracts water—together with its dissolved gases, inorganic salts, and organic materials—into the matrix. In this way materials necessary for normal metabo-lism are made available to the cartilage cells. The amount of fluid drawn into the cartilage depends on the concentration of glycoproteins in the matrix.

The entry of materials into the cartilage matrix is possible only when no compression forces are being applied to the cartilage. When compression is applied, water and the various substances dissolved in it are squeezed out.

To provide for regular movement of materials into and out of the cartilage moderate compression needs to be alternatively applied and released. In the absence of compression metabolites remain in the matrix and the oxygen content will be lowered. The chondroblasts respond by reducing the secretion of glycoproteins, and possibly increasing their production of procollagen. Thus, over time, the lack of normal activity results in the progressive conversion of hyaline cartilage to fibrocartilage.

Hyaline cartilage covers the articular surfaces in synovial joints. Lubrica-tion between the two surfaces of hyaline cartilage is facilitated by the secretion of hyaluronic acid by the chondroblasts. A layer of hyaluronic acid molecules forms a viscous covering on the surface of the cartilage with a reserve store of these molecules being retained in the cartilage matrix. When compression is applied to the joint, more of these molecules are squeezed onto the surface of the articular cartilage. The trapping of synovial fluid in gaps between these molecules ensures that lubrication of the joint is maintained even during weight-bearing activities.[19]

Aging Changes in Cartilage

After the age of 30, a variety of age-related changes have been reported in cartilage. There is a gross alteration from a bluish, translucent structure to a yellowish, opaque one, with surface cracking, fraying, and fibrillation.[20]

The earliest stages of degeneration of cartilage probably results from a progressive reduction in the ability of the chondroblasts to secrete adequate amounts of glycoproteins. Proper lubrication of the joint during movements will become more difficult as the hyaluronic acid secretion is reduced; greater friction and heat will be generated during movements. A reduction in the secretion of chondroitin sulfate will result in a reduced ability of the matrix to retain fluid, and the movement of materials into and out of the cartilage will be hampered.

Owning to the lower oxygen concentration in the fluids surrounding the chondroblasts, an increase in their production of procollagen will occur. Increased amounts of collagen will become deposited in the matrix, progressively converting the previous hyaline material into fibrocartilage.

The chondroblasts may respond to their reduced ability to secrete adequate amounts of specific glycoproteins by undergoing a process of cellular proliferation. Cell division increases the number of cells capable of secreting the necessary materials and increases the surface-to-volume ratio of the secretory mass. In older cartilage the cell clusters each contain more cells than in younger specimens. As the nutrient supply to these degenerating cells becomes worse, death and disintegration of the chondroblasts may follow, leaving empty cavities within the cartilage.[21]

The thickness of the articular cartilage diminishes over time as first its fluid content is reduced and then as more material that has been worn away is not replaced by the chondrocytic activity.

Clinical Problems of Aging in Cartilage

Although moderate intermittent compression is required to remove metabolic waste materials from the cartilage, the effects produced by heavier compression or by impact loading are somewhat unclear. On the one hand a group of long-distance cross-country runners showed no increase of pain or other symptoms associated with joint degeneration when compared with a matched group of long-distance swimmers.[22] However, a recently published study of histologic changes in the knee cartilage of experimental animals following a treadmill running program showed evidence of focal damage within the cartilage, and death of cartilage cells, even though no gross surface changes were visible to the naked eye and no undue narrowing of the joint space could be detected.[23]

The degenerative changes of aging in cartilage are not reversible. Until further evidence is available, the physical therapist planning activity programs for elderly patients would be advised to exercise caution over the use of prolonged jogging or other impact-type activities in these programs, particularly if any joint symptoms exist and if accelerated degeneration of the cartilage in weight-bearing joints is to be avoided. The impact forces on weight-bearing joints when jogging are three times greater than while walking.[24] The optimum degree of compression to the articular cartilage is probably close to the forces generated by full-range isotonic movements.

BONE

Normal Development and Function

All types of connective tissue develop from a common type of primitive mesenchymal cell. If these primitive mesenchymal cells are subjected to mechanical tension in conditions of low oxygen concentration they become fibroblasts, whereas the application of compression under similar conditions of low oxygen concentration will result in their transformation into chondroblasts. When compression is applied in the presence of higher concentrations of oxygen, the primitive mesenchymal cells become osteoblasts.

The development of bone takes place in two stages:

Stage 1. In the first stage the organic component of the bone is laid down. The undifferentiated mesenchymal cells migrate ahead of the capillaries; the leading cells therefore exist in conditions of low oxygen concentration. The application of tension to these cells at this time results in the production of procollagen by the ribosomes within the cells, providing that vitamin C is present. Once liberated from the cells the procollagen will be converted first into tropocollagen and then into collagen fibers. These collagen fibers will be laid down predominantly along the lines of mechanical stress to become the organic component of the developing bone. Within a given plate (lamella) of bone the collagen fibers pass in a single direction; the lamellae on either side of this will have their collagen fibers aligned in a different direction.

When compression forces are applied to this area while the oxygen concentration within the tissue remains moderately low, the mesenchymal cells respond by secreting chondroitin sulfate. This substance passes into the surrounding area to fill the spaces between the collagen fibers that were previously laid down. A progressive hardening of this cartilaginous matrix follows, although inorganic salts and small protein molecules may readily permeate this matrix.

Stage 2. The second stage of bone development begins when an improved oxygen content of the tissue occurs after the capillary network has caught up with the migratory mesenchymal cells. A delay of approximately 8 to 10 days exists, after the collagen has been laid down, before this second stage commences. As the oxygen concentration in the area increases, parts of the active mesenchymal cells tend to break away from the general mass of the cell bodies. These cellular fragments, with many enzyme-containing mitochondria, pass into the intercellular matrix.

The most significant enzyme for bone development contained in these fragments is alkaline phosphatase. The presence of alkaline phosphatase in the matrix causes inorganic calcium and phosphate ions to react together to form crystals of hydroxyapatite, or bone crystals. Initially, the hydroxyapatite crystals are attracted to a particular point on the collagen fiber by electrostatic forces created both piezoelectrically and by the flow of blood through neighboring vessels.[25] The piezoelectric charges are developed as the result of intermittent compression of the developing tissue.[26] Growth of these bone crystals by surface aggregation continues within the matrix until all the spaces between the collagen fibers have been filled, providing that the oxygen concentration of the tissues remains high and intermittent compression is maintained. The availability of calcium salts to the developing bone mass is increased through the action of vitamin D.

The deposition of calcium and phosphate ions in the developing bone is regulated through hormonal control. Calcitonin produced by the thyroid gland encourages the deposition of calcium salts in the matrix and their development into bone crystals; the secretion of parathormone by the parathyroid glands tends to have the opposite effect. The balance of activity between these two hormones controls the rate and degree of calcification of the matrix.

Bone is a very active tissue; a constant exchange occurs in both the organic and inorganic components of the bone. Bone is therefore subject to a constant remodeling process, which continues throughout life in response to changes in the functional forces to which the bone is subjected, alterations in the availability of calcium and phosphate ions, and shifts in the hormonal balance. These changes are more apparent in the trabecular bone than in the cortical bone.

Aging Changes in Bone

The bones of older persons invariably are less dense than the bones in younger persons. The reduction in density may be the result of failure in the development of either the organic or inorganic components of bone, a condition known as *osteopenia,* or through defective or abnormal mineralization of the matrix—*osteomalacia.* In the past the term *osteoporosis* tended to be applied to any condition where reduction in bone density had occurred, but now it tends to be used to indicate a condition in which, although the bone density is reduced, the chemistry of the bone remains normal.

Pathologic osteoporosis has been related to diets chronically deficient in calcium[27] and to those high in dietary acid derived from meat and poultry.[28] Osteoporosis follows neoplastic infiltration of bone[29] and increased secretion of parathormone[30] and ACTH.[31]

Senile (or involutional) osteoporosis, on the other hand, would appear to be an extension of the developmental process rather than a degenerative disease of old age.[32] The usual reduction in bone density found in older persons whose general activities have been progressively restricted may be compounded by a wide variety of pathologic problems. The term *involutional osteoporosis* is preferable to senile or postmenopausal osteoporosis. Although the majority of sufferers are elderly women, the problem is not restricted either to older persons or to females.

During aging, osteocytes undergo degenerative changes—reduction in RNA production, protein synthesis, and mitochondrial activity. The functional activity of the cells is reduced, and glycogen, lysosomes, and age pigment accumulate in the cell bodies.[33] Aging does not alter the ability of these cells to respond to trauma, but their degree of response is reduced.

Cells responsible for bone resorption and removal are known as *osteoclasts*. These are large, multinucleated cells, having large numbers of mitochondria and containing large amounts of acid phosphatase, that are formed by fusion of cells in the osteogenetic layer.[34] Osteoclastic activity does not appear to be greatly affected by aging. The progressive loss of bone that occurs during aging is primarily the result of a reduced ability to produce new bone, rather than an increase or acceleration in the rate of bone resorption.

In both sexes the bone density begins to decline after the age of 30. In males, the rate of loss throughout life is approximately 0.5 percent per year. In females, a similar rate of loss occurs until the age of 50 and after the age of 65; a more rapid rate of bone loss of 2.5 to 3.0 percent per year occurs between the ages of 50 and 65.[35]

In men of all ages, and in women over the age of 65, similar reductions occur in the density of both cortical and trabecular bone. In contrast, the loss of bone in women around the time of the menopause appears to affect the trabecular bone selectively, with the horizontal trabeculae showing the greatest reduction in both thickness and number.[36]

Any reduction in bone density weakens the bone. Osteoporosis achieves clinical importance when the density and mechanical strength of the bones have been reduced to such an extent that the weakened bones may fracture when minimal trauma is applied. Unless such fractures occur, the condition is usually symptomless.

It is possible that, apart from the bone loss associated with hormonal changes at the menopause, the reduced density of bone in the elderly of both sexes may be primarily attributed to age-associated decreased activity of daily living.[37] Decreased activity, which reduces both the normal mechanical stresses and strains placed on the bone and the blood circulation within the bone, appears to be a major factor in the development of osteoporosis in the elderly. During the first stage of bone development a reduction of the stresses and strains on the tissues results in lowered secretion of procollagen and chondroitin sulfate; if these forces are reduced in the second stage, attachment of bone crystals to the collagen fibers will be hampered.

Two mechanisms, weight bearing and muscle action, have been described as being important in maintenance of normal bone density.

In patients who are confined to bed, a decrease in their bone mass can be detected within 2 weeks; the calcium lost from the bones is excreted in the urine. This loss of calcium occurs in all bedridden persons, whether healthy or ill, male or female, young or old. Once the bedridden patients resume their normal up-and-about activities, both the nitrogen and calcium excretion rapidly decrease below the baseline level for each person.[38] The performance of exercises, from a supine position using a bicycle ergometer for up to 4 hours a day, does not alter the rate of calcium loss.[39] Rapid decalcification has also been reported from the bones of astronauts during weightless spaceflights, even though stringent exercise programs were undertaken during these flights.[40]

Weight bearing alone, although helpful, is not necessarily adequate cither. Patients with poliomyelitis affecting muscles of the calf, who were involved in a program of standing on the affected limbs for 3 to 4 hours a day failed to demonstrate any increased density in the bones of the calf and foot.[39] From these findings it would appear that *the simultaneous compression of the bone and activity of the overlying muscles are necessary to maintain the bone density and to stimulate bone growth.*

A general relationship exists between the bone mineral content in the axial skeleton and the general physical performance capacity of older men and women.[41] It has been shown that the bone mineral content of the lumbar vertebrae correlates closely with both the force of the maximum voluntary contraction of the back extensor muscles[42] and the cross-sectional area of the muscle belly of the psoas major muscle.[43] A similar strong correlation also exists between physical work capacity and the mineral content of bones in the lower limb and trunk.[44]

Muscle action is important to the bones not only by producing some of the electrical potentials required for its regrowth and remodeling, but also by protecting the bone from damage during the performance of activities. This protection comes from both the direct cushioning effect the muscles may give to the underlying bone in the event of a fall and a protective hydraulic supporting effect to the bone during activity created by contraction of the overlying muscles.[45]

When bones are compressed, some of the blood contained in the cancellous endosteal bone and some of the other fluids present in the marrow cavity are forced out of the bone through small foramina in the bone surface. If the muscles surrounding the bone are contracted at the time the compression force is applied, the expulsion of these fluids is slowed or prevented entirely, depending on the degree of muscle contraction; the bone marrow pressure will be raised. The presence of fluid at an increased pressure in the marrow cavity absorbs some of the potentially damaging and destructive forces that would otherwise have fallen on the bone tissue when the compression was applied. These potentially damaging or destructive forces are dissipated and resisted by this hydraulic support.[46]

The forces developed by maximum voluntary muscle contractions in males are consistently higher than for females of similar age. The rate of force development during a muscle contraction is also greater in males.[47] Because the time taken to generate a given force of muscle contraction (and consequently, the time to develop an effective level of hydraulic support) is longer in females, their bones will remain at risk for a longer period during falls or impact activities than in males. Differences between males and females in both the strength and speed of muscle contraction may explain, at least in part, why the fracture rate in a given bone is invariably higher in women than in men in situations where the bone density in the two groups is the same.

When compression forces are applied to the osteoporotic bone, damage to the horizontal trabeculae occurs first, followed by injury to the oblique and vertical trabeculae, and finally to the bone cortex.[48] Fractures associated with osteoporosis occur most frequently in the vertebral bodies and at the upper end of the femur, but may also occur elsewhere. The lower the bone density, the greater will be the ease with which a bone fractures during the performance of an everyday activity, or as the result of minor trauma.[49]

Clinical Problems of Aging in Bone

Osteoporosis

Osteoporosis is an almost inevitable accompaniment of old age in both men and women.[50] It would appear advisable, then, to regard osteoporosis as a normal feature of the aging process. If this concept is accepted, the approach should be directed toward reducing, halting, and possibly even reversing the progressive bone loss. Basically, this amounts to ensuring that regular and adequate electrostatic forces continue to be generated in the bones by the use of weight-bearing activity programs.

In general, the greater the amount of weight-bearing physical activity performed over time, the greater will be the effect on the bone density.[51,52] Jogging, tennis and other racquet sports, aerobic classes, and dancing have all been shown to be beneficial,[53] and, undoubtedly, skating and cross-country skiing would prove equally helpful. For less active elderly people a regular daily program of walking and stair climbing should be considered.

Whatever type of weight-bearing activities are recommended to patients, one common feature—enjoyment—needs to be emphasized. Unless enjoyment is obtained from participation in these activities, ongoing compliance is unlikely. Only if these activities are continued for many months will any effect on bone development be produced, although improvement of muscle function will be evident much earlier. Clearly, enjoyment of the physical activities and the social contacts made through the program increase the likelihood that these will be continued.

Most geriatric patients, as well as nursing-home residents, participate in group exercise and activity programs for their physical and social benefit. These activity sessions need to include as much weight-bearing activity as possible if the best effects on bone are to be produced.[54] Exercises that alter the amount of weight on each foot, attempts to balance on one foot, arm-swinging exercises from the standing position, raising the heels from the floor, ball-catching activities, and passing articles between standing group members all involve shifts of position, changes in the forces applied to the weight-bearing bones, and alterations in the patterns of activity in the muscles that ensheath these weight-bearing bones. During all these activities electrical potentials to encourage the continuing redevelopment and reorganization of bone are being produced through both piezoelectric and flow-potential mechanisms.

Care should always be taken to select a program of activities in which the mechanical forces developed during those activities are not likely to lead to compression and fracture. In cases where osteoporosis is extensive or severe, it may be necessary to have the patient enroll in a preactivity exercise program of non-weight-bearing exercises to increase both the force and speed of contraction of muscles in the lower limb and trunk, before allowing progression into the weight-bearing activities program. This preactivity exercise program is intended to first improve muscle function, and therefore increase the effectiveness of the muscle-produced hydraulic support needed to protect the weakened bone, before subjecting the weight-bearing bones to increased impact-compression forces. It would appear that supervised activity programs produce greater increases in bone density than the performance of unsupervised exercises.[55,56]

Patients with osteoporosis are treated medically with a variety of drugs, in addition to their planned program of physical activity. Low dosages of estrogen—even when continued for long periods—are now considered to be safe by many physicians and are reported to have a beneficial effect in reducing bone loss and, in some cases, to restore some of the bone previously lost.[57] Fluoride has also been shown to be helpful in increasing bone density in many patients.[58]

It is not yet known whether these increases in bone density of osteoporotic patients leads to a significant reduction in the subsequent fracture rates. Indeed, some evidence indicates that bone produced through the use of fluoride treatments, although more dense, may be more brittle than usual. Further studies are required to determine the interactive effects between the use of exercise and various drug regimens.

Fractures in Osteoporotic Patients

In patients with advanced osteoporosis acute compression fractures often occur during the performance of an everyday activity, such as bending forward to pick up an object from the floor, tying a shoelace, coughing or sneezing. Alternatively, these fractures may result from a minor slip or twist or from a fall that would be unlikely to cause a fracture in persons with normal bone density. Osteoporotic fractures are most often found in the vertebral bodies and at the upper end of the femur. In some cases the damage to the bone may be limited to the internal trabeculae, in which case there will be no overall deformation of the bone; if the damage is more extensive, and the bone cortex is damaged as well as the trabeculae, the affected portion of the bone will show displacement and wedging.[59]

If the damage is limited to the trabeculae the patient will complain of discomfort at the site of the injury, and spasm of the surrounding muscles is usually evident. Unless other injuries are present, the patient usually responds well to a program of bed rest for 1 to 2 days with liberal use of mild analgesic drugs, followed by a resumption of normal activity. Obviously, it is necessary to shorten the period of bed rest as much as possible in order to reduce further bone loss to a minimum.[60] If compression of the femoral head has resulted, a hip replacement prosthesis is likely to be needed, and a lengthy period of rehabilitation will be necessary.

Where wedging of one or more vertebral bodies has occurred, but the fracture is stable and no further displacement is likely, the patient is usually kept in bed for 2 weeks or so before reactivation is attempted. Problems associated with orthostatic hypotension may occur if the crush fracture has affected the upper lumbar area. Some form of spinal support—normally a semirigid corset rather than a plaster cast—is used to protect the damaged and painful area until the fracture has healed. Flexion exercises increase the likelihood of producing further fractures in the weakened spine and should be avoided.[61]

Osteomalacia

Osteomalacia results from a lack of vitamin D. Humans can synthesize vitamin D in the presence of sunlight; many people also supplement their diet to provide an adequate intake. Osteomalacia is found less frequently in people living in areas with long hours of sunshine. In a city in northern England, where the total number of hours of sunshine each year is low, a high incidence of osteomalacia has been noted.[62] A lower incidence is likely in most parts of the United States because of adequate sunshine and vitamin D supplementation of food.

As it is not possible to distinguish by means of x-ray examination among senile osteoporosis, pathologic osteopenia, and osteomalacia, vitamin D is often given to all patients with reduced bone density, although its use will lead to improvement only in patients with osteomalacia.[63]

THE NERVOUS SYSTEM AND AGING

Aging is often characterized by reductions in sensibility, coordination, cognitive abilities, and ability to react to changing circumstances. A general assumption is made that loss of nerve tissue is a predominant feature of aging. In reality, although some loss of nerve cells does take place during the aging process, the extent to which this loss occurs is less than usually assumed. The reduced level of nervous system functioning in the elderly is better explained in terms of biochemical and functional changes that take place in neurons during aging and senescence.

There are, however, many functional losses in the human nervous system that are accepted as age-related, yet little is known of the intracellular changes that cause these losses. Part of this problem is due to the fact that in life nerve cells always exist as a system in communication with, and affected by, activity in other types of tissue. The story is still incomplete.

The functional deficits of aging in the nervous system may be explained in terms of a combination of

1. Loss of neurons
2. Loss of dendrites
3. Loss of synapses
4. Microscopic changes in senescent neurons
5. Changes in nerve conduction
6. Changes in neurotransmitter mechanisms

Loss of Neurons

The weight of the brain is reduced in old age; there is a 5 percent loss in weight by age 70, 10 percent by age 80, and 20 percent by age 90.[64] It is also accepted that the volume of the brain is reduced to a similar degree.[65]

Reduction in weight and size of the brain has usually been assumed to result from a progressive loss of nerve cells in the brain over a period of time. In an early study it was shown that there was an early loss of Purkinje cells from the cerebellar cortex[66] and that a definite loss of cells from the hippocampus also occurs.[67] In most areas of the brain, however, it has not been possible to demonstrate age-related neuronal loss.[68]

From these studies it would appear that although some neuronal loss does occur as part of the normal aging process, this loss does not affect all nerve cell populations to the same degree, and some cells remain unaffected. The extent of neuronal loss is certainly much less than previously assumed. No regular or predictable pattern of neuronal degeneration has been established. The loss of neurons that has been demonstrated is insufficient to account for the reduced ability for control and coordination seen in the nervous systems of elderly people. The accompanying reduction in size of the brain with age is due primarily to the progressive dehydration of the brain over time.

Loss of Dendrites

Although the number of neurons in most parts of the brain may not be reduced significantly during aging, it has been found that a reduction in the number of dendrites associated with a particular neuron is a generalized feature of the aging process. The mechanism of this progressive dendritic loss is unknown, although it has been suggested that the dendritic atrophy begins in the most distal parts of the dendritic branches and gradually works its way toward the cell body of the neuron.[69]

Loss of Synapses

It has been suggested that a typical motor neuron in the spinal cord has perhaps 10,000 synaptic contacts on its surface, of which about 2000 are on its cell body and 8000 are on its dendrites. This does not mean that 10,000 intermediate neurons impinge on the motor neuron; each intermediate neuron tends to make multiple synaptic connections with each of its target cells. It is evident, then, if the dendritic tree of a neuron is reduced during aging, there will be a loss of synaptic connections with other cells.[70] The number of synaptic connections will also be reduced if similar degeneration has affected the terminal branches of the axons.[71] It is not known which of the different afferent systems lose their synaptic connections during aging and senescence.

It is probable that the number of synaptic connections is not static in normal persons at any age. Synapses may be constantly remodeled during adult life, and the change in the number and distribution of synapses in adulthood may be irregular and may be a reflection of changing functional capacity.[72] In older persons the capacity for remodeling is retained, but is usually somewhat reduced. It may be that synapses are lost in the aged brain as a normal part of the turnover process but that they are less easily replaced.

When new synaptic connections are made, some appear to aid in the restitution of function, whereas others oppose this.[73] Misplaced synaptic connections may increase the noise level in the system and decrease the precision of information processing along the abnormal pathways. One theory to account for the decline in functional capacity with aging is that the turnover and cell loss increase the number of inappropriate new synaptic connections.[74]

Microscopic Changes in Senescent Neurons

A number of changes are regularly found in senescent neurons when these are examined under the microscope. Granules of lipofuscin pigment accumulate in the cell bodies of neurons as a function of age. Traditionally, this pigment has been regarded as resulting from the wear and tear processes in those cells with a high level of oxidative activity. Lipofuscin appears to be formed from lysosomal material within the cell. There is no evidence, however, to support the notion that the presence of lipofuscin granules within the cytoplasm has a detrimental effect on the normal functioning of the cell. Indeed, one of the heaviest accumulations of lipofuscin pigment occurs in the inferior olivary nucleus, which appears to function normally, and from which no neurons are lost during senescence.[75]

Evidence of degeneration of the neurofibrils in the cell body is predominant in some types of senile dementia, but such degeneration is also to be found in brain cells of persons who have not exhibited any symptoms of dementia. It is possible that the stimuli that lead to the production of neurofibrillary tangles in cells of the hippocampus, frontotemporal cortex, and reticular formation may cause different degenerative changes in other types of nerve cells.[76] No evidence has been presented to demonstrate that the presence of neurofibrillary tangles causes a decrease in the axoplasmic transport, as is often assumed.

Other changes that have been reported—alterations in the Golgi complex, reduction of ribosome concentration in the endoplasmic reticulum, and lowered fluid content of the cells—are not restricted to nerve cells but are generalized characteristics of degenerating and senescent cells of all types.

Changes in Nerve Conduction

In the resting state the interior of the nerve cell and its processes are rich in potassium ions and low in sodium ions, whereas on their exterior the concentration of these ions is reversed. Because of this unequal distribution of ions, together with the fact that the membrane in its resting state is much more permeable to potassium than sodium ions, the nerve has a resting potential of approximately 70 mV, the outside being electrically positive with respect to the interior.

A nerve impulse is created by the temporary depolarization of the nerve membrane. Channels in the membrane open up to allow the flow of sodium ions into the cell, with a second set of channels allowing for the outward flow of potassium ions from the cell after a slight delay. A wave of depolarization is conducted over the whole surface of the neuron from the point at which it was originally generated. In myelinated nerve fibers the nerve impulse jumps quickly from one node of Ranvier to the next. The conduction velocity of nerve impulses along myelinated fibers is up to 25 times greater than along unmyelinated fibers of similar diameter.

The ionic exchange across the nerve membrane to produce a nerve impulse is a relatively simple biochemical mechanism.[77] It is altered little during the normal aging process. In normal older people there is no significant change in the conduction velocity along a specified portion of a nerve trunk when compared to that found in younger adults. In the elderly, as in younger persons, if a reduction in conduction velocity is found, some narrowing of the fiber, or some impairment of blood flow to the nerve sheath, or some degree of demyelination of the fiber should be suspected.

Changes in Neurotransmitter Mechanisms

The arrival of a nerve impulse at an axon terminal causes the sudden release of molecules of a transmitter substance from the terminal. The transmitter molecules then diffuse across the fluid-filled gap between the two cells and act on specific receptors on the surface of the adjacent neuron. The electrical activity of the receptor neuron is altered by this action of the transmitter substance. To date, more than 30 different transmitter substances have been identified; each has a characteristic excitatory or inhibitory effect on the postsynaptic cell. There are three types of neurotransmitter substances: (1) those affecting the ionic gate mechanisms, (2) monoamine transmitters, and (3) neuropeptides.

Changes in Ionic Gate Activity

At the nerve–muscle junction and between many neurons in the brain and spinal cord, the transmitter substance liberated from the terminals of the presynaptic cell is acetylcholine. Molecules of acetylcholine are stored in the vesicles within the axon terminal. When the nerve impulse arrives at the terminal, calcium ions flow into the depolarized membrane, causing several hundred synaptic vesicles to fuse with the presynaptic membrane. Each vesicle load of acetylcholine causes some 2000 ionic channels to open up in the postsynaptic membrane. Movement of sodium ions into the postsynaptic cell and outflow of potassium ions from the cell then occurs.

The acetylcholine molecules in the synaptic gap are rapidly broken down by the enzyme acetylcholinesterase. Most of the molecules resulting from this deactivation process will be reabsorbed back into the axon terminal of the presynaptic neuron, to be resynthesized back into acetylcholine and re-stored in the terminal for future repeated use. The relative simplicity of this process, combined with the regular resynthesis of acetylcholine molecules, means that this process is not affected to any degree by the aging process.[78]

At synapses in the central nervous system where acetylcholine is liberated a second group of presynaptic neurons terminate. The transmitter substance liberated from the axon terminals of this second set of neurons is gamma-aminobutyric acid (GABA). GABA acts on a second set of receptors on the surface of the postsynaptic cell to open pores in that membrane that are selectively permeable to negatively charged chloride ions. As the chloride ions pass through the open pores into the postsynaptic cell they increase the voltage across the membrane and temporarily inactivate the cell. Approximately one-third of all cells in the central nervous system are thought to use GABA as their neurotransmitter. No GABA-producing neurons terminate at the nerve–muscle interface.

The actions of acetylcholine and GABA on the postsynaptic cell are complementary. Whether the postsynaptic cell fires or fails to fire when both neurotransmitters are liberated simultaneously is determined by their summated or cumulative effect on the resting potential of the postsynaptic membrane. If the membrane is depolarized because of the stronger acetylcholine effect, activity will be created in the postsynaptic neuron; if the inhibitory action of GABA is greater than the excitatory influence of acetylcholine, the postsynaptic cell will not fire. Like acetylcholine, GABA is rapidly broken down and inactivated in the synaptic gap and reabsorbed into the presynaptic neuron.

During aging there appears to be a 15 percent reduction in the GABA content of the brain.[79] A reduction in GABA secretion and liberation throughout the nervous system results in progressive deterioration of fine coordination of motor activities. When the GABA neurons of the corpus striatum degenerate selectively, Huntington's chorea is produced, a hereditary condition in which uncontrolled movements are a predominant feature.

Changes in Monoamine Transmitter Activity

At many synapses the neurotransmitter substance is a monoamine, a substance synthesized within the nerve cell via changes in amino acid molecules absorbed from the bloodstream. For example, molecules of tyrosine (an amino acid) are taken into the nerve terminal from the bloodstream and are acted on by enzymes contained within the mitochondria of the axon terminals. In some cells the tyrosine is converted first into dopa and then into dopamine; in other cells, where different enzymes are present, the tyrosine is converted into norepinephrine. As the molecules of both dopamine and norepinephrine contain a single amino radical, they are termed *monoamine transmitters*. Other monoamine transmitters have also been identified.

Molecules of monoamine transmitters from the axon terminal interact with specific receptor sites on the postsynaptic membrane. The receptor molecules are coupled in the cell membrane to an enzyme that converts adenosine triphosphate (ATP) into cyclic adenosine monophosphate (cyclic AMP; cAMP). Cyclic AMP then acts on the biochemical machinery of the cell to initiate a further response; for this reason, cAMP is often termed a "second-messenger" substance.

The postsynaptic cell responds to cAMP in two stages. In the first stage depolarization of the membrane occurs instantaneously; in the second stage the cell body of the postsynaptic cell is triggered into a bout of synthetic activity that begins after some period of delay but may continue for some time thereafter.

Once the monoamine transmitter has set off the second-messenger activity its molecules are reabsorbed from the synaptic space into the presynaptic neuron. Some are repackaged in synaptic vesicles for repeat use; other molecules are inactivated and destroyed by the enzyme monoamine oxidase in the terminal.[80]

These transmitters are not evenly distributed regularly throughout the brain but are highly localized in discrete centers and pathways. The cell bodies of most of the dopamine-producing cells are located in the substantia nigra of the midbrain, from where many of their axons project into the corpus striatum, where they play an important part in the control of voluntary movements. Other axons pass into the forebrain to assist in the control of emotional responses. The cell bodies of the norepinephrine-producing neurons, on the other hand, are located mostly in the brainstem, with their axons radiating to the hypothalamus, the cerebellum, and parts of the forebrain where they are important in maintaining arousal and regulating mood.

The enzymes associated with the metabolism of the different monoamine transmitters are particularly vulnerable to aging changes. If the monoamine pathways degenerate, there will be impairment of motor, emotional, and mood control.

Selective degeneration of one or more of these pathways may occur. Where the degeneration selectively affects the dopamine system neurons, symptoms of parkinsonism will develop, whereas selective degeneration of the norepinephrine pathways will result in depression. The presence of degenerative changes in the monoamine-producing neurons tends to be more pronounced than degenerative changes in other types of neurons.

Changes in Neuropeptide Activity

Transmitters affecting the ionic gate mechanisms and the monoamine transmitters are manufactured in the axon terminals of different neurons; a third group of neurotransmitter substances—the neuropeptides—are produced in the cell body.[81] Peptides are chemical substances produced when a number of amino acid molecules are linked together in a particular order to form a single large molecule. The sequence of amino acid components in peptide molecules is fixed, encoded by a gene; thus a strand of DNA in the cell nucleus is required. The genetic encoding mechanism in the nucleus is transcribed onto a strand of messenger RNA, which carries the code to the ribosome. Ribosomes in the cell body are the sites at which peptide synthesis occurs. The original peptide molecules synthesized by the ribosomes is very large; enzymes in the cell body cleave the larger peptide strand into a number of shorter chains. Different groups of nerve cells contain different enzyme systems, and thus the neuropeptide transmitter substances produced will vary.

Once the neuropeptides have been synthesized in the cell body they must be transported along the whole length of the axon to its terminals. Those substances that are relatively small may be carried in the fast-transport mechanisms of the neuron; the larger neuropeptides will be carried in the slow-transport mechanism. The action of cAMP as the second messenger in the cell body will stimulate the production of the neuropeptide and its transport to the axon terminals. The effect of stimulation, triggering the production of neuropeptides in the cell body and the eventual release of the substance at the terminals, may continue for minutes or hours. The mechanisms involved in the encoding, synthesis, transport, storage, liberation, and inactivation of neuropeptides are obviously more complex than those involved with other types of neurotransmitters. As a result, these mechanisms are more affected by the aging process.

Two neurotransmitters produced through this mechanism—P substance and endorphin—are of particular interest because they can directly affect the ease of movement. *P substance* is a chain of amino acids produced in and liberated by nerve cells along the pain pathways. Ribosomes in some of the cell bodies in the posterior root ganglion produce molecules of P substance, which are then transported through the neuron. The generation of a nerve impulse along the pain fibers causes P substance molecules to be liberated from the axon terminals of these fibers in the substantia gelatinosa. The second-stage neurons in the lateral spinothalamic tract, which pass upward in the central nervous system to the thalamus, liberate further amounts of P substance in the thalamus. Re-uptake of P substance from the presynaptic cleft into the presynaptic terminal is a slow process compared with the uptake of cholinergic or monoamine transmitters. While molecules of P substance remain, pain sensation will persist.

Another neuropeptide substance, similar in composition to morphine, is liberated from other axon terminals in the proximity of synapses along the pain pathway. This substance is known as *endorphin*. Endorphin appears to have an action on the axon terminals of the pain fibers by inhibiting their ability to release P substance, and so result in a reduction of the number of pain impulses being transmitted to the brain.

Normally, the secretion and activity of P substance and endorphin are well coordinated. During the aging process the production and activity of one or both of these substances may be impaired. In some elderly people a generalized reduction in sensory activity may occur, largely owing to a raised threshold of stimulation being required to trigger off activity in the sensory nerves. In this situation, and when the pain pathways themselves selectively degenerate, the sensitivity to painful stimulation is reduced. In other older persons selective degeneration of the endorphin-producing neurons will result in increased sensitivity to pain and possibly the development of certain types of chronic pain states. Acupuncture is thought to produce its pain-relieving effect largely through stimulation of increased secretion of endorphins. Older persons are less responsive to treatment by acupuncture, possibly as the result of a decreased ability to produce endorphins.[82]

MUSCLE TISSUE

Skeletal muscle fibers are large, cylindrical multinucleated cells with a diameter between 10 and 100 μm and a length of up to 40 cm. Each fiber is surrounded by a plasma membrane, the sarcolemma. The fiber contains a number of segments, called *sarcomeres,* arranged end to end along the length of the fiber. The sarcomere is the basic contractile unit of the muscle fiber. It contains thick and thin fibers of myosin and actin arranged in a regular fashion to produce the characteristic cross-striations of the fiber in an alternate light and dark pattern. Enzyme-filled mitochondria and ribosomes for protein synthesis exist within the fluid matrix of the fiber.

Forming a network around the sarcomere is a closed system of tubules, the sarcoplasmic reticulum, in which calcium ions are retained. Nerve impulses cause the liberation of calcium ions from the sarcoplasmic reticulum into the sarcomere, and cross bridges are established between the myosin and actin filaments. The formation of these cross bridges causes a sliding movement to occur between the two sets of filaments, with subsequent shortening of the sarcomeres and therefore of the muscle fiber. The calcium ions then return into the sarcoplasmic reticulum, the cross bridges are broken, and the muscle reverts to its original length.

Energy to produce the movement between the myosin and actin filaments comes largely from the breakdown of adenosine triphosphate (ATP) into adenosine diphosphate (ADP). As only a small amount of ATP is available in the muscle fibers, the ADP will need to be rebuilt into ATP as quickly as possible. Most ATP production and reconstitution takes place in the mitochondria, which are found close to the myofibrils where the ATP is required.

Mitochondria in type I fibers contain enzymes that work relatively slowly on free fatty acids under aerobic conditions to produce the energy required to restore ADP to ATP. In type II fibers different enzymes act on carbohydrate materials under anaerobic conditions to produce this restoration more quickly. Type I fibers are often termed slow fibers, and type II fast fibers. Some muscle fibers, termed type IIa fibers, possess both oxidative and glycolytic enzyme systems.

To maintain aerobic functioning as long as possible, aggregations of myoglobin exist in the sarcoplasm of type I fibers. The presence of myoglobin in the fiber facilitates the passage of oxygen into the fiber and also provides for some oxygen storage.

In some animals all the muscle fibers in a particular muscle belly are of the same type, but in humans type I and type II fibers are intermingled in each muscle belly, although the proportion of each type varies from one muscle to another. All muscle fibers in a particular motor unit (i.e., one supplied by the same nerve fiber) are of the same type, however.

Aging Changes in Muscle Tissue

The direct effects of age on skeletal muscle are difficult to assess because increasing age and decreasing physical activity are highly correlated. If skeletal muscles are used frequently, they show remarkably few structural and functional changes with age in most people. It may be more reasonable to define most of the changes found in the muscles of elderly persons more as characteristics of disuse rather than of age.

Chemical Changes During Aging

The changes that occur during aging may involve

1. Loss of fluid and inorganic salts
2. Changes in enzyme activity

3. Reduction in contractile proteins
4. Cellular disintegration and death

Loss of Fluid and Inorganic Salts. Under normal conditions the sarcolemma acts as a selectively permeable membrane, resulting in an imbalance in the concentration of sodium and potassium ions on the two sides of the membrane. Sodium ions are largely prevented from entering the muscle fiber, whereas potassium ions pass readily through the sarcolemma into the muscle fiber and are then retained within the cell. This results in a high intracellular concentration of potassium ions.

A rapid loss of fluid from the muscle fibers, together with the loss of dissolved inorganic salts occurs when injury or disease affects the locomotor system. Within the space of an hour or two, a reduction in size of the affected muscles may be noted. During aging a slow but progressive loss of fluid and potassium salts occurs from the muscle fiber, as the result of degenerative changes in the sarcolemma.[83] It is possible that this problem may be compounded by a lack of potassium in the diet of older people, who tend to select foods low in potassium.[84]

Lack of potassium ions in the aging muscle reduces the force of the maximum voluntary contraction the muscle is capable of generating. The patient complains of tiredness and lethargy. The characteristic day-to-day variations often found in older persons most likely results from fluctuations in the potassium ion content of the tissues, particularly if that patient also exhibits pronounced dehydration.

Many patients are admitted to chronic-care institutions suffering from dehydration and with low potassium levels and are referred to the physical therapist for strengthening exercises and general activity programs. Little improvement can be expected if the tissue dehydration and the lack of potassium are not corrected. If the blood chemistry is attended to by the physician, a dramatic improvement in the physical capabilities of the patient will usually result. Careful monitoring of dehydrated patients receiving potassium ion supplements is necessary to detect any signs of cardiac arrhythmia that may be produced.[84]

In most cases reduction in muscle bulk in elderly patients is more likely to be due to dehydration and altered ionic concentrations in the tissues rather than resulting from other more complex degenerative changes within the muscle.

Changes in Enzyme Activity. Most enzymes in the muscle fiber are contained in the mitochondria. The mitochondria in type I fibers contain oxidative enzymes; in type IIa fibers some mitochondria contain oxidative enzymes and others glycolytic enzymes; only glycolytic enzymes are present in the mitochondria of type IIb fibers.

Changes begin to occur in muscle enzyme function within 2 or 3 days of cessation of normal activity. These changes first occur, and are most apparent, in the glycolytic enzyme systems of type II fibers, although if inactivity persists the oxidative enzyme systems of the type I and type IIa fibers may also become involved.

Reduction in enzyme activity results in a reduced capacity of the muscle to break down food materials to provide energy. This lessening in enzyme activity is reflected in a reduction of the enzyme content of the mitochondria within the muscle fibers. The number of mitochondria is not reduced, however.[86]

Degenerative changes in the mitochondria are reversible. If activity is commenced or increased, improvements in the enzyme concentration of the muscle mitochondria may begin to appear within a few days, even in the muscles of elderly patients, although the rate of redevelopment is slower in older persons when compared with that of younger persons.[86]

Reduction in Contractile Proteins. Changes to the contractile protein complex in the muscle fibers—true atrophy—only occur to a limited extent, and then only as the result of extremely prolonged inactivity or a loss of the nerve supply. Although true atrophy of muscle fibers is most unlikely in normal persons before the age of 65, there is some evidence to suggest that after that age atrophy may appear in some muscle fibers in some elderly persons. In these cases it is suggested that although the nerve cell and axon in a motor unit may be structurally unaffected, some of the terminal axon filaments may cease to conduct nerve impulses, or fail to liberate effective amounts of neurotransmitter substance. Thus some, but not all, of the muscle fibers within the motor unit are left in a functionally denervated condition.

In those muscle fibers that have lost their nerve supply, breakdown of the contractile elements will result. The unaffected fibers in that and other motor unit in the muscle will be required to carry an increased load and may undergo hypertrophy.[87] Examination of a cross section of such a muscle under the microscope reveals considerable variation in the diameter of the muscle fibers, whereas in normal muscle the diameters of muscle fibers within a single area of a muscle are remarkably similar. Breakdown of the contractile complex tends to occur first, and is most apparent, toward the outside of the muscle fiber, with those filaments closer to the center of the fiber being relatively unaffected.

Neuropathic changes in the muscle appear to be the most common finding in muscles of persons over the age of 65. The most important factor in the changes of senile muscle is a progressive decrease in the number of functioning motor units.[88] These changes have been reported in approximately 30 percent of persons over the age of 60, with no increase found in those over 80. In contrast, the selective atrophy of type II fibers that occurs in conditions of disuse and malnutrition, increases from 30 percent in the 60- to 70- and 70- to 80-year-old groups to 50 percent in persons over 80.[89]

Disintegration of the Muscle Cell. In the event of fluid loss, changes in electrolyte balance, reduction of mitochondrial enzyme activity, and breakdown of the contractile elements the muscle fiber gradually reverts to a more primitive form of connective tissue cell. Ribosome function in the degenerating cell shifts from a production of specialized actomyosin to an increase in the procollagen secretion. Waste materials accumulate progressively within the cell. If the changes are especially severe, breakdown of the nuclei within the muscle fiber may follow, and the abnormal nuclei may be extruded from the fiber. In either case, death of the fiber will occur, and the debris left behind will be gradually absorbed by migrating reticuloendothelial cells.

Changes in Neural Activity

Muscle fibers within a motor unit all possess similar characteristics; all are either type I or type II fibers. This finding suggests that the chemical composition of a muscle fiber is dependent on neural control, at least to some degree. Neural control is exercised over the muscle fiber through two mechanisms: (1) the pattern of nerve impulse activity in the motor end-plate area, and (2) by the exudation of neurotrophic substances across the neuromuscular junction, independent of impulse activity.

There is a difference in the frequency of impulse activity to slow and fast muscle—the frequency of impulses required to produce a tetanic contraction in type I fibers is approximately half that needed to produce a tetanic contraction in type II fibers.

In animal experiments it has been shown that when type I fibers are subjected to chronic stimulation at high frequency they come to resemble type II fibers more closely. Conversely, chronic application of low frequency stimulation to type II fibers results in a lengthening of their contraction time.[90] Although this type of experiment has not been conducted on humans, it appears reasonable to conclude that impulse activity has some influence on the chemical composition of a muscle fiber. However, as the patterns of impulse activity to both type I and type II fibers do not alter significantly with age, it is unlikely that the chemical changes that occur in the fibers of elderly humans can be related to impulse activity changes.

Acetylcholine and other neurotransmitters are liberated in small amounts from the end plates, independent of impulse activity in the nerve. These substances have a trophic, or nutrient, effect on the muscle fiber. Although some of these neurotransmitters may be manufactured and stored in the end-plate region, others are thought to be produced in the cell body or other parts of the neuron, from where they move slowly along the axon to the end plate and across to the muscle fiber. Some of these trophic substances move along the axon at speeds as low as 1 mm/day, although others move more quickly. These trophic neurotransmitters are of particular importance in regulating the enzyme activity for the rebuilding of ATP in the muscle following contraction. If this enzyme activity is reduced, the contraction times lengthen.

If denervation occurs, both impulse activity and neurotrophic influences on the muscle fiber will be lost. Loss of innervation leads to a dedifferentiation between type I and type II fibers, with each reverting to a more primitive form of cell. In type I fibers the most profound change is in the loss oxidative enzymes; in type II fibers an equivalent loss of glycolytic enzymes occurs. The differences between type I and type II fibers are progressively reduced.

There is little or no evidence that degeneration of the end plates takes place as the result of aging, even when extensive changes are found in the muscle fibers. Some reduction may be noted in the number of mitochondria and vesicles in the end plates, especially in those that terminate on the surface of type II fibers, but this reduction is not extensive. A reduction in the size, depth, and number of the junctional folds at these end plates may reduce the capacity for materials to pass across the membrane.

Changes in Blood Flow Through the Muscle

The transfer of metabolites across the capillary membranes within the muscle is reduced in senescent muscle because of an increased thickness of the basement membrane of the capillaries, a decrease in the density of the capillary network, and a diminished reaction of blood vessels in senescent muscle to chemical and nervous stimulation.

Degeneration of the basement membrane of cells that form the capillary wall follows the same pattern as that noted previously for muscle and nerve cell membranes. Changes in the surrounding connective tissue add further to the difficulties of transfer of metabolites to and from the muscle fibers.

Three sets of blood vessels, each separately controlled, exist in skeletal muscle bellies. One set of vessels is responsible for the nutrition of the supporting connective tissue, and two sets are responsible for the nutrition of the muscle fibers. The muscle fiber vascular bed consists of two parallel pathways, one of which is influenced by changes in the concentration of hormones in the circulating blood and one that is controlled by autonomic stimulation.[91]

Vasodilation occurring in muscles at or before the commencement of exercise is a response to alterations in the concentration of various hormones in the circulating blood, unaccompanied by any change in the metabolic rate of the muscle. During exercise, further vascular changes result from changes in the pattern of autonomic nerve activity in the working muscles. In the elderly both these mechanisms become less effective, resulting in a decrease in the degree of circulatory response possible in the working muscle when exercise is performed. It therefore is evident that older persons are able to perform less work than younger persons before anaerobic conditions develop in the working muscles.

Commentary

Preventive care is the key to reducing aging changes in muscle tissue. If skeletal muscles are used frequently, they show remarkably few structural changes, even in advanced age. The majority of changes noted in muscles of elderly persons are characteristics of disuse rather than age. Even though degenerative changes may have occurred as the result of aging and disuse, some degree of restoration of muscle bulk, aerobic capacity, and contractile strength can be expected from properly designed exercise and activity programs.

CONTROL MECHANISMS AND AGING

General Physiologic Principles

Claude Bernard pointed out many years ago that all physiologic mechanisms are designed to facilitate one goal—that of maintaining constant the composition of the internal environment of the body. Two basic principles are involved in all physiologic control mechanisms: (1) the Arndt-Schulz Principle and (2) the Law of Initial Values.

The Arndt-Schulz Principle

The Arndt-Schulz principle is as follows:

1. The application of a subthreshold level of stimulation produces no changes in the physiologic system.
2. The application of a suprathreshold level of stimulation will result in an increase in physiologic function.
3. The application of a supramaximal level of stimulation will reduce the level of function and may cause destructive changes to occur.

Although this general principle applies to persons of all ages, it has five special clinical implications when dealing with elderly patients. First, a greater amount of stimulation is required by an elderly person before any physiologic response is obtained (i.e., the threshold level for stimulation is raised). This means that if the therapist only uses the same level of stimulation as that required to produce a minimal response in younger patients, in many cases no physiologic response will be obtained at all in elderly patients, and thus the treatment will be ineffective. A lack of response of an older person to a standard test or procedure designed for use with younger persons may be misinterpreted by the therapist as an indication that rehabilitation potential is lacking.

Second, the level and type of response resulting from the application of any suprathreshold level of stimulation is usually lower and less predictable for the aged than with younger patients.

Third, in elderly patients the peak level of physiologic and therapeutic response is usually produced by a level of stimulation less than that required to produce a maximum response in younger persons.

Fourth, the use of a strong stimulus that produces beneficial effects when applied to a younger person may result in detrimental effects when applied to an elderly patient, if this patient's supramaximal level is exceeded.

Fifth, the range of levels of stimulation that produces beneficial responses in older persons is considerably narrower than that for younger persons. The therapist is required to exercise greater judgment on the intensity and duration of the stimuli to be applied during a treatment program for older patients than with younger patients if an effective result is to be produced.

Law of Initial Values

The Law of Initial Values states that with a given intensity of stimulation, the degree of change produced tends to be greater when the initial level of that variable is low; and that the higher the initial value, the smaller will be the change produced.

If the composition of the internal environment (the homeostatic level) is maintained at a completely steady level, the application of a given stimulus would tend to produce a similar degree of response to each stimulus. In life, the homeostatic level fluctuates up and down over time. Some physiologic functions vary in a regular cyclic fashion over time; these are referred to as biorhythms. Those biorhythms with 24-hour cycles are termed diurnal variations. In normal young adults the sequence of the many diurnal variations and other biorhythms is highly coordinated.

In older persons the biorhythm cycles become less regular, and greater variations occur between the high and low values of particular variables over time than would be found in younger persons. As the result of increasingly irregular fluctuations in the level of physiologic activities in older persons, the amount of response following the application of a particular stimulus becomes more variable, and thus less predictable.

Clinically, the law of initial values has considerable implications for the organization of rehabilitation care for the elderly disabled person. It becomes obvious that the evaluation of a patient's current abilities and capacity for improvement should not be based on a single evaluation if those abilities are likely to vary considerably from one day to the next, or from hour to hour. In addition, the timing of treatment sessions during the day should be scheduled at the time of each patient's greatest physiologic efficiency; this time is likely to be a different one for each patient. The success of a treatment program for older persons, particularly those with unusually long-standing or especially severe or complex problems, may well hinge on the appropriateness of the scheduling of treatment sessions to meet their individual needs.

Diurnal variations of physiologic function are controlled, at least to some degree, by the regular alternation of light and dark periods during the 24-hour cycle. This form of control becomes less effective during aging, as the result of progressive loss of visual function. Attempts have been made to make use of repeated short periods of high intensity light (at intensities up to six times greater than normal daylight) to help restore the normal pattern of diurnal rhythms. A second approach to improvement of this metabolic disorientation of interest and value to physical therapists is through the use of general physical activity programs.

The whole structure of rehabilitation programs needs to be examined to assure that it supports the stabilization of biorhythms of each individual patient. Customized scheduling may be difficult to arrange in an institutionalized environment and is a strong argument for an increasing emphasis to be given to home-based rehabilitation for the elderly whenever possible.

Hormonal Control Mechanisms and Aging

In a small number of neurons in the central nervous system the major peptide produced within the cell body is ACTH. Liberation of ACTH from the axon terminals of these neurons produces different effects on different groups of postsynaptic cells. ACTH and a number of other peptide transmitter substances that have been identified are substances also produced outside the nervous system by cells of the endocrine system. When produced by endocrine cells, these substances are termed *hormones*.

At neuron-to-neuron connections the transmitter substances are liberated in moderate amounts from the axon terminals. The small amount of transmitter substance liberated is rapidly deactivated at the release site. The effect of release of neurotransmitters is limited to a very localized area for only a very short period of time.

Movement of molecules between capillaries and extracellular spaces in the central nervous system is more difficult than in other tissues. Nerve cells have become more sensitive than other types of cell to their immediate chemical environment; thus, the nerve needs to be protected from the presence of stray molecules of other substances that may arrive by change in the area. This protection is obtained by increased resistance of the capillary walls to the passage of many substances contained in the blood plasma. The passage of food-derived peptide molecules across the capillary wall, in particular, would obviously grossly upset the peptide-controlled neurotransmitter mechanisms.[79]

The capillary wall thickening is achieved partly by a thickening of the basement membrane of the epithelial cells that form the capillary wall, and party as the result of glial activity. The glial cells are connective tissue cells responsible for producing the connective tissue packing material for the nerve cells and their fibers. The protein glial membranes that are produced contain finer fibers than those contained in other connective tissues. The presence of the glial membrane around the small blood vessels and capillaries in the brain produces the so-called blood-brain barrier, which reduces the possibility of stray peptide movement.

During aging the glial cells often become more active, with the result that the glial membrane is thickened. If this occurs the passage of materials across the blood-brain barrier becomes progressively more difficult. The volume of the extracellular space will be reduced.

Although these changes make it less likely that the nerve cell function is affected by diffusion of stray peptide molecules, passage of other materials necessary for the continuing proper functioning of the nerve cells is also made more difficult. It is possible that at those sites in the brain at which selective neuronal degeneration has been demonstrated, the degeneration may be linked, at least in part, to thickening of the blood-brain barrier at these locations.

An increased hydrostatic blood pressure will be required in those locations where thickening of the glial membrane has occurred if adequate amounts of nutrients are still to be moved across the thickened blood-brain barrier from the capillaries to the nerve cells in that area. This increase in blood pressure is vital if normal activity of the nerve cells is to be maintained. Often, the use of hypotensive drugs in the treatment of older patients precipitates a sudden decrease in the brain's ability to function, as indicated by confusion or loss of motor control. Care needs to be exercised in the use of hypotensive drugs in this type of situation (see Ch. 6).

Although all neuron-to-neuron connections in the brain are protected by the blood-brain barrier, some nerve connections are made with cells outside the nervous system. Such connections form the neuroendocrine system.[92] Connections from the hypothalamus to the posterior lobe of the pituitary gland belong to this system. The cells in the posterior lobe of the pituitary gland lie outside the blood-brain barrier. Stimulation of cells in this area will result in the liberation of peptide molecules from the cells. These molecules will pass into the bloodstream as it flows through the area.

Cells in the true endocrine glands (anterior lobe of the pituitary, thyroid gland, etc.) respond to stimuli from chemicals in the blood flowing through the gland rather than from chemical stimulation from direct neurotransmitter activity. The exercise of some control in the activity of the anterior lobe of the pituitary gland by the hypothalamus is not through direct neuronal connections; neurohormones are liberated from the nerve endings in the hypothalamus, enter the pituitary portal vessels, and then pass directly into the anterior lobe of the pituitary where they help to regulate its secretions.[93]

As the result of specific patterns of neural activity, neurotransmitter substances are liberated at particular sites to produce localized changes for short periods of time. To complement this, the endocrine system of the body provides for simultaneous regulation and coordination of activities to modify the structure and function of different organs and tissues of the body over longer periods. This is achieved through the action of chemical substances secreted by certain collections of cells and transported throughout the body via the blood and lymph. Normally, the activity of many endocrine glands is finely balanced and highly coordinated. In the elderly this coordination is progressively disrupted.

Much of this disruption is the result of the body's reaction to increasing stress. When a person is exposed to stress—whether physical, psychological, sociologic, socioeconomic, or emotional—changes take place in the body in an attempt to deal with the stress. Many of these changes involve a shift away from the normal endocrine balance. Selye referred to this reaction as the general adaptation syndrome (GAS), and he divided the response into three distinct phases: the alarm reaction, the stage of resistance, and the stage of exhaustion.[94]

Aging is a period of chronic and increasing stress. The development of the GAS in elderly persons differs somewhat from the reaction in younger subjects. In the alarm reaction and the stage of resistance the degree of response tends to be much reduced. As the result of chronic stress from multiple causes the body's defense mechanisms may not be able to continue to cope, and the stage of exhaustion ensues. In the stage of exhaustion physiologic responses become increasingly unpredictable; these may be greater or less than the usual responses in younger persons, may fluctuate greatly from day to day, or may be opposite in direction—paradoxical—to the normal reaction.

IMPLICATIONS OF BIOLOGIC CHANGES OF AGING ON EXERCISE AND ACTIVITY PROGRAMS FOR THE ELDERLY

In developing exercise and activity programs for the elderly, special considerations apply to this population if appropriate modifications are to be taken in respect to (1) preactivity warm-up, (2) development of coordination, (3) endurance training, (4) muscle-strengthening programs, (5) power exercises, and (6) psychological benefits.

Preactivity Warm-up

The importance of proper warm-up before engaging in purposeful exercise is well recognized. Failure to pay attention to this concept will not only result in reduced effectiveness in the performance of exercises and activities but will also lead to an increased incidence of injuries in persons of all ages.[95] In the elderly this concept is even more important than for younger persons.

The temperature of any tissue at rest depends on the heat delivered to the tissue via the circulating blood, on heat produced from the chemical reactions of metabolism of that tissue, and on the extent to which the heat produced by these metabolic reactions is lost from the tissue, either directly through conduction or radiation or indirectly via the bloodstream passing through the tissue.

In normal aging both the heat production and heat loss mechanisms are affected. On the one hand, less heat is produced in the tissues of the elderly person owing primarily to a progressive reduction of the metabolic rate of all body tissues with aging and partly to a reduced flow of blood through these tissues. On the other hand, heat loss through the skin tends to be proportionately greater in the elderly. The result when these three factors are combined is an overall lowering of tissue temperatures from the level found in younger persons. In winter conditions hypothermia in the elderly may produce a life-threatening situation.

Reference has been made previously to the fact that three sets of blood vessels supply the skeletal muscles—one supplying the connective tissue matrix and two separate sets of vessels supplying the muscle fibers themselves.[91] In the elderly those vessels previously controlled by hormone concentrations in the circulating blood become less able to respond, with the result that the circulatory increase that occurs in younger persons as an anticipation of exercise is progressively lost. Once this responsiveness has disappeared, only vascular reflexes triggered by accumulation of metabolites from muscle activity can be brought into play. The degree of responsiveness is considerably lowered. The time taken for the muscle to reach its most effective working temperature is delayed in the elderly.

The lower temperature in the muscle fibers in elderly persons is reflected in the muscle connective tissue. The lower the temperature of this connective tissue, the less will be its capacity for stretch. Static stretching procedures are less effective when attempted on older persons for this reason[95] and need to be performed with increased care if damage is to be avoided.[96] To reduce the possibility of damage, hold-relax procedures should be incorporated with heat and passive stretching to achieve the greatest increase in muscle length and flexibility.[97]

Although the importance of application of heat as a preparation for exercise may be of questionable value in the management of younger patients whose vascular supply to the working muscles remains sensitive to changes in circulating hormone levels, its value for older persons would appear to be well established. A recent study of the effects of preheating muscles in the calves of elderly men showed that immersion in hot water at a temperature of 44° C for 30 minutes before exercising resulted in significant increases in the speed of development of maximum contraction, the height that could be jumped from a standing start, and the capacity to generate power, although there was no difference between their performance and that of a control group in the maximum tension that could be developed in the muscles during an untimed contraction.[98]

Development of Coordination

A significant loss of coordination is noted in the elderly, although whether this is due to disuse, lack of fitness, normal aging, or a combination of these factors in a given individual is difficult to determine. The loss of coordination with advanced age need not always affect self-care capacity.

A decrease in coordination is noted early in adult life and continues progressively from that time. The performance of an efficient, skilled movement that is properly coordinated depends on a three-part, but continuous, sequence of appropriate perception of sensory information from a variety of sources; effective decision making as to what action or sequence of actions is necessary to deal with the perceived situation; and the correct performance of those actions.[99]

Appropriate perception may be improved by the use of eyeglasses and hearing aids. The difficulty of picking out visual cues from an indistinct background may be overcome by imaginative decorating schemes in the home to make important objects stand out more clearly from the background through the use of contrasting colors. Accurate perception may also be improved if the level of lighting in the room is increased, if the attention of the older person is specifically directed toward the appropriate cues, if spoken instructions from the therapist are given more slowly, if the pitch of the voice is lowered, if clear demonstrations of what is wanted are performed, if the patient is unhurried, and if the overall stress of the situation can be reduced.[100]

The decision-making component in the performance of skilled motor activities usually presents the greatest difficulties, particularly if the cues from the environment are continuing to change. It appears that the brain, like a computer, is programmed to deal with one set of information, and to make a decision on a suitable response to that information, before a new set of information can be processed. With the general slowing of transmission at the many synapses involved in the decision-making pathways in the brain, the processing of perceptual information becomes progressively more difficult. Slowing of the decision-making processes in older persons is usually more pronounced than reductions in either the perceptual or action stages.[101]

Inappropriate perception, combined with reduced decision-making ability, will inevitably result in performance of a poorly coordinated movement. The performance of an efficient, skilled movement that is properly coordinated incorporates three components: avoidance of unnecessary muscle activity, an almost perfect replication of the activity on succeeding attempts, and a resting posture where muscle activity returns to near normal levels and the joint alignment is natural.

When a movement is performed in an uncoordinated fashion a considerable amount of unnecessary muscle activity is performed. Muscles not required to function at all in the activity are brought into action, and those muscles essential to the performance of the activity may work more than necessary. As a training effect is produced, the amount of unnecessary activity is progressively reduced.

When an untrained person makes repeated attempts to perform an activity, considerable variation occurs between one attempt and the next in the way the movement is executed. In a trained person the degree of variation is reduced; a well-trained person is able accurately to reproduce the movement on succeeding attempts.

Both reduction of extraneous muscle action and perfect replication of movements result from the development of new patterns of activity in the central nervous system. The training of coordination involves a training of central nervous system activity. The synaptic resistance along the frequently used pathways in the central nervous system is reduced, thereby facilitating repeated accurate performance of that activity at some later time. As the synaptic resistance in older persons is generally higher than in younger people, the development of new coordinated patterns of movement in geriatric patients will be more difficult to achieve and the maximum degree of skill in the performance of an older trained person will be less than in a similarly trained younger person.[102]

In dealing with geriatric patients and others with a particularly low exercise tolerance (as measured by cardiopulmonary response), it is often preferable to commence the coordination training program with attempts to improve the efficiency of those functions the patient is able to perform before progressing to training of new activities, the development of increased endurance, and improvement in the strength and power of muscle contractions.

In the elderly there is not only an overall slowing down of performance but also greater irregularity and unevenness. Practice brings greater uniformity of performance, but some reorganization of the task may be needed to distribute the older person's resources more effectively over the whole task. The therapist should not limit training to patching up of an existing performance but can consider reorganizing the whole pattern of activity.

Any complex activity is composed of a number of separate actions, each performed as part of a total sequence. When training younger persons to perform a new task or improve the level of performance of an existing activity, it is usually found to be more effective to ask the young person to attempt the whole complex movement sequence and then add appropriate corrections to different elements of the imperfectly performed complex task. When dealing with older persons, and particularly geriatric patients, more satisfactory results are usually obtained by first teaching each component of the activity separately, and then progressively linking the different component together.[103]

Other general points that have been identified with regard to skill training for older persons include observations that the process will be most successful if it is gradual; if the trainees can approach the task in their own way at their own speed; if mistakes in performance can be avoided, especially in the early stages of learning; and if the activity is valued by the learner.[104]

Endurance Training

An endurance exercise is characterized by the performance of an activity over a period of time with moderate loading of the working muscles. An increase in endurance occurs when a person can continue to perform a given activity at the same load for a longer time without fatigue. In other words, there has been an increase in the aerobic capacity.

During activity the different types of muscle fibers are recruited in a regular order: the slow oxidative type I fibers are recruited first, the fast oxidative/glycolytic type IIa fibers are recruited next, and the fast glycolytic type IIb fibers are recruited last. It is evident, then, that the recruitment of type IIa and type IIb fibers will only occur if the load applied is sufficiently high.[105]

The progressive reduction in aerobic capacity during aging in normal older persons results from a combination of reduced oxidative enzyme content in the type I and type IIa muscle fibers,[106] reduction in the blood flow through the muscles,[107] and reduction in cardiopulmonary efficiency.[108]

Improvement in the oxidative enzyme and myoglobin content have been reported within 2 or 3 days of commencement of an activity program in experimental animals. Similar effects have been difficult to demonstrate in humans.[109]

The degree of improvement and the rate at which aerobic capacity improves depends on the loading applied and the duration of the training program. Considerable differences have been found in changes to VO_2max resulting from various training programs.[110-113] These differences possibly reflect the use of subjects of different ages, differences in the intensity and form of exercise, and differences in the duration of the programs. Although each of these studies showed a significant gain in performance of experimental over control subjects, considerable differences were found between subjects in each group.

For younger subjects a training level of 50 to 80 percent of VO_2max is usually regarded as an appropriate endurance training stimulus. A recent study has reported that the responses of groups of men over 60 to programs requiring three sessions per week, over a period of 9 weeks, of cycle ergometer training at intensities of 30 and 70 percent VO_2max produced similar improvements.[114] Consistent with the Law of Initial Values, the amount of increase in aerobic capacity of men in both groups was greater in those whose initial VO_2max level was low and less in those whose original aerobic capacity was higher than average. Geriatric patients referred for physical therapy are likely to have a lower, and usually a considerably lower, than average aerobic capacity for their age group. The lower this initial capacity, however, the greater is the chance of significant improvement in aerobic function resulting from a properly designed treatment program, providing this is continued for a sufficiently long period.

Endurance training not only produces an increase in the oxidative enzyme content of the type I and type IIa muscle fibers, but also results in an increased density of the capillary bed in the working muscles. Exchange of materials—respiratory gases, metabolites, food materials, and hormones—between the blood and tissue fluid across the capillary wall is improved and facilitates the aerobic activity. This improvement in the peripheral aerobic mechanisms may be developed in the calf muscles of patients complaining of intermittent claudication from peripheral vascular disease, as well as in normal older persons.[115]

Endurance training for young persons involves total body activity; many muscles are used in the performance of that activity. When the muscles contract, blood is pumped into the venous side of the circulatory system. An increased venous return to the heart is produced; in normal elderly persons this will result in an increase first in the stroke volume of the heart, followed by an increase in the heart rate. In patients with coronary artery disease little increase in stroke volume is produced when the venous return is increased;[116] in elderly patients with this condition it is possible that no change in stroke volume will result from exercise.

The increase in heart rate produced by a given level of activity in an older person is greater than the increase created by the same level of activity in a younger person, owing to lack of adjustment in the stroke volume. Thus the cardiac reserve in elderly persons is less than in younger people, and the likelihood of undesirably high cardiac rates being produced by exercise is progressively increased with age. Especially careful monitoring of the heart rate of elderly persons during exercise is therefore necessary.

To avoid undue strain on the heart, activity restricted to one part of the body, rather than a general body activity, may have to be the starting point for general exercise in severely debilitated patients. In general, lower limb activities place less strain on the heart than equivalent exercise to the upper limbs.[110] Jogging or fast walking produce less strain on the heart than is developed by exercise on the static cycle at the same VO_2max level. If a well-heated pool is available, water-resisted calisthenics provide a useful group activity.[117] It is often advisable to begin with a regimen of upper and lower limb functional endurance exercises on alternate days, with progression to general body activity only after some improvement of aerobic capacity and cardiac reserve has been obtained. The exercise potential of daily living should be used to supplement the formal exercise sessions. Within the home many simple chores have an appropriate training intensity for an older person, although care should be taken to avoid performing tasks such as fixing shelves and painting ceilings because of a possible undesirable rise in blood pressure from the upper limb isometric activity.[118]

The risk that inappropriate exercise may precipitate cardiac arrest or ventricular fibrillation is small. For men 65 to 70 years old this risk has been estimated at 1 in 27,000, whereas risks for elderly women are approximately one third of those for men.[119] As the risk appears to be greatest in those persons with a highly competitive type A personality, the chance of this problem in geriatric patients is extremely remote. In dealing with geriatric patients, an unfounded fear of heart attack by either the patient or the therapist often precludes the development of an effective training program.

The initial exercise program is usually planned to keep the maximum heart rate during exercise below that calculated from the formula (200 minus the age of the person). Thus the maximum heart rate of a 70-year-old patient should not be allowed to exceed 130 beats per minute.

For most geriatric patients, fast walking is usually adequate to produce an increase in heart rate to the maximum permitted level. As improvement occurs it may be possible to progress to a regimen in which equal distances of approximately 400 meters be covered by alternating fast and slow walking over a 30-minute period. This type of program for elderly people has been shown to result in a 20 percent increase in VO_2max over a period of 21 weeks.[110] The largest increase was found in those subjects who followed a high intensity/high frequency exercise regimen. These subjects also showed a faster recovery of heart rate following submaximum and maximum exercise efforts. Slowing of the resting pulse rate is not always found when older people undergo physical conditioning.[120] Those who show an improvement in physical fitness also show decreases in ST abnormalities on ECG records.[121]

Muscle-strengthening Programs

The amount of force developed by a muscle during contraction depends on the number of motoneurons that are activated and the tensile force developed by each of the contracting muscle fibers. If muscles continue to be used fully, they show surprisingly few degenerative changes with aging. In miners and others employed in heavy manual occupations there is little or no loss of muscle bulk; enzymatic action remains high; and the maximal contractile force the muscle is able to generate shows only a minor reduction.

When a strong contraction is attempted, there is a progressive recruitment of fibers within the muscle—first, an activation of the type I (oxidative) fibers, then a spread of activity to the type II (oxidative/glycolytic) fibers, and, finally, should the demand be sufficiently high, to the type IIb (glycolytic) fibers. In later life fewer strong contractions are ever attempted by most people, so the type IIb fibers are seldom recruited, the type IIa fibers are only activated occasionally, whereas most activities can be performed adequately by the type I fibers alone. Although degenerative changes resulting from disuse may be found to some extent in all types of fibers, these changes are greatest and most extensive in the type IIb fibers, which tend to be used least of all.

A recent review summarized the findings of a number of studies on the effectiveness of strength training programs for elderly people.[122] The investigations showed significant increases in leg strength,[123–125] index finger strength,[126] and little finger strength.[127] The gain reported in these studies varied from 10 to 72 percent; the variability was believed to be due to differences in the types of subjects, the training programs used, the duration of the programs, and the motivational methods employed.

In these studies the greatest gains in muscle strength were produced following a program of progressive resistance exercises done at high intensity levels. In those studies that had used isometric exercise as both the training stimulus and the test measure, the average gain in strength following a 6-week training program was around 50 percent. In those studies that had used isotonic exercise as the training stimulus, but used isometric or isokinetic test measures, the gains reported varied between 7 and 33 percent, with an average gain of approximately 20 percent.

Two conclusions may be drawn from these published data: (1) that some increase in muscle strength in older men and women may be expected to result from a training program of progressive isometric or isotonic resistance exercises, but (2) that most of the gain produced was specific to the training stimulus used (i.e., whereas the use of isotonic exercise over a 6-week period led to a 20 percent gain in isometric strength, the use of isometric exercise as the training stimulus produced a 50 percent increase in isometric strength over the same period). No studies were reported in which the training stimulus used was isometric exercise and the test measured isotonic function. All the studies that were reviewed used healthy older people as experimental subjects; similar studies to examine whether the same responses might be expected from the frail elderly or elderly persons with specific clinical problems have not been undertaken.

Isometric exercise is the most effective approach with younger persons to increase muscle bulk as well as contractile strength.[128] The generation of progressively increasing tensile forces within the muscle, and the increasing demand on the glycolytic enzyme systems of the fast-contracting fibers, leads in younger persons to development of additional amounts of actomyosin, providing that appropriate stimulation of this process by the anabolic steroid endocrinal secretions is available.

In older persons, little or no increase in muscle bulk normally accompanies the increase in contractile strength. This is probably related to the reduction in anabolic steroid secretion and metabolism in older people. Under certain conditions the potential for true hypertrophy continues to exist. When functional denervation results in the loss of neuronal connections to some muscle fibers in a motor unit, the remaining muscle fibers in that same motor unit may develop a compensatory hypertrophy.

Increases in contractile force resulting from strength training programs in elderly subjects are better explained in terms of improved motoneuron recruitment in the central nervous system than by changes within the muscles. This view is reinforced by the fact that increases in maximum contractile forces occur quickly in elderly persons and that cross transfer of training effects to the contralateral limb are produced.

Some anatomic loss of motor units in muscles of the hand and feet has been found in normal elderly people;[129] some of the motoneurons that remain function poorly, intermittently, or not at all.[130,131] However, an increase in the compound electromyogram (EMG) signal developed during attempted maximum voluntary contraction is found to occur as the result of training. As little or no increase has been demonstrated in the evoked potentials from single-motor unit firing, the increase in the total voluntary EMG signal is best explained in terms of an increase in the number of motor units being recruited.

During the early part of each training session the maximum tension should be developed slowly, with the patient concentrating as fully as possible on the contraction; the use of multiple feedback (visual, auditory, proprioceptive, and possibly biofeedback) will assist this. Later, the speed of attempted contractions may be increased, although the therapist must be careful to avoid any increase in speed being accompanied by a reduction in the tensile forces produced. Static holdings of the maximum contraction against increasing resistance should also be practiced. The increased loading of the muscles results in increased feedback to the central nervous system and is likely to increase motoneuron recruitment. In trained elderly persons no difference is noted between the evoked EMG potentials generated by a muscle during supramaximal electrical stimulation and those generated through maximum voluntary activity.[132]

For maximum development of strength, exercise at very high intensity is required. Although each muscle contraction should be repeated, the number of repetitions need only be low; two or three bouts of six to ten repetitions performed once a day (after the muscles have been properly warmed up) is usually considered sufficient.[133] In younger persons, the increase in isometric tension developed during a strength-training program will usually be retained for up to 2 months following completion of the program and discontinuation of supervised exercise. In older persons, the improved ability is rapidly lost if exercise is not maintained.

In those elderly persons in whom muscle weakness is produced through functional denervation as well as from simple disuse, the application of high loads to the contracting muscles may result in further weakening and damage to the muscle. In younger persons the appearance of tenderness and soreness in a muscle following exercise, and the development of overwork weakness, are temporary problems that are usually followed by a productive gain in exercise capacity or performance. In many geriatric patients, especially those with neurologic deficits or circulatory problems, the probability of anatomic and/or functional motoneuron loss exists. If the muscles of these patients are overworked and overwork weakness follows, this could result in rapidly accelerated degeneration of the affected muscles, similar to that reported in patients with poliomyelitis[134] and muscular dystrophy.[135]

Power Exercises

As a means of increasing power (rate of working), isokinetic forms of exercise are the most effective. Certain devices (e.g., the Cybex apparatus) have been designed for isokinetic training. The apparatus can be adjusted to allow movements to be performed at various speeds, with the angular velocity of the movement remaining constant throughout the whole range once the controls have been set. The patient exerts maximum effort throughout the movement.

Few studies have examined the usefulness of isokinetic devices in assisting in the development of power in muscles of older persons. The sparse evidence tends to show that the decrease in isometric strength and the decrease of isokinetic ability at low angular velocities are similar during normal aging; however, at higher angular velocities the decrease in isokinetic activity is significantly greater than the reduction in isometric function.[136] Increases of 7 to 22 percent in isokinetic ability of the quadriceps in older men and women have been claimed following training programs.[124,125] The increases found in women were half that of men, and the results were less satisfactory in treating subjects over 70 than in the 65- to 70-year-old groups. In each of these studies general calisthenic exercises were given to the healthy older subjects as the training stimulus, with the isokinetic device merely measuring their level of isokinetic performance before and after completion of the training. No studies have been reported in which the effectiveness of isokinetic training at specific angular velocities on isokinetic function has been evaluated. Reliable data are also lacking on responses of geriatric patients to specific isokinetic training using these devices. The isokinetic mechanical devices may have less attraction for older persons and geriatric patients than they do for younger, more athletically inclined persons.

Special equipment is not necessary to train isokinetic activity. When using manual resistance, whether against isolated or pattern movements, therapists tend to vary their resistance in different parts of the total range in such a way that the movement is performed smoothly at a constant speed. It is evident that therapists have regularly used the concept of isokinetic training in their rehabilitation exercise programs quite unknowingly.

Another approach to power development is the use of the principles of circuit training.[137,138] A series of different activities is designed, and the patient is asked to complete this series of activities in the shortest possible time. Using the principle at its simplest level, an elderly patient may first be asked to walk a given distance at their own pace; the time taken to cover this distance is noted. Then the patient is asked to complete the same distance in a shorter time on succeeding attempts. The patient will need to generate more power in order to complete the task in a shorter time.

The number of tasks performed and the energy required to perform each task is progressively increased, while the time allowed to complete the sequence is progressively reduced. Rather than artificial exercises being used in a program of this type, timed everyday functional activities are recommended with geriatric patients. Therapists working in home-care programs will find this approach invaluable in the rehabilitation of their clients.

Power is defined as the rate at which work is being performed; an increase in power is made when a given task is performed in a shorter period, or if more work is performed in the same time. Power differs from endurance, which is the ability to continue to perform a given task over a longer time period. Both effective power and endurance capacities are needed to perform the many tasks of daily life. Therapists must recognize the differences between the two and ensure that both endurance and power training are addressed when rehabilitation programs are being developed for geriatric clients.

Only if the particular deficits are properly identified and appropriate strategies devised to deal with these can significant functional improvement be expected. The lower exercise tolerance of older persons makes it necessary to plan each component of the total program with extreme care, so that maximum effectiveness is obtained.

Psychological Benefits

Under normal circumstances most persons "feel good" or "feel better" following vigorous exercise.[139] These subjective reports made by normal people have been supplemented by the use of various psychometric instruments measuring changes in anxiety,[140] depression,[141] and self-esteem[142] associated with exercise and activity programs. In general, temporary improvements lasting 2 to 5 hours have been shown on each of these variables in response to acute physical activity. When the effects of long-term activity are evaluated, although reduction in anxiety still results, the ongoing benefits on measures of depression and self-esteem are limited to those persons who scored low on these variables before commencing the exercise program. A position statement from the National Institute of Mental Health[143] claims:

(a) Exercise is associated with the reduction of stress emotions such as state anxiety;

(b) Anxiety and depression are common symptoms of failure to cope with mental stress, and exercise has been associated with a decreased level of mild to moderate depression and anxiety;

(c) Long term exercise is associated with reductions in traits such as neuroticism and anxiety;

(d) Appropriate exercise results in reductions of various stress indices such as neuromuscular tension, resting heart rate, and some stress hormone levels;

(e) Current clinical opinion holds that exercise has beneficial effects across all ages and in both sexes.

Four general hypotheses may be put forward in an attempt to explain the affective benefits of exercise: the distraction hypothesis, the metabolic reorganization hypothesis, the amine hypothesis, and the endorphin hypothesis.

The Distraction Hypothesis

This hypothesis claims that the affective benefits are not the direct result of the exercise itself, but rather occur as the result of the exercising person being distracted during and by the exercise from attention to stressful stimuli. Evidence has been shown that a number of distraction strategies (including exercise) all lead to reductions in tension and anxiety, but the use of exercise tends to be followed by a greater reduction in these and a more prolonged effect than produced by other strategies.

In geriatric patients the stress level is usually high, owing to the variety and severity of stresses to which this population is especially subject. Although some geriatric patients, especially those suffering from predominantly psychosocial or psychiatric problems, may benefit from the distracting effect of attempted exercise, others with painful locomotor problems or who suffer from dyspnea will not be as likely to regard exercise as the most effective form of distraction.

The Metabolic Reorganization Hypothesis

Note has been made earlier in this chapter that as the result of increasing stress, and particularly following reduced visual input, there may be considerable disturbance of the "metabolic clock." Disorganization of the normal carefully regulated and controlled sequences of metabolic activity occurs, particularly in those processes that undergo diurnal variation. The metabolic disturbance is similar to that produced in jet lag.

In normal young adults the effects of jet lag may persist only for a few hours or last for a number of days; the time taken to restore the system to normal depends on the degree of disorganization produced by the flight— predominantly by the number of time zones crossed and the degree of dehydration of the tissues. Participation in jogging or racquet sports as soon as possible following the flight, and early resumption of normal activities are usually recommended for travelers to assist with restoration of normal metabolic activity.

Metabolically disoriented geriatric patients often find similar benefits from general activity programs, and in those cases where psychological disorientation has been produced by disturbances of the metabolic clock, improvements in both mental function and affect can be expected. Once the improvement has occurred, regression may occur if the level of physical activity is not maintained; this underscores the particular importance that exercise and activity have in maintenance programs for the bedridden or institutionalized elderly.

The Amine Hypothesis

There is considerable evidence that a number of the monoamine neurotransmitters, particularly norepinephrine, serotonin, and dopamine, are involved in depression[144] and schizophrenia.[145] In older adults the secretion of these neurotransmitters is altered; depression and schizophrenia are therefore more likely to be found among the elderly.

Experimental studies on rats have shown that the levels of norepinephrine and serotonin are both increased following a program of treadmill exercise.[146,147] To date, no consistent studies have demonstrated similar effects on humans, although the altered behavior patterns of humans following long-term exercise are similar to those shown by rats in the studies reported.[139]

The type of exercise used in those studies which increases in catecholamines have been recorded was either treadmill running or swimming. These exercises all involve the use of a moderate load, repetitive movements, and moderate duration (15 to 20 minutes) of the activity period.

The deliberate use of this strategy by therapists in the activity programs they design for use with depressed and anxious elderly patients would appear advisable. The link between depression and difficulty in initiating and continuing smooth repetitive movements is demonstrated in many patients suffering from Parkinsonism. Both the locomotor signs and the mood change are regulated by reduction in the catecholamine secretion mechanism. Treatment designed to improve mood is likely to produce improvement in locomotor control and function; conversely, attempts to improve locomotor function are likely to also influence mood.

The Endorphin Hypothesis

A great deal has been written recently on the affective benefits of exercise though the operation of changes in endorphin secretion during prolonged exercise.[148,149] Endorphins—chemicals similar to morphine—occur naturally in the body and are produced by certain nerve cells along the pain pathways in the spinal cord and brain stem. In these locations the specific purpose of these substances appears to be to reduce or prevent the liberation of another peptide neurotransmitter—P substance—from the nerve endings in the substantia gelatinosa of the spinal cord and at other synapses along the ascending pain pathway and also possibly to deactivate those amounts of P substance that have been liberated. The activity of endorphin reduces the possibility of pain stimuli being passed to the brain and also governs the time pain will continue to be experienced once P substance has been liberated.

Although part of the endorphin material will remain in the localized area in which it was liberated, some will pass into the bloodstream and be transported throughout the body. Claims have been made that this is the physiologic mechanism involved in both the runner's high and second wind mechanisms in athletes and highly active younger adults. As these phenomena have only been related to the performance of high levels of activity maintained for a considerable time, it is unlikely that it can have any bearing on the mood of geriatric patients involved in activities as part of their total rehabilitation program.

CONCLUSION

The biology and physiology of older persons should not be viewed as a simple continuation of those processes operating in younger individuals. It needs to be recognized that the responses of the elderly often differ both qualitatively and quantitatively from the reactions of younger adults. These differences are due to varying patterns of change and degeneration in the multiple mechanisms involved in maintaining the body's homeostasis, and, although we remain ignorant on many points, a great deal is known about these changes. This information can greatly assist the physical therapist working with geriatric patients to understand why the signs and symptoms presented by the elderly often differ from those in younger people—that they are due to superimposition or interaction of aging changes with the pathological changes of disease. A better knowledge and understanding of these differences will enable physical therapists to understand the limitations of their older clients more fully, to appreciate the fascinating diversity among their elderly patients a little better, and to plan even more effective treatment programs for them.

REFERENCES

1. Goldberg B, Green H: Collagen synthesis on polyribosomes of cultured mammalian fibroblasts. J Mol Biol 26:1, 1975
2. Gross J: Organization and disorganization of collagen. Biophys J 4:63, 1964
3. Chapman JA, Kellgren JH, et al: Assembly of collagen fibrils. Fed Proc 25:1811, 1966
4. Ramachandrau GN, Saisakharan V: Refinement of the structure of collagen. Biochem Biophys Acta 109:314, 1965
5. Vais A, Anasey J: Modes of intermolecular crosslinking in mature insoluble collagen. J Biol Chem 240:3899, 1965
6. Hayflick L: The biology of human aging. Am J Med Sci 265:433, 1973
7. Barnes MJ: Function of ascorbic acid in collagen metabolism. Ann NY Acad Sci 258:264, 1975
8. Ehrlich P, Hunt TK: Effects of cortisone and vitamin A on wound healing. Ann Surg 167:324, 1968
9. King AL: In Remington JW (ed): Tissue Elasticity. Waverly Press, Baltimore, MD, 1957
10. Meyer K, Hoffman P, et al: Mucopolysaccharides of costal cartilage. Science 128:896, 1958
11. Jehens EW, Monk-Jones ME: On the viscosity and pH of synovial fluid and the pH of blood. J Bone Joint Surg 41B:388, 1959
12. Lazardies E, Revel JP: The molecular basis of cell movement. Sci Am 248:100, 1979
13. Johns RJ, Wright V: Relative importance of various tissues in joint stiffness. J Appl Physiol 17:824, 1962
14. Sapega AA, Quedenfeld TC, et al: Biophysical factors in range-of-motion exercise. Physician Sports Med 9(12):57, Dec 1981
15. Lehmann JF, Masock AJ, et al: Effect of therapeutic temperatures on tendon extensibility. Arch Phys Med Rehab 50:481, 1970
16. Lehmann JF, DeLateur B, et al: Selective heating effects of ultrasound in human beings. Arch Phys Med Rehab 47:331, 1966
17. Ryan GB, Cliff WJ, et al: Myofibroblasts in human granulation tissue. Hum Pathol 5:55, 1974
18. Hjertquist SO, Lampberg R: Identification and concentration of glycosaminoglycans of human articular cartilage. Calcif Tissue Res 10:203, 1972
19. Caillet R: Mechanisms of joints. p. 17. In Licht S (ed): Arthritis and Physical Medicine. Waverly Press, Baltimore, MD, 1969
20. Sokoloff L: The Biology of Degenerative Joint Disease. University of Chicago Press, Chicago, 1969
21. Stockwell RA: The cell density of human articular and costal cartilage. J Anat 101:753, 1967
22. Sohn RS, Michell LJ: The effect of running on the pathogenesis of osteoarthritis of the hips and knees. Clin Orthop 88:106, 1985
23. Walker JM: Exercise and its influence on aging in rat knee joints. J Orthop Sports Phys Ther 8:310, 1986
24. Cavanaugh PR, Lafortune MA: Ground reaction forces in distance running. J Biomech 13:997, 1980

25. Johnson MW, Chakkalakal RA, et al: Fluid flow in bone in vitro. J Biomech 15:881, 1982
26. Bassett CAL: Effect of force on skeletal tissues. In Downey JA, Darling RC (ed): Physiological Basis of Rehabilitation Medicine. WB Saunders, Philadelphia, 1971
27. Lutwak L: Continuing need for dietary calcium throughout life. Geriatrics 29:177, 1974
28. Bargel US: Osteoporosis. Grune & Stratton, Orlando, FL, 1970
29. Mundy GR, Raisz LG, et al: Evidence for the secretion of an osteoclast stimulating factor in myeloma. N Engl J Med 291:1041, 1974
30. Berlyne GM, Ben-Ari J, et al: The aetiology of senile osteoporosis. Q J Med 44:505, 1975
31. Storey E: Bone changes associated with cortisone administration in the rat. Br J Exp Pathol 41:207, 1960
32. Atkinson PJ: Structural aspects of aging bone. Gerontologia 15:171, 1973
33. Towne JA: Electron microscopic evidence of altering osteocytic-osteoclastic activity in perilacunar walls of aging mice. Connect Tissue Res 1:221, 1972
34. Burstone MS: Histochemical demonstration of acid phosphatase activity in osteoclasts. J Histochem Cytochem 7:39, 1959
35. Meema S, Meema HE: Menopausal bone loss and estrogen replacement. Isr J Med Sci 12:601, 1976
36. Gordon GS, Genant HK: The aging skeleton. Clin Geriat Med 1:95, 1985
37. Khairi MRA, Johnston CG: What we know and don't know about bone loss in the elderly. Geriatrics 33:67, Nov 1978
38. Issekutz B, Blizzard JJ, et al: Effect of prolonged bed rest on urinary calcium output. J Appl Physiol 21:1013, 1966
39. Geiser M, Trueta J: Muscle action, bone rarefaction and bone formation. J Bone Joint Surg 40B:282, 1968
40. Mack PB, La Chance PA, et al: Bone demineralization of the foot and hand of Gemini-Titan IV, V, and VII astronauts during orbital flight. Am J R 100:503, 1967
41. Yeater RA, Martin RB: Senile osteoporosis—effects of exercise. Postgrad Med 75:147, 1984
42. Sinaki M, McPhee MC, et al: Relationship between bone mineral density of the spine and strength of the back extensors in healthy postmenopausal women. Mayo Clin Proc 61:116, 1986
43. Pogrund H, Bloom FA, et al: Relationship of psoas width to osteoporosis. Acta Orthop Scand 57:208, 1986
44. Oyster N, Morton M, et al: Physical activity and osteoporosis in postmenopausal women. Med Sci Sports Exerc 16:44, 1984
45. Kumar S, Davis PR, et al: Bone marrow pressure and bone strength. Acta Orthop Scand 50:507, 1979
46. Roaf R: A study of the mechanisms of spinal injury. J Bone Joint Surg 42B:810, 1960
47. Bell DG, Jacobs I: Electromechanical response times and rate of force development in males and females. Med Sci Sports Exerc 18:31, 1986
48. Courpron P: Bone tissue mechanisms underlying osteoporoses. Orthop Clin N Am 12:513, 1981
49. Newton-John HF, Morgan DB: The loss of bone with age, osteoporosis and fractures. Clin Orthop 71:229, 1970
50. Jaworski ZFG: Physiology and pathology of bone remodelling. Orthop Clin N Am 12:485, 1981

51. Falch JA: The effect of physical activity on the skeleton. Scand J Soc Med Suppl 29:55, 1982

52. Jacobson PC, Beaver W, et al: Bone density in women—college athletes and older athletic women. J Orthop Res 2:328, 1984

53. Brewer V, Meyer BM, et al: Role of exercise in the prevention and treatment of osteoporosis. Med Sci Sports Exerc 15:445, 1983

54. Chow RK, Harrison JE, et al: Physical fitness effect on bone mass in postmeno- pausal women. Arch Phys Med Rehabil 67:231, 1986

55. Krolner B, Toft B, et al: Physical exercise as a prophylactic against involutional bone loss—a controlled trial. Clin Sci 64:541, 1983

56. Chow RK: The study of a structured exercise program for osteoporotic patients— in hospital versus home program. Arch Phys Med 66:530, 1985

57. Aloia JF: Estrogen and exercise in prevention and treatment of osteoporosis. Geriatrics 27:81, 1982

58. Chow RK, Harrison JE, et al: The effect of exercise on bone mass of osteoporotic patients on fluoride treatment. Clin Invest Med 10(2):59, 1987

59. Johnston CC, Norton J, et al: Heterogeneity of fracture syndromes in postmeno- pausal women. J Clin Endocrinol Metab 61:551, 1985

60. Sinaki M: Postmenopausal spinal osteoporosis—physical therapy and rehabilita- tion principles. Mayo Clin Proc 57:699, 1982

61. Frost HM: Clinical management of the symptomatic osteoporotic patient. Orthop Clin N Am 12:671, 1982

62. Aaron JE, Gallagher JC, et al: Frequency of osteomalacia and osteoporosis in fractures of the proximal femur. Lancet 1:229, 1974

63. Slovik DM: The vitamin D endocrine system, calcium metabolism and osteopo- rosis. Spec Topics Endocrinol Metab 5:83, 1983

64. Ordy JM, Brizee KR: Neurobiology of Aging. Plenum, New York, 1975

65. Himwich HE: Biochemistry of the nervous system in relation to the process of aging. In Birren JE, et al: The Process of Aging in the Nervous System, Charles C Thomas, Springfield, IL, 1975

66. Corsellis JAN: Some observations on the Purkinje cell population and on brain volume in human aging. In Terry RD, Gershon S (eds): Neurobiology of Aging, Raven Press, New York, 1976

67. Ball MJ: Neuronal loss, neurofibrillary tangles and granulovacuolar degeneration in the hippocampus with aging and dementia. Acta Neuropathol 37:111, 1976

68. Konigsmark BW, Murphy EA: Neuronal populations in the human brain. Nature 228:1335, 1970

69. Vaughan DW: Age related degeneration of pyramidal cell basal dendrites in the rat auditory cortex. J Comp Neurol 171:501, 1977

70. Nauta WJH, Feirtag M: Organization of the brain. Sci Am 241:88, Sept 1979

71. Bondareff W: Synaptic atrophy in the senescent hippocampus. Mech Aging Dev 9:163, 1979

72. Sotelo C, Palay SL: Altered axons and axon terminals in the lateral vestibular nucleus of the rat—possible example of remodelling. Lab Invest 25:653, 1976

73. Schneider GE: Synaptic remodelling. Neuropsychol 17:557, 1979

74. Cotman CW: Synaptic structure and plasticity. In Schimke RJ (ed): Biological Mechanisms of Aging. National Institutes of Health, Bethesday, MD, 1981

75. Brody H: Aging in the vertebrate brain. In Development and Aging of the Nervous System. Academic Press, Orlando, FL, 1972

76. Wisniewski WM, Terry RD: Morphology of the aging brain—human and animal.

Prog Brain Res 40:167, 1973

77. Keynes R: Ion channels in nerve cell membranes. Sci Am 240:126, March 1979
78. Hollander J, Barrows CH: Enzymatic studies in senescent rodent brains. J Gerontol 23:174, 1968
79. Iversen LL: The chemistry of the brain. Sci Am 241:134, Sept 1979
80. McGeer EG, McGeer PL: Age changes in humans for some enzymes associated with the metabolism of catecholamines, GABA and acetylcholine. In Ordy JM, Brizzee KE (eds): Neurobiology of Aging. Plenum, New York, 1975
81. Bloom FE: Neuropeptides. Sci Am 245:148, Oct 1981
82. Sodipo JOA: Therapeutic acupuncture for chronic pain. Pain 7:359, 1979
83. Yiengst MJ, Barrows CH, et al: Age changes in the chemical composition of muscle and liver cells in the rat. J Gerontol 14:400, 1959
84. Anderson F: Practical Management of the Elderly (3rd Ed). Blackwell, Oxford, 1978
85. Drahota Z, Gutmann E: Long term regulatory influence of the nervous system— some metabolic differences in muscles of different function. Physiol Biochem 12:339, 1963
86. Finch CE: Enzyme activity, gene function and aging in mammals. Exp Gerontol 7:53, 1972
87. Tomonek RJ, Woo JK: Compensatory hypertrophy of the plantaris muscle in relation to age. J Gerontol 25:23, 1970
88. Campbell MJ, McComas AJ, et al: Physiological changes in ageing muscles. J Neurol Neurosurg Psychiatr 36:174, 1973
89. Tomonaga M: Histochemical and ultrastructural changes in senile human skeletal muscles. J Am Geriatr Soc 25:125, 1977
90. Vrolova G: Factors determining the speed of contraction of striated muscle. J Physiol 185:17, 1966
91. Walder DN: Vascular pathways in skeletal muscle. In Hudlicka O (ed): Circulation in Skeletal Muscle. Pergamon, Oxford, UK, 1968
92. Everitt AV, Burgess JA: Hypothalamus, Pituitary and Aging. Charles C Thomas, Springfield, IL, 1976
93. Harris GW: Neural Control of the Pituitary Gland. Arnold, London, 1955
94. Selye H, Prioreski B: Stress in relation to aging and disease. In Everitt AV, Burgess JA: Hypothalamus, Pituitary and Aging, Charles C Thomas, Springfield, IL, 1976
95. Devries H: Evaluation of static stretching procedures for improvement of flexibility. Res Q 33:222, 1962
96. Cooper DL, Fair J: Stretching exercises for flexibility. Physician Sports Med 5(3):114, 1977
97. Tanigawa MC: Comparison of hold-relax procedure and passive mobilization on increasing muscle length. Phys Ther 52:725, 1972
98. Davies CTM, Young K: Effect of heating on the contractile properties of triceps surae and maximal power output during jumping in elderly men. Gerontology 31(1):1, 1985
99. Marteniuk RG: Motor skill performance and learning—considerations for rehabilitation. Physiother Can 31:187, 1979
100. Welford AT: Sensory, perceptual and motor processes in older adults. In Birren JE, Sloane PB: Handbook of Mental Health and Aging. Prentice-Hall, Englewood Cliffs, NJ, 1980
101. Fitts PM, Posner MI: Human Performance. Brooks/Cole, Belmont, CA, 1967

102. Sullivan RJ: When the get up and go has got up and went. J Am Geriatr Soc 34:323, 1986
103. Singer RF: Motor Learning and Human Performance. Macmillan, New York, 1968
104. Bromley DB: The Psychology of Human Ageing. Pelican, Harmondsworth, UK, 1966
105. Desmedt JE: Size principle of motoneuron recruitment and the calibration of muscle force and speed in man. In Desmedt JE (ed): Motor Control Mechanisms in Health and Disease, Raven Press, New York, 1983
106. Moller P, Brandt R: The effect of physical training in elderly subjects with special reference to energy rich phosphagens and myoglobin in leg skeletal muscles. Clin Physiol 2:307, 1982
107. Bass A, et al: Biochemical and histochemical changes in energy supply and enzyme functions of muscles of the rat during old age. Gerontologia 21:31, 1975
108. Bancroft H: Blood flow and metabolism in skeletal muscle. In Hudlicka O (ed): Circulation in Skeletal Muscle. Pergamon, Oxford, UK, 1968
109. Astrand P, Rodahl K: Textbook of Work Physiology. McGraw-Hill, New York, 1970
110. Sidney KH, Shephard RJ: Maximum and minimum exercise tests on men and women in the seventh, eighth, and nineth decades of life. J Appl Physiol 43:280, 1977
111. Buccoli VA, Stone WC: Effect of jogging and cycling programs on physiological and personality variables in aged men. Res Q 46:134, 1975
112. Suominen WE, Heikkinen E, et al: Effects of eight weeks of physical training on muscle and connective tissues in vastus lateralis in 69 year old men and women. J Gerontol 32:33, 1977
113. DeVries HA: Physiological effects of an exercise training regimen upon men aged 52–88. J Gerontol 25:325, 1970
114. Badenhop DT, Cleary PA, et al: Physiological adjustments to high and low intensity in elders. Med Sci Sports Exerc 15:496, 1983
115. Pritikin N, Pritikin R, et al: Diet and exercise as a total therapeutic regimen for rehabilitation of patients with peripheral vascular disorders. Arch Phys Med Rehabil 56:558, 1975
116. Froelicher V, Jensen D, et al: Cardiac rehabilitation—evidence for improvement in myocardial performance and function. Arch Phys Med Rehabil 61:517, 1980
117. Lawrence G: Aquafitness for Women. Wiley/Everest, Toronto, 1981
118. Pendergast D, Cerretelli P, et al: Aerobic and glycolytic metabolism in arm exercise. J Appl Physiol 47:754, 1979
119. Shephard RJ: Sudden death—a significant hazard of exercise? Br J Sports Med 8:101, 1974
120. Stanford BA: Physiological effects of training upon institutionalized geriatric men. J Gerontol 27:451, 1972
121. Costill DL, Branam GE, et al: Effects of physical training in men with coronary heart disease. Med Sci Sports Exerc 6:95, 1974
122. Vandervoort A, Hayes KC, et al: Strength and endurance of skeletal muscle in the elderly. Physiother Can 38:167, 1986
123. Perkins LC, Kaiser HL: Results of short term isotonic and isometric exercise programs in persons over sixty. Phys Ther Rev 41:663, 1961
124. Aniansson A, Gustafsson E: Physical training in elderly men with specific reference to quadriceps muscle strength and morphology. Clin Physiol 1:87, 1981

125. Aniansson A, et al: Effects of a training program for pensioners on condition and muscle strength. Arch Gerontol Geriatr 3:229, 1984

126. Chapman EA, de Vries HA, et al: Joint stiffness—effects of exercise on young and old men. J Gerontol 27:218, 1972

127. Kaufman TC: Strength training effect in young and aged women. Arch Phys Med Rehabil 65:223, 1985

128. Hansen JW: The training effect of repeated isometric muscle contractions. Int J Angew Physiol 18:474, 1961

129. McComas AJ, Upton ARM, et al: Motoneuron disease and ageing. Lancet 2:1477, 1973

130. Campbell MJ, McComas AJ, et al: Physiological changes in aging muscles. J Neurol Neurosurg Psychiatr 36:174, 1973

131. Brown WF: Functional compensation of human motor units in health and disease. J Neurol Sci 20:199, 1973

132. Belanger AY, McComas AJ: Extent of motor unit activation during effort. J Appl Physiol 51:1131, 1981

133. Hislop HJ: Quantitative changes in human muscle strength during isometric exercise. J Am Phys Ther Assoc 43:21, 1963

134. Bennett RL, Knowlton GC: Overwork weakness in partially denervated skeletal muscles. Clin Orthop 12:22, 1958

135. Johnson EWJ, Braddon R: Overwork weakness in spino-scapulo-humeral muscular dystrophy. Arch Phys Med Rehabil 52:333, 1971

136. Larsson L, Grimby G, et al: Muscle strength and speed of movement in relation to age and muscle morphology. J Appl Physiol 46:451, 1979

137. Morgan RE, Adamson GT: Circuit Training. GT Bell, London, 1962

138. Royal Canadian Air Force: Exercise plans for physical fitness. This Week Magazine, Mount Vernon, NY, 1962

139. Morgan WP: Affective beneficence of vigorous physical activity. Med Sci Sports Exerc 17:94, 1985

140. Bahrke MJ, Morgan WP: Anxiety reduction following exercise and mediation. Cog Ther Rev 2:323, 1978

141. Greist JH, et al: Running as treatment for depression. Comp Psychiatr 20:41, 1979

142. Morgan WP: Physical activity in mental health. In Eckert H, Montoye FJ (eds): Exercise and Health, Human Kintics Pub, Champaigne, IL, 1984

143. Morgan WP: Coping with Mental Stress—the Potential and Limits of Exercise Interaction. National Institutes of Health, Bethesda, MD, 1984

144. Weiss JM: A model for neurochemical study of depression. American Psychology Association Convention, Washington, DC, 1982

145. Hollister LE: Clinical Pharmacology of Psychotherapeutic Drugs. 2nd Ed. Churchill Livingstone, New York, 1983

146. Brown BS, van Huss WD: Exercise and rat brain catecholamines. J Appl Physiol 34:644, 1973

147. Barthan J, Freedman D: Brain amines—response to physiological stress. Biochem Pharmacol 12:1232, 1962

148. Pargman D, Baker MC: Running high—enkephalin indicated. J Drug Issues 10:341, 1980

149. Farrell PA, Gustafson AB, et al: Enkephalins, catecholamines and psychological mood alterations. Med Sci Sports Exerc 19:347, 1987

3 | Older Adult Learning

David A. Peterson

Educational intervention in the lives of older adults has been a subject of rapidly increasing interest over the past 15 years. This interest originates not only from a recognition that people have learning needs at every age, but from an appreciation of the plasticity of human intelligence and the conviction that people can continue to grow and change throughout life. Literature on the intelligence and learning abilities of older persons, although sometimes inconclusive, tends to support the conviction that intellectual aging is modifiable and that learning at any age is possible and valuable. Furthermore, it suggests that there may be specific instructional strategies that facilitate the learning of persons in their later years.

Any comprehensive discussion of how to help older adults learn, however, must be more than merely prescriptive; an understanding of the derivation of useful strategies is equally important. Such basic knowledge will assist therapists to use these strategies more successfully and perhaps guide them in generating innovative strategies of their own. This chapter, consequently, attempts to provide the reader with both practical suggestions to facilitate the learning of older adults and their foundation in psychological and educational research.

The chapter is divided into two major sections, research on intelligence and learning performance and implications of this research for practice. Although a certain amount of overlap exists between these two areas, they are sufficiently distinct to indicate that such a separation is reasonable. The chapter proceeds from the more abstract concerns of research studies on intelligence to the more practical application of instructional strategies for dealing with older people.

INTELLIGENCE

Many studies have attempted to determine the intelligence of individuals and to ascertain if change typically occurs in this attribute over the course of the life span. The literature describing these findings offers a massive accumulation of data on the basic questions. However, definitive answers are not yet available, and researchers still differ on some points concerning the relationship of intelligence and age. A review of these studies provides insight into the intellectual potential and performance of middle aged and older persons as well as indicating several significant implications for those who would provide instruction to persons in these age groups.[1]

The Meaning of Intelligence

As with most fundamental concepts, intelligence is difficult to explain. It is usually considered to be the cognitive capacity of the individual, the ability to learn, the facility at manipulating and understanding common and unique items. This cognitive potential is impossible to measure directly, so all research on intelligence has inferred the underlying traits of an individual by measuring performance in a number of settings. Performance and innate ability are not necessarily synonymous because numerous factors (health, perceptual acuity, motivation) can affect performance. Thus, IQ, the performance measure, may closely approximate the ceiling potential of the individual or may greatly underestimate it.

Likewise, high IQ scores do not assure an individual success, do not indicate social or vocational competence, and may not lead to adaptation to the society or any particular role. IQ historically was developed as a means to predict success in educational endeavors. Because it deals with cognitive abilities and these are closely related to any learning enterprise, it has proved to be a fairly reliable indicator of performance in an educational setting. It is also very useful in estimating success in employment that has high educational prerequisites. However, there are many areas of life in which learning is not particularly relevant. In these areas (interpersonal relations, adjustment, physical strength, beauty, commitment, self-esteem, motivation, and wisdom), other variables may prove to be substantially more powerful determinants of success than intelligence. Thus, intelligence should be considered as an important attribute of each individual, but high or low scores do not automatically determine the quality of performance that can be expected from that individual.

Although intelligence is a singular noun, most psychologists would agree that there is no single entity that can be thought of as intelligence. It is probably more accurate to think of "intelligences," which each individual has and which can be measured in a variety of ways.[1] One conceptualization of intelligence that has received wide acceptance over the past 25 years is that of fluid and crystallized intelligence.[2] *Crystallized intelligence* depends on sociocultural influences; it involves the ability to perceive relations, to engage in formal reasoning, and to understand the intellectual and cultural heritage. It is measured through culture-specific items such as number facility, verbal comprehension, and general information. Thus, the amount the individual learns, the diversity and complexity of the environment, the openness to new information, and the extent of formal learning opportunities are likely to be influential in the score of the individual. In general, crystallized intelligence continues to grow slowly throughout adulthood as the individual acquires increased information and develops an understanding of the relationships of diverse facts and constructs. Continued acculturation through self-directed learning and education can encourage the growth of crystallized intelligence even after the age of 60.[3]

Fluid intelligence, on the other hand, is not closely associated with acculturation. It is generally considered to be independent of instruction or environment and depends more on the genetic endowment of the individual. It consists of the ability to perceive complex relations, use short-term memory, create concepts, and undertake abstract reasoning. Items that are included in tests of fluid intelligence are memory span, inductive reasoning, and figural relations, all of which are assumed to be unresponsive to training or expertise. Fluid intelligence involves those items that are the most neurophysiologic in nature and are generally assumed to decline after the individual reaches maturity. However, the decline that results before age 60 or 65 in most people is small.[1]

Intellectual Changes over the Life Span

The earliest studies of adult intelligence showed an increase in IQ until the late teens or early twenties and then a slow decline throughout the rest of the adult years. These studies used a cross-sectional design that tested people of several ages and then compared the scores of current younger people with those of persons who were older. The differences in the scores were assumed to be related to age. Later studies have used longitudinal designs in which the same persons were tested at various points over the life span and changes in scores were compared so that trends in intellectual performance could be observed. These studies have reported a somewhat different pattern of change, with less decline occurring and IQ peaking in the thirties or forties.[4]

Before examining these trends, however, we must consider once again the great individual differences that exist in intellectual functioning. Any general description of the relationship of age to intellectual change will obscure some of the variation that is observable in a large population. Thus, knowing the age of an individual is insufficient to estimate whether that person is intelligent or not; or whether because of age, any individual has suffered such decline that he/she is no longer capable of learning or functioning successfully. Age does have some effect on intelligence, but it does not override many other influencing factors.

Botwinick[5] has described the "classic aging pattern of intelligence." Over the adult portion of the life span, verbal abilities decline very little if at all whereas psychomotor abilities decline earlier and to a greater extent. Thus, on the Wechsler Adult Intelligence Scale (WAIS) tests, the verbal subtests show virtual stability throughout the years from age 20 to 60 whereas the performance subtests show decline from the late twenties on. After age 65 to 70, decline in both areas increases but does not reach a point where the individual is incompetent. This pattern holds for men and women, black and white adults, persons from various economic strata, and persons in both mental hospitals and the community. These findings are consistent with the notion that crystallized intelligence is maintained over the adult life span whereas fluid intelligence declines. Taken together, this decline in fluid intelligence and growth in crystallized intelligence is assumed to approximately balance out, so that the loss of biological potential is offset by the wisdom, experience, and knowledge that the older adult has acquired. Stability of intellectual performance over the greatest part of the typical life span would appear to be normal, and persons in their fifties will have maintained learning ability equal to what they had in their twenties, when they can control the pace. Although ability may begin to fall off between the ages of 60 and 70, the tasks that become most difficult are those that are fast-paced, unusual, and complex.[6]

The amount of deficit that occurs after age 70, however, is unclear. Although a fairly sharp decline is typically shown, this may be caused by what has been called *terminal drop*. This phenomenon, first reported by Riegel and Riegel[7] is a decline in the IQ scores of individuals a few years before death and is thought to be caused by physiologic deterioration. For some reason, intellectual functioning appears to be one means of predicting approaching death. If the older sample in any study included a preponderance of persons who were nearing death, their IQ scores would indicate a substantial decline compared to younger persons; however, this may be traced to their nearness to death and not to some other change that occurs around age 70. Increased medical treatment, preventive health care, and improved public health may prolong the healthy portion of life and consequently extend the period in which intelligence remains basically stable.

Schaie[8] has suggested an alternative view of life-span IQ change. By designing a study that was both longitudinal and cross sectional, he has shown that performance of older adults is maintained through the adult years with minimal decline occurring before age 60 to 70. However, each generation scores slightly higher on the IQ measures than the preceding one, and thus cross-generational comparisons disadvantage older cohorts. His conclusion is that each generation is slightly more intelligent than the preceding ones and that comparisons of 20-, 40-, and 60-year-olds do not show declines in IQ scores but generational differences. Each generation maintains its scores, but succeeding generations score slightly higher, so that any comparison makes it appear that decline has occurred.

Persons who were initially tested when they were aged 25 or 32 have the highest scores. Those first tested at 39 or 46 have the next highest scores, and those who entered the testing situation at age 53, 60, or 67 have the lowest scores. However, scores for the youngest group show slight change over the 21-year period, scores for the middle group show no change at all, and scores for the oldest group decline substantially only after age 74. Schaie's data suggest clearly that intelligence as measured by the Thurstone Primary Mental

Abilities Test is quite stable over the life span and that subsequent cohorts score better than preceding ones.

Age, of course, is not the only variable that affects IQ. Education, socioeconomic status, and cohort are also major factors in determining the intelligence of any individual. Birren and Morrison[9] analyzed a large amount of data from the WAIS test and concluded that education is much more important than age in determining the IQ of the individual. With increased education the IQ scores rise sharply; this does not necessarily mean that education increases IQ. It may mean that people with high IQ are more prone to attend school longer or enjoy it more; or it may mean that there is some third factor involved that affects IQ and education. Regardless of the causative relationship, increased education and higher IQs appear to be positively associated.

Likewise, greater socioeconomic status is associated with higher IQ scores. As noted earlier, crystallized intelligence is sensitive to experience and acquired information. These are likely to increase with higher socioeconomic status because travel, a stimulating environment, availability of books, or encouragement of continued learning are likely to be available. Whichever of these is involved, they are more available for persons who are at a higher level of income, occupation, and education—the components of socioeconomic status.

We may conclude that intellectual potential is maintained throughout the major portion of the life span. People even into their eighth decade have the ability to learn and change. However, they often have not cultivated that ability and must expend additional energy to succeed despite growing infirmities and difficulties. The role of the therapist is to understand the areas where additional help is needed and to design content and process so that learning can be maximized.

Implications

What implications may be drawn from research on intellectual performance? Studies of intelligence in later life show clearly that in the verbal and sociocultural areas, decline is least and comes latest. This suggests that the cognitive abilities that are of greatest relevance to the daily lives of older learners are those that evidence the most resistance to decline with age. Acquisition of knowledge or skill that is relevant to the older person's interests, needs, and wants should be learned quickly and efficiently. The *usefulness* of the content to the learner should be given special emphasis. If the topic is of interest and can be used in some important manner, the older person will be likely to learn.

Individual differences in intellectual performance (as well as practically every other variable) increase throughout the adult years. Thus, in attempting to help older people learn, the therapist must expect that the intellectual range will be great, experience will be diverse, and individual learning skills will differ extensively. The therapist must be flexible and frequently individualize instruction.

LEARNING ABILITY AND PERFORMANCE IN LATER LIFE

Learning occurs throughout life. People continually learn through study, incidental contact with others, their jobs, and analysis of their reactions and feelings. This learning process does not abruptly change when a person reaches old age, but differential performance and ability between older and younger people have been reported. This section emphasizes the measurement of learning performance and the means by which learning efficiency can be improved.

An immediate caveat must be presented. Learning and performance are not the same. Because an item has been learned does not necessarily mean that it can be recalled or recognized in every situation. In other words, poor performance on a learning task may mean that insufficient learning has occurred or it may mean that the performance does not accurately reflect the extent of the learning achieved. However, it is only through the observation or measurement of performance that we can infer learning. Consequently, throughout this chapter when learning is discussed it is the observable results of the learning that are measured and not some internal change that has taken place.

Over the past three decades, a large number of laboratory studies of learning performance have been undertaken that provide extensive and reliable data on the changes that occur with age and are especially amenable to intervention. The purpose of those studies has been to explore the age-related differences in learning performance (i.e., the differences between older and younger learners). The review of these studies, therefore, will be selective in an attempt to abstract those that are of greatest relevance to the therapist. In doing this, it will be necessary to extrapolate from the findings in an attempt to suggest some instructional applications or principles. Thus, the intent will be to provide a general understanding of the research, to report the more relevant findings, and to identify the implications and insights that are salient to persons attempting to help older people learn.

Laboratory Study of Learning

Studies of learning performance have been largely conducted in a laboratory setting. Several experimental procedures have been used in which subjects either see or hear words, letters, or symbols and then are asked to recall or recognize them. In some studies paired words are presented and the subject is expected to recall which word was matched with which other word. The specific design and method have varied widely depending on the type of hypothesis being tested, but in general the subject attempts to memorize several words and to recall them after the passage of a short period of time.

Performance on learning tasks is affected by several factors. The intelligence of the individual, the learning skills that the person has acquired over the years, and the flexibility of learning styles are, of course, key variables. There are, however, several other variables, often called noncognitive factors, that can also have a significant effect on learning. These do not involve the intellectual ability but nevertheless have a great bearing on the individual's performance. Noncognitive factors include the visual and auditory acuity of the learner, the health status of the individual, the motivation to learn, the level of anxiety, the speed at which the learning is paced, and the meaningfulness of the material to be learned.

Several of these noncognitive factors are treated as major variables in research on learning performance. Others such as perceptual acuity and health status are not. It should be obvious, however, that persons who are unable to see or hear well are not likely to perform at an acceptable level. They will misunderstand directions, fail to adequately take in the material, and have a difficult time responding in written or oral form. These hindrances to learning do not relate to the individual's innate ability, but they interfere to such an extent that any learning performance is likely to be severely affected.

Likewise, poor health can be a major detriment in any learning situation. If the individual is not able to concentrate on the instruction because of pain, if physical stamina and strength are lacking, or if the senses are dulled through illness or medication, the learner will not be productive. Because the number of days of illness per year increases with age, physical health of the individual must be considered in any measurement of learning performance and especially in any attempt to teach individuals or groups. Thus, attention to the noncognitive factors as well as the cognitive ones are important considerations in laboratory and field learning settings.

Findings from Laboratory Studies

Laboratory studies of learning in adulthood and later life have provided a wealth of data on the changes that occur in learning performance over the life span, the characteristics of this change, and the means by which learning performance can be improved in old age. These conclusions are reported in the following sections.

Interference. Interference can cause a learning task to be less efficiently accomplished. Most researchers seem to believe that interference can keep the individual from learning the new materials or substantially impede the learning process. There are several ways interference can occur. First, it can result from the conflict of present, personal knowledge with the new knowledge to be learned. Second, two learning tasks undertaken at the same time can interfere with each other. Third, subsequent learning can interfere with the intended learning. Each of these can prove to be a difficulty in the learning process.

Interference from prior events or knowledge has occurred in studies where older people were asked to learn nonsense words or symbols. On occasion, some of these symbols are contrary to common knowledge; for instance, $6+2=3$. Arenberg and Robertson[10] report studies in which this type of learning proved to be substantially more difficult for older people than were nonsense symbols that did not conflict with present knowledge, for instance, $A+D=F$. From a research point of view, these equations are comparable, so differences in the scores are attributed to conflict with present knowledge.

The therapist working with older people could use this understanding by emphasizing new knowledge that will be consistent with previous learning, minimizing any conflicts between new and old knowledge, and helping the older person unlearn incorrect knowledge. A specific implication of this understanding is that the therapist can benefit from a familiarity with the older person and the beliefs, experiences, and knowledge the older person brings to the learning setting. If the new information is likely to be in sharp contrast with present knowledge, the therapist needs to proceed in a slow and careful manner because overt or implicit resistance to the new information can be expected.

On the other hand, it is possible to use the past knowledge and experience of the older learner in a very positive and beneficial fashion. Studies have shown that older people benefit more than young adults when the material is familiar or consistent with what they already know.[10] The past experience and knowledge of the older person can be either positive or negative, depending on its consistency or conflict with the new learning being undertaken, and needs to be given special consideration by the therapist.

A second type of interference occurs when the older learner is expected to attend to two things at once. In laboratory studies this often occurs when subjects are expected to listen to different word lists in each ear simultaneously, remember which light was flashed a few seconds ago, or repeat some words while listening to other words. In those studies where older people must divide their attention among intake, attention, and retrieval processes, they seem to be especially disadvantaged.[6] When the older person is required to shift attention from one learning task to another, efficiency of learning suffers.

The implication of concurrent interference is that the therapist needs to concentrate on one task at a time and assure that one item is satisfactorily learned before the next is undertaken.[5] If a second task must be learned, it needs to be postponed as long as possible and needs to be clearly distinctive so that it is possible to know when one has completed the first task and is moving on to the next. Apparently, older people need more time to integrate the new learning and to rehearse it before it is well set in their long-term memory. Additional stimulation during this period is likely to result in premature forgetting or inability to retrieve the information adequately.

Another type of concurrent interference occurs from distractions at the time of learning. These may come from background noise, room conditions, personal anxiety, or numerous other factors. Whatever the cause, if the older person divides attention between the learning task and something else, the learning speed and accuracy will decline. Thus the therapist is well advised to reduce the potential for distraction whenever possible and to help the older person concentrate exclusively on the learning at hand. This may not be easily done, but it is an effective means of increasing learning performance.

A third type of interference, retroactive, occurs when the individual completes one learning task and then must concentrate on some other task. This subsequent diversion may have a negative effect on retrieval, although this is not as well documented as are other types of interference.[11]

Older people are well advised to space the learning experiences sufficiently to allow time for integration, to assure that the content of the subsequent learning does not conflict with the previous learning, and to follow up at a later time to evaluate the quality of the knowledge retained. The possibility of retroactive interference is sufficient to encourage the therapist to incorporate review, reflection, and application of the learning in order to avoid forgetting.

Pacing. Laboratory studies have consistently shown that older people perform less well when the learning task needs to be completed under the pressure of time.[12] Paired-associate tasks have proved to be especially difficult for older persons, who do less well than younger persons when tasks are to be completed quickly.[5] Canestrari[13] reported, however, that the learning deficiency can be somewhat overcome if the older learner is provided additional time and will almost disappear when the subject can control the learning pace. Thus, when self-pacing by the older learner is allowed, the learning performance appears to be optimized.[5,14]

One implication of fast pacing in learning experiments is that older persons make more errors of omission, errors in which they make no response at all rather than risking a wrong answer. Omission errors are much more common to older learners and may result in part from inadequate time to determine the preferred response; therefore, no response is made. Arenberg and Robertson-Tchabo[11] suggested that additional time was useful in reducing the amount of nonresponse. When extra time is available, it can lead to a successful search of long-term memory so that correct answers are forthcoming.

The application of this insight from laboratory research is very direct in a learning setting. Instruction needs to be self-paced, or if that is not possible, needs to be paced rather slowly in order to provide time for both intake and retrieval.[5,14] Because a presentation (even to a single individual) is a form of timed instruction, it needs to be structured in such a manner that material is presented, reviewed, and examined. This may be effectively supplemented by an opportunity for questions and discussion, which allows it to be related to previous knowledge, offers time for consideration of the material, and can reduce the psychological pressure of speeded learning.

The importance of controlling the pacing of instruction cannot be overemphasized. The laboratory learning studies, research on adult intelligence, and practical experience clearly indicate the need for slowly paced or self-paced instruction for older people. This will typically require the therapist to reduce the amount of content to be presented and to offer greater clarity, specificity, and depth rather than cover a number of diverse topics. In posing questions to older persons, increased time needs to be allowed for response and greater care taken in framing the questions so that they are specific and directed.

Organization of Material. Learning performance depends in part on whether the individual is able to retrieve what has been learned. Within the information-processing model of learning, retrieval is primarily dependent on the manner in which the information is organized or "filed" in the brain. By organizing information into categories and sequences, or by using some type of visual or mnemonic device, the individual is generally able to increase the quality of retrieval.

This has been shown to be especially applicable to older persons. Older adults typically do more poorly than younger adults on learning tasks. In an attempt to provide explanations for this in addition to pacing and interference effects, the extent to which persons use some kind of organizing strategy has been studied.[15] Evidence is persuasive that older persons are less likely than others to organize spontaneously as a way to help memory.[4,5] When investigators have encouraged older people to categorize words to be learned, scores have improved, but when the organizing strategy is provided by the researcher, then scores improved significantly. This appears to be especially true for older people who have poor verbal skills; for highly verbal older people, the weaknesses in their organizing strategies are less pronounced, so improvement is minimal with this type of assistance.

Learning performance of older people can be improved by assisting them to organize the material in better ways and by encouraging alternatives to rote memorization. This can be done through the provision of *advance organizers,* aids to help the learner appropriately direct attention. Many older learners have difficulty following the content because they cannot anticipate what will be taught and do not see the whole that is being presented. It is often helpful to provide an introductory overview in which the entire lesson is given in outline form. This provides an early opportunity to see the "map" that is being followed, an insight that is especially useful for older people.[5]

Advance organizers can also provide the bridge between what the older person already knows and what is intended to be learned in the present session. They can indicate the size, shape, extent, and orientation of the content to be covered so that dimensions can be appreciated in advance. Specific examples of advance organizers include the provision of an outline of the session; sets of notes to follow; initial summaries of the content; or lists of facts, concepts, or issues to be examined. These, of course, need not be provided in written form, but when that is the procedure, it does offer a guide that can be reviewed by the learner at any time.

A related aspect of this topic may be seen in studies in which older people are asked to reorganize the knowledge before responding. For instance, they are read a list of words or numbers and then asked to repeat them in reverse order. Studies have shown that older people do significantly poorer on this type of activity than younger persons[16] because they must not only remember the material but also reorganize it. Thus, the older person faces not only the learning problem but the interference effects of two different processes.

There are clear implications from this finding for instruction of older people. If the content is presented in one way and the older person is expected to apply it some other way, the transition may cause difficulty. This would generally mean that older people should not be expected to acquire abstract information and to make the transition to practical application themselves. The instruction needs to be provided in the format that is to be used whenever possible. Most therapists are probably familiar with the situation in which the older person takes what is said too literally and is unable to generalize or apply the material to comparable settings. The reorganization process is not an easy one; it needs to be minimized whenever possible.

Another means of improving learning performance is through the use of mediators, that is, the association of the word or information to be learned with some other word, image, or story that can be remembered easily. As with other organizing strategies, older people are less likely than younger ones to consciously and regularly employ some type of mediators. Rather, they are likely to use rote memorization in order to remember the new information. Studies have shown that when older persons are assisted in using mediators, their scores improve. Some researchers have hypothesized that visual mediators (such as forming a picture of the word or information) are more effective in improving learning performance than verbal mediators; however, both were helpful in improving the organization and remembering of the new information.

Mediators are useful in showing the relationships between facts that are known and those that are being learned. They can tie the new information to the old and help to show where the new knowledge fits in the individual's scheme of organizing information. Because older people are not likely to employ these mediational devices automatically, their learning efficiency can be improved by helping them form pictures, stories, analogies, or examples in order to make the tie and find the organizing variable. This can be done through encouragement of note taking so that the individual will indicate the new information and where it fits with the old. It can also occur by helping the individual develop little stories or pictures that help recall specific information.

Although not particularly useful in many situations, the chaining of words or ideas is helpful in recalling lists. Each item of a list is related by a story or picture to the next. Thus, when the first word is recalled, it needs to be possible to recall the whole list by remembering the tie (picture) to the next word. Another method is to relate the words in a list to a numbered series of learned words. For instance, if you remember that one is "fun" and relate the first word to fun, it can be remembered easier. If two stands for "shoe" and the second word is related to shoe by a small story, it too may be more easily recalled.

The implication from these data on the use of organization and mediative devices in learning is that the therapist needs to provide the time and opportunity for the learners to apply the new information, either in a mnemonic or nonsense way, or to relate it to previous knowledge. This provides not only the additional time that has been identified earlier as necessary, but also the possible reduction of interference with previous knowledge. By use of these strategies and devices, it is possible to improve the quality of learning even though the amount of content covered may need to be reduced because of the time involved in the application process.

Motivation. It is generally accepted that older people are less motivated when approaching a learning task than are younger people. Obviously, a desire to succeed and a commitment to conscientiously address the task are important elements in successful learning performance. Because older people are known to have less general interest in learning, and because many of the tasks involved in the various studies have relatively little meaning or relevance to the older person, it has been assumed that older learners do less well because they are less motivated. Hulicka[17] reported that older persons refused to continue to attempt learning tasks that involved "such nonsense." This type of reaction has been reported by other researchers and has been interpreted as indicating low motivation or self-esteem.

One means of increasing motivation is to make the learning undertaken more meaningful to the individual learner. Calhoun and Gounard[14] reported that older people learned significantly more highly meaningful material than they did medium or low meaningful material. They concluded that understanding the needs and wants of the older learner and directing the content toward those meaningful areas will result in greater motivation as well as greater learning by the older learners.

Another approach to meaningfulness may be through the level of concreteness of the material. Several studies have pointed out the decline in abstract behavior with increased age[5], so older people may be unable or unwilling to deal with problems, even in the laboratory, that are distant from present reality. Arenberg[18] reported that when learning tasks were presented with abstract elements (forms, colors, numbers), older people had an extremely difficult time completing the tasks. However, when the elements were changed to more concrete items, specific beverages, meats, and vegetables, the older learners accomplished the task much more easily. Thus it would appear advisable to present instructional components in ways that are as concrete as possible and as personally meaningful to the older learner.

Other researchers have found contradictory results when measuring the motivation of older people in a learning task. Powell, Eisdorfer, and Bogdonoff[19] took blood samples and measured galvanic skin response and heart rate of older subjects involved in a learning study and reported that older persons had higher levels of arousal, indicating greater involvement than younger subjects. Older people experienced greater stress in the learning situation and performed the learning task more poorly than did younger persons.

Subsequent studies[20] have shown that if the degree of arousal is reduced by medication, the older learners improved their performance. This suggests that the older learner may be so motivated or involved in the study that his/her emotional state interferes with the cognitive processes. By overreacting to the stress of the situation, the subject may withhold responses, score poorly on the learning task, and further increase anxiety in a vicious cycle.[21]

One means of overcoming this overarousal is by providing a supportive learning environment. If older people are placed in a situation in which they are expected to compete with others or be evaluated on their performance, they are likely to be overaroused and to do less well. Ross[22] reported a study in which three different sets of instructions were given to older subjects. One was considered to be supportive, one neutral, and one challenging. Older persons did substantially better when given the supportive instructions, less well with neutral instructions, and least well with challenging instructions. The conclusion was drawn that a positive expectation and supportive learning situation are likely to reduce the threat of the learning experience and to result in greater learning.

It has long been assumed that by rewarding correct responses and not rewarding incorrect ones, subjects will learn most quickly. A study by Leech and Witte[23] indicated that by rewarding all responses, although correct ones more strongly than incorrect ones, older persons could be persuaded to make some responses and thus reduce the errors of omission. Learning tends to be poorer when the learner does not respond in some way, and the method of rewarding every response assists older persons to take a chance and perhaps learn something in that process.

The implications of these motivation studies are important for teaching of older adults. First, it is obvious that older people will be more highly motivated if they are learning meaningful material. Their interest will be heightened, and their commitment is likely to be better. It is thus imperative that the relevance of the information presented is made clear and that its usefulness be emphasized.

Second, if anxiety causes a decrease in learning efficiency, then the instruction needs to be carried out in a way that will reduce the fear of failure. This can occur primarily through the attitude and approach that the therapist brings to the learning setting. By presenting material at an appropriate level of complexity, setting a relaxed pace, and reducing the threat of failure, the learning experience can become more successful and enjoyable.

Third, the reward for participation in the learning setting needs to be clear and regular. To assume that the older person is able to stand defeat and has the necessary self-confidence to persevere regardless of the results may be inaccurate. The need for constant monitoring of the supportiveness of the climate, the extent to which the older people feel a part of the situation, and the extent to which they are appreciated and valued regardless of their achievement is necessary for continued involvement and progress. Most important, however, is the clarity and meaningfulness of the learning undertaken. To maintain motivation, the outcomes must be clear and closely related to the wants and interest of the older participants.

Sensory Modality. Several studies have attempted to determine whether visual or auditory input is most effective in learning. Although all of us learn both by seeing (reading) material as well as by hearing (listening) the spoken word, questions have been raised about the extent to which one is superior to the other. McGhie, Chapman, and Lawson[24] reported that auditory means are generally slightly superior than visual when the information is to be retrieved within a very short time. Visual, on the other hand, may be superior if the information is to be held in the long-term memory for some period.[25]

Several studies have attempted to determine if learning is improved when one type of presentation (visual or verbal) is supplemented with the other. If the learner is provided both visual images and hears the same material simultaneously, learning is usually improved. In general, this has proved to be the case.[17] If subjects are provided with one of three experimental conditions: looking at a list of words, looking at the words while the experimenter reads them (passive), or looking at the words and reading them aloud (active), the results support the hypothesis that supplementation in either the active or passive form was valuable, and that active supplementation was the most helpful.

These studies suggest that therapists may facilitate learning by using both of the major senses, especially when this can be done simultaneously. By providing written material for the learner to follow while a presentation is being made, increased learning is likely to result. However, there is also a caution that needs to be added. If the verbal and the visual presentations are not similar, the older person may experience the interference that occurs when they divide their attention. Thus, if the written materials are quite different from the verbal presentation, less rather than more learning may result. The teacher needs to choose the material to be presented in written form carefully so that it closely conforms to the presentation. Simply finding a pamphlet or other handout may not be helpful unless it is adhered to closely.

Another inference that may be drawn from the studies of modality relates to the active/passive aspect of the learning. Persons who were active in the learning process, even in such a minimal way as saying aloud the words to be learned, succeeded to a much greater extent. Most therapists have assumed that activity was a valued part of the learning enterprise, but this underscores the need to continue involvement of the older client, to seek ways for activity related to the new learning, and to encourage the older person not to passively soak up the knowledge.

Feedback. Studies have shown that older persons are assisted in their learning when they are provided feedback on their performance.[26,27] Because the older person often continues to use improper or ineffective means to address problem-solving or learning situations even after these have proved to be unproductive, feedback is especially useful when it includes suggestions for alternative approaches.

The implications for instruction include the obvious value of allowing the older learner an opportunity to rehearse the behavior or learning under the guidance of the therapist so that corrective feedback can be provided. Because the older person typically requires longer time and a greater number of trials to achieve the desired learning, feedback on the amount of progress being made and the current level of functioning is generally of value.

As with most suggestions, negative results can occur. Older people are typically less able to accept negative feedback and continue to do well. Because they often have less interest, greater anxiety, and lower self-concept, they are likely to experience greater detrimental results from negative feedback. Thus, every attempt needs to be made to avoid a judgmental, critical position; a more supportive, helpful posture needs to be taken whenever possible.

Similarly, older people need to be helped to avoid errors to the extent possible. Because they tend to remember errors and repeat them, it is most advisable to design the situation so that successful completion of the task is likely.[10] With mistakes, the self concept of the older person is likely to fall and continuing commitment to the learning experience is reduced.

CONCLUSION

The central premise of this chapter is that older adults can and do learn effectively. Helping them to do this is both an art and science and will be most successfully accomplished when knowledge of intelligence, learning ability, and teaching techniques is combined with personal judgment that is characterized by flexibility and a positive attitude toward the learning potential of older persons.

The research reviewed in this chapter leads to several conclusions of relevance for the therapist working with older persons. First, although there are some aspects of intelligence that do indeed decline with age, other aspects appear to improve. In general, it seems that intelligence typically remains fairly stable until late in life, and differences in intelligence among individuals are likely to be far more significant than differences in intelligence based merely on age.

Second, learning ability does not abruptly change in old age, but a modest decline in performance appears to occur owing, in part, to noncognitive factors. Older persons requiring therapeutic intervention may experience, at the outset, even greater difficulty in learning owing to such factors. Performance may be affected by depression, poor health, sense of losing autonomy, or fear and unfamiliarity with the treatment setting, in addition to other noncognitive factors noted in this chapter.

Understanding such factors and their implications for the learning performance of older persons can help the therapist to modify this decline. Techniques suggested by these implications include minimizing the effects of interference from prior knowledge, by basing new knowledge on old; allowing for self-pacing of instruction; facilitating the organization of materials; ensuring the relevance of materials presented; using both visual and verbal modes of instruction; and providing constructive feedback.

Despite changes in intelligence and learning performance, it is evident that older persons can learn and that well-planned instruction can facilitate learning efficiency and effectiveness. Understanding both the limitations and potentials of older adults and integrating that understanding with specific techniques will help therapists design quality instructional experiences for their clients.

REFERENCES

1. Labouvie-Vief G: Intelligence and cognition. In Birren JE, Schaie KW (eds): Handbook of the Psychology of Aging. Van Nostrand Reinhold, New York, 1985
2. Cattell RB: Theory of fluid and crystallized intelligence: a clinical experiment. J Educ Psychol 54:1, 1963
3. Knox AB: Adult Development and Learning. Jossey-Bass, San Francisco, 1977
4. Willis SL: Towards an educational psychology of the older adult learner: intellectual and cognitive bases. In Birren JE, Schaie KW (eds): Handbook of the Psychology of Aging. Van Nostrand Reinhold, New York, 1985
5. Botwinick J: Aging and Behavior: A Comprehensive Integration of Research Findings. Springer Publishing, New York, 1978
6. Hayslip B.,Jr., Kennelly KJ: Cognitive and non-cognitive factors affecting learning among older adults. In Lumsden BD (ed): The Older Adult as Learner. Hemisphere Publishing, Washington, DC, 1985
7. Riegel KF, Riegel RM: Development, drop, and death. Devel Psychol 6:306, 1972
8. Schaie KW: The Seattle longitudinal study: a twenty-one year investigation of psychometric intelligence. In Schaie KW (ed): Longitudinal Studies of Adult Psychological Development. Guilford Press, New York, 1983
9. Birren JE, Morrison DF: Analysis of the WAIS subtests in relation to age and education. J Gerontol 16:363, 1961
10. Arenberg D, Robertson EA: The older individual as a learner. In Grabowski SM, Mason WD (eds): Education for the Aging. ERIC Clearinghouse on Adult Education, Syracuse, NY, (n.d.)
11. Arenberg D, Robertson-Tchabo EA: Learning and aging. In Birren JE, Schaie KW (eds): Handbook of the Psychology of Aging. Van Nostrand Reinhold, New York, 1977
12. Salthouse TA: Speed of behavior and its implications for cognition. In Birren JE, Schaie KW (eds): Handbook of the Psychology of Aging. Van Nostrand Reinhold, New York, 1985
13. Canestrari RE, Jr: Paced and self-paced learning in young and elderly adults. J Gerontol 18:165, 1963
14. Calhoun RO, Gounard BR: Meaningfulness, presentation rate, list length, and age in elderly adult's paired associate learning. Educ Gerontol 4:49, 1979
15. Hultsch D: Adult age differences in the organization of free recall. Devel Psychol 1:673, 1969
16. Craik FIM: Age differences in human memory. In Birren JE, Schaie KW (eds): Handbook of the Psychology of Aging. Van Nostrand Reinhold, New York, 1977
17. Hulicka IM: Age differences in retention as a function of interference. J Gerontol 22:180, 1967
18. Arenberg D: Concept problem solving in young and old adults. J Gerontol 23:279, 1968
19. Powell AH, Jr., Eisdorfer C, Bogdonoff MD: Physiologic response patterns observed in a learning task. Arch Gen Psychiatry 10:192, 1964

20. Eisdorfer C, Nowlin F, Wilke F: Improvement of learning in the aged by modification of autonomic nervous system activity. Science 170:1327, 1970
21. Elias MF, Elias PK: Motivation and activity. In Birren JE, Schiae KW (eds): Handbook of the Psychology of Aging. Van Nostrand Reinhold, New York, 1977
22. Ross E: Effect of challenging and supportive instructions in verbal learning in older persons. J Educ Psychol 59:261, 1968
23. Leech S, Witte KL: Paired-associate learning in elderly adults as related to pacing and incentive conditions. Dev Psychol 5:180, 1971
24. McGhie A, Chapman J, Lawson JS: Changes in immediate memory with age. Br J Psychol 56:69, 1965
25. Taub HA: Mode of presentation, age, and short term memory. J Gerontol 30:1975
26. Hornblum JN, Overton WF: Area and volume conservation among the elderly: assessment and training. Dev Psychol 12:68, 1976
27. Schultz NR, Hoyer WJ: Feedback effects on spacial egocentrism in old age. J Gerontol 31:72, 1976

4 | Psychosocial Dysfunction in the Aged: Assessment and Intervention

Kenneth Solomon

The elderly suffer from a greater incidence of psychopathology than any other age group. More than 50 percent of the elderly are at risk for developing a major psychopathologic dysfunction at some point in their life after age 65. The incidence of psychopathology in the institutionalized elderly may be greater than 75 percent. Major physical illness with chronic limitation of function further increases the risk of the older person developing a psychopathologic disorder. The older person's mental status will have major ramifications for functional prognosis and response to physical therapy and rehabilitation.

Physical therapists are more likely than most other health professionals to spend a good portion of their professional time with the elderly population. Because physical therapists come into frequent contact with older people, accurate assessments become necessary for the appropriate treatment of the older patient. Being able to identify psychological and social consequences of functional deficits and psychosocial factors that influence outcome will allow the physical therapist to function in a more productive and clinically successful manner. Most physical therapists know, for example, that the depressed patient is less likely to be motivated in physical therapy and is less likely to respond to interventions.

Knowledge of other stresses and resources in the psychosocial environment may make a world of difference in the outcome of treatment of the older person. For example, two men in their eighties suffered from severe functional disabilities, including apraxias, aphasias, and hemiparalyses, after a series of cerebrovascular accidents. One man was a childless widower whose only relative in the area was an older and frail sister. The other man had a devoted wife who was willing and capable of learning basic physical therapy skills. The first man was placed in a long-term-care institution following his discharge from the hospital. Despite active rehabilitation and nursing interventions, he developed recurrent decubiti and secondary infections and died within 2 years after his stroke. The second man went home with his wife and received outpatient physical therapy. His wife made sure that he exercised daily, both actively and passively, and took care of his basic psychosocial and biological needs. His family visited frequently, and with the help of some stronger family members he was able to be carried downstairs to a chair outdoors in the springtime. Although he suffered from several minor setbacks, this man stayed at home until his death in his sleep 7 years after discharge from the hospital.

Knowledge of psychogeriatrics also will help clear up misconceptions about and stereotypes of elderly patients that get in the way of appropriate treatment. Terms such as paranoia, depression, and acting out have become virtually meaningless jargon because usage of these terms has moved beyond their specific scientific meaning.[1] Other terms, such as senility or cerebral arteriosclerosis, have no place in the language of the health care professional, as these words are totally meaningless; indeed, they represent myths. Other words (e.g., manipulative) may be used for their pejorative connotation without the realization that its usage is a staff reaction to and labeling of certain disliked patients.[2]

This chapter presents an overview of psychogeriatrics. Issues and techniques of assessment of the elderly patient with psychosocial dysfunctions are discussed, and common psychopathologic syndromes that are seen in older people are reviewed. Principles and techniques for intervention are also discussed. Throughout the chapter the orientation is for the clinical physical therapist and members of the rehabilitation team, emphasizing the types of problems with which these health care providers come into contact.

NORMALITY AND PSYCHOPATHOLOGY

Normality, although a word used glibly every day, is virtually impossible to define. It has been used in many ways by a variety of clinicians with different approaches. The four major conceptualizations of normality used in health care, based on the work of Offer and Sabshin,[3] are presented here.

The first concept is normality as average. Normality used this way is based on statistics—mean, median, mode. For example, normal laboratory values for certain bodily components are expressed as a range derived from the mean plus or minus two standard deviations for the person's age and sex in that laboratory. Sociologically, this translates to behavioral norms, which are behaviors expected of an individual (actor) in a given role in a specific social situation based on expectations of behaviors that most people in such a setting would display.[4] However, judgments based on societal values bias the labeling of "statistical deviations" as pathology. For example, most people who are intelligent are statistically abnormal—their IQs are outside the range of two standard deviations—but are not considered pathologic. Similarly, people who behave in a societally deviant way are also abnormal because their behavior does not conform to the social norms; these individuals, however are labeled "mentally ill."[5-7]

A second concept of normality is that of normality as utopia. It was embodied by Freud in his legendary statement that the goals of psychological functioning are *lieben und arbeiten,* to love and to work. By this he meant that the psychologically "normal" adult is involved in a long-term, committed, one-to-one, intimate, heterosexual relationship and lifelong meaningful work, both conditions free of conflicts from previous stages of psychologic development. More recently, the "human potential movement" has translated this into self-knowledge and awareness of all one's conflicts, so that one can "work through" them and "grow" to a higher level of functioning; this process is called self-actualization.[8]

A third concept of normality is normality as the absence of disease. Using the broader World Health Organization definition, it would be the absence of dis-ease or physical, emotional, or social discomfort. This concept fits most acute medical or emotional dysfunctions but not other situations. For example, a person may repeatedly behave in a socially maladaptive way but not be uncomfortable. Although this behavior might be considered evidence of a personality disorder, it is also the absence of disease. Similarly, a patient with hypertension who is asymptomatic and totally unaware of the pathologic process in his or her body would be considered healthy by this concept. It also does not take into account a variety of common and not uncomfortable physical entities such as birthmarks (which are considered by dermatopathologists to be "abnormal").

The fourth concept of normality is normality as alloplasticity. Alloplasticity is the ability to manipulate both oneself and one's environment to meet one's needs and to manipulate one's needs to meet the needs of the environment. It includes the ability actually to create a new psychosocial environment if necessary. (In some ways this definition differentiates human beings from other forms of animal life). Alloplasticity involves not only self-knowledge and growth but the development of skills of coping with an unpredictable biopsychosocial environment with subsequent flexibility and adaptability. In some ways it is related to normality as utopia, but it does not involve or demand the goal of conflict-free experience. On the contrary, it assumes that although many areas of ego functioning are conflict free, human beings as complex animals can never be completely conflict-free but can learn to use the results of these conflicts to manipulate their environment and themselves to get their needs satisfied. This is an important concept for physical therapists, involving as it does the basic goals of rehabilitation.

Based on the alloplasticity concept of normality, psychopathology can be defined as follows: Psychopathology includes all forms of behavior [action, affect (or emotion), and cognition (or thought)] that interferes with or blocks an individual's alloplastic capabilities, causes discomfort for the individual and/or those around that person, and is not a self-limited response to transitions and crises in the life cycle. It thus excludes responses to "problems of daily living" or adjustment disorders but includes most major disturbances as defined in the *Diagnostic and Statistical Manual, Third Edition, Revised*[9] of the American Psychiatric Association (DSM-III-R).

TYPES OF ASSESSMENT

There are four major types of psychosocial assessments of the elderly. Each follows a different model. Each was developed by different disciplines, and each gives important information about the older person. The first three major types of assessment are quite traditional in orientation and conceptualization. These are the diagnostic assessment, psychodynamic assessment, and the assessment of needs. The fourth, the comprehensive psychogeriatric evaluation, is discussed below. The information obtained by all four assessments overlaps to some degree, and the process of getting this information is identical for all four. They differ primarily in comprehensiveness of data collection and in how the data are organized and translated into intervention.

The Diagnostic Assessment

The diagnostic assessment is based on the medical model. In it, objective signs and subjective symptoms, along with other objective data, are combined under as few labels as is necessary to explain the entire clinical picture (syndromes). For example, a person who was previously in good health develops changes in level of consciousness over a period of several minutes, with symptoms of confusion and anxiety, dizziness, and loss of motor power in one-half the body. Objective signs include a hemiparesis, a hemianopsia, and a variety of other neurologic findings. Ancillary data would include increased uptake on a radioisotope brain scan, an area of increased radiolucency on computerized axial tomography of the head, an increased density on magnetic resonance imagery, and focal slowing on the electroencephalogram. A diagnosis can be made of a cerebrovascular accident, probably from an embolism.

In the psychosocial sphere, a similar diagnostic process leads the examiner to combine signs, symptoms, and other ancillary data in labels codified and defined in DSM-III-R. Familiarity with this work is necessary in communicating with psychiatrists and in order to understand the diagnostic shorthand and jargon embodied in DSM-III-R. It should be remembered that any diagnosis is just a label, a metaphor, to allow clinicians to communicate simply, a clinical shorthand used so that one does not have to list all the signs and symptoms of each patient each time.[10] It may also lead to specific biological/medical interventions. For example, a diagnosis of a major depressive disorder is an indication for treatment with antidepressant medication and psychotherapy, whereas a diagnosis of an adjustment disorder with depressed mood is an indication for treatment with psychotherapy alone.

The Psychodynamic Assessment

The psychodynamic assessment embodies another way of looking at a person's behavior, one derived from the work of psychodynamic theorists. Rather than examining the end results of the psychologic problems as a medical syndrome with a diagnosis (e.g., depression or schizophrenia), the psychodynamic assessment attempts to evaluate some of the unconscious and interpersonal motivations for the person's behavior in an attempt to understand the roots of this behavior. It dictates psychological/interpersonal interventions based on uncovering, clarifying, and gaining mastery over these unconscious and interpersonal motivations, with secondary change in behavior. Although psychoanalysis is the prototype of this modality, almost all psychotherapies, regardless of theoretical backbone, follow this model.

Assessment of Needs

A third model is derived from an assessment of needs. Based on the work of social workers, it conceptualizes the person from a functional point of view. It examines the needs that people have and how well they are satisfying these needs. Maslow[8] has identified three types of needs: basic needs (food, water, touch, love), esteem needs (interpersonal interactions, caring, validation from others), and metaneeds (self-actualization).

In some ways needs assessment is very simple. In physical therapy, for example, if a person with a need to be mobile suffers from a hemiparesis, this need is not being satisfied. The physical therapist has certain skills to help a person satisfy a given need, the satisfaction of which will also affect the satisfaction of other needs (such as, in our example, the need to be autonomous and independent and the need to have a meaningful role). These become secondary issues to the immediate task at hand (improving mobility), although they have major psychosocial importance to the patient.

THE PSYCHOGERIATRIC EVALUATION

The fourth kind of assessment, and most comprehensive, is the psychogeriatric evaluation. It is an attempt to gather and integrate biological, psychological, and social data so that a comprehensive understanding of the person's psychosocial state can be achieved. Problems are then delineated along a hierarchy of needs, and appropriate interventions are developed.

The psychogeriatric evaluation has 11 components. It is presented in its entirety in this chapter, but the physical therapist, as a member of the rehabilitation team, is neither expected nor required to be responsible for the entire evaluation. Many authors[11-20] have examined the roles of various mental health professionals and have divided them into two major categories: generalist and specialist roles. Generalist roles are those clinical roles not limited by disciplinary boundaries or training. Rather, these roles are used by all professionals in the fulfillment of various professional tasks. They are discussed in more depth elsewhere.[11,12,18-20] Specialist roles differentiate among different professionals on the team and utilize specific skills, knowledge, and personality traits of these professionals in the total care of the patient.

Most work accomplished in the psychosocial aspects of caring for the elderly person in a rehabilitation setting uses generalist skills of all members of the rehabilitation team. The psychogeriatric evaluation is one task that can be completed using only generalist skills. Thus physical therapists need to be able to complete a psychogeriatric evaluation, if necessary, and be able to use that information to formulate a treatment plan that maximizes the rehabilitation potential of the individual. Physical therapists should be able to understand the work of other professionals on the team so as to be able to interact professionally and communicate effectively, thus maximizing team functioning.[21-23] This procedure does not minimize the specialist roles of the physical therapist, roles that involve the various techniques used in physical therapy and rehabilitation.

The components of the psychogeriatric evaluation are discussed in turn.

History of the Present Episode

One needs to know exactly what the person is feeling and experiencing, how long it has been going on, what seemed to trigger it, what makes it better (even temporarily), what seems to make it worse, and what interventions the patient and family and mental health personnel have tried hoping to improve this particular problem. It is in the history of the present episode that one asks the specific questions regarding the various symptoms—including presence or absence of vegetative, depressive, psychotic, phobic, and obsessive-compulsive symptoms—needed to make a diganosis as well as to assess blocks in need satisfaction.

Psychiatric History

Onc not only needs to ask if the person has had inpatient or outpatient psychiatric treatment in the past, but whether or not the person has received intervention for emotional problems from other personnel, such as psychologists, social workers, psychiatric nurses, and clergy. In addition, knowledge of any history of receiving "nerve pills" or other psychotropic drugs from a family physician is important. This information will help clarify a person's ability to cope and the coping mechanisms. The presence of a history of a severe psychiatric disability would be an indication for a prescription of specific interventions (especially psychopharmacologic) that have been successful in the past[24] or the avoidance of interventions that have been previously proved unsuccessful.

Past and Present Medical Status

Knowledge of the person's medical history is necessary to assess the person's overall functional capabilities and to know what problems to expect in the future. The presence or absence of certain medications may impair or enhance the overall rehabilitation process. This history may also hint at certain somatic disorders or medications that may be causing the psychopathology noted (e.g., depression secondary to hypothyroidism or toxic psychosis secondary to antidepressants).

Drug History

The patient's use of drugs must be ascertained, including not only prescription medications but also over-the-counter drugs and street drugs. Many older people have problems with alcohol or drugs that may interfere with the patient's overall functioning as well as with the rehabilitation program or may otherwise cause specific psychiatric disorders. Besides alcohol, the most commonly abused drugs in the elderly are over-the-counter "nerve pills," benzodiazepines, marijuana, barbiturates, amphetamines, and legal narcotic analgesics; any use of these drugs must be specifically ascertained.

Psychosocial Evaluation

The purpose of the psychosocial evaluation is to gather information about the person's past coping skills and about factors that may enhance or inhibit psychiatric and physical rehabilitation and to assess other stresses and resources in the patient's environment.

The psychosocial evaluation begins with a family history, including information about the patient's parents, siblings, and children. It also includes the medical and psychiatric history of these individuals and what kind of relationships these people had and have with each other and with the patient. In addition, the family history includes occupational and social-class background of the patient's parents (and whether or not they were immigrants) and the relationship between the parents.

In the developmental history, the person's meeting of developmental landmarks is assessed. The examiner also gathers information about the person's childhood.

In the educational history, one asks questions about the person's level of education and use of this education. Why a person stopped or continued educational pursuits at different times is ascertained, and interest in lifelong learning, vocational rehabilitation, and attitude toward education are assessed.

In the person's occupational history the examiner looks at jobs held, ability to hold a job, and the kind of work the person is interested in. One also examines for exposure to occupational hazards that might have diagnostic or therapeutic implications.

In the marital and sexual history one examines these relationships as a major resource and/or stress regardless of marital status, sexual orientation, or sexual exclusivity or nonexclusivity. If the patient has never married or cohabited with someone, the reasons for this need to be assessed. The entire spectrum of the individual's interpersonal relationships is examined in this way. One also ascertains the patient's interest in and level of sexual activity, with its obvious implications for rehabilitation.

One then looks at the person's current financial situation. This includes examination not only of sources of income but includes other social services that substitute for income (e.g., health insurance coverage and nutrition programs).

The examiner then investigates the patient's current housing for the presence and absence of barriers and to see how the house can be made barrier-free. Thus housing can be both a stress and a resource to the individual.

How the person uses leisure time is also assessed. This assessment is important not only in planning relaxation for the patient but also for gathering information about the patient's ability to relax, experience positive affects, and develop meaningful rather than just time-consuming activities.

In planning a rehabilitation program as well as psychotherapy, knowledge of the person's premorbid personality is crucial. This information will tell the therapist what kind of defenses and coping mechanisms the person uses. The examiner will also learn how the person has satisfied various needs in the past and whether or not the person has been capable of adapting to stress in the past. This information will clarify other psychologic stresses and resources the individual brings into the rehabilitation situation and will help to assess the risk of the individual developing major psychopathology in the future. For example, people with labile personality disorders are at risk for developing depression, and those with stable personality disorders are at risk for developing either depression or paraphrenia when stressed in old age.[25-27] People without personality disorders are more likely to cope successfully with stress. At the same time that one assesses the premorbid personality of the patient, one examines the entire environment to assess other stresses and resources present.

Review of Systems

Although such review has traditionally been part of the medical examination, it can be done by any health professional. The examiner asks about various symptoms of disease, including pain, visual problems, bowel habits, diet and appetite, sleep, and sexual functioning. Formal guides to a review of systems have been published elsewhere.[28-31]

Physical Examination

The physical examination should be complete, including rectal and pelvic examination. Although this must be done by a physician, nurse practitioner, or physician's assistant, the physical therapist must be apprised of this information in order to understand the problems of the older person and plan appropriate interventions.

Neurologic Examination

Because many older patients in the rehabilitation setting have or are suspected to have neurologic disease, a thorough neurologic examination must be done. This does not have to be done by a neurologic consultant, as all physicians and other health professionals who do physical examinations are trained to perform neurologic examinations. The information garnered must be transmitted to the members of the rehabilitation team.

Mental Status Examination

There are 15 parts of the mental status examination. Part of the mental status examination involves observation of the patient during the conduct of the psychogeriatric examination rather than as a separate part of the formal examination.

Delineation of psychopathologic symptoms is necessary for an accurate assessment of the psychosocial status of the older patient. Accurate, value-free descriptions of behavior, without labels, are the backbone of the mental status examination. In reviewing the mental status examination, one can easily see many forms of behavior varying from the expected normative behavior of the patient. These variations are not necessarily psychopathologic. For example, a sad affect would be very appropriate to someone who has recently had a cerebrovascular accident but would not be appropriate for someone who has just won a lottery. There are several descriptions of the conduct of the mental status examination.[32-34]

Appearance

First, one notes the patient's appearance. How is he or she dressed? Is she or he in a bed or wheelchair or ambulatory? What is his or her posture? Are there any other signs that might indicate the possibility of physical disease?

Appearance is either appropriate or inappropriate for the patient's medical condition and social setting. For example, it generally would not be considered appropriate for a patient to wear pajamas to an outpatient appointment, but it is appropriate to wear them in a hospital. The social context of a patient's appearance must be taken into account. The same holds true for posture, which may be relaxed, tense, indicative of physical pathology, or bizarre and unusual as in some psychotic patients.

Level of Consciousness

One then notes the patient's level of consciousness and alertness. The level of consciousness may be normal, or the patient may be hyperalert with wide eyes scanning the environment. The patient may be hypoalert or may be drowsy, sleeping, obtunded, semicomatose, or comatose.

Attention Span

The third part of the examination is evaluation of the patient's attention span. The patient may have marked difficulty paying attention because of distractibility or hearing deficit. On the other hand, a patient may be demonstrating denial or selective inattention or may for unconscious reasons not attend to the examiner. Selective inattention is usually under some conscious control but denial is not. Distractibility is usually noted in those with severe psychotic or cognitive disorders.

Mood

Mood is ascertained by asking the patient how she or he feels and what the underlying mood is. For example, is the patient happy, sad, or angry? Mood may be happy or sad within the realm of human experience, or the patient may experience extremes of mood, including elation or euphoria on the one hand or severe depression on the other. The person may be angry or hostile or experiencing anxiety or fear.

Affect

Associated with mood is the fifth parameter of the mental status examination, affect. This is the behavioral manifestation of the underlying mood, and it is usually ascertained through examination of the patient's facial expressions. Is the facial expression angry, sad, happy, dull, or blunted? Also, the examiner wants to know if the affect corresponds to the expressed thought content. The patient's affect may be appropriate or inappropriate. Inappropriate affect is affect that does not fit the underlying mood of the content of the person's thoughts. If inappropriate, it may also be blunted or flattened, which is when the person does not facially express underlying feelings.

Level of Activity

Sixth, one examines the level of activity. Is it normally active, hyperactive, or hypoactive? Are there tremors or other abnormal movements? The patient may demonstrate psychomotor retardation, in which all physical functions are slowed up, or psychomotor agitation, in which there is restlessness or agitation. Mild agitation may be manifested by mild finger-tapping and hand-wringing. Severe agitation is manifested by a person having difficulty staying still for more than a few moments. This condition must be differentiated from akathisia, which is a common parkinsonian symptom.

Speech

One then examines the quality of the patient's speech. One looks at the quantity, volume, tone, inflection, speed, and understandability (coherence) of speech. Speech may be incoherent or indistinct on the basis of aphasia or dysarthria. It may be rapid or slow, monotonous in tone and inflection, or too low or loud volume. It may or may not be appropriate to the situation, content, or affect.

Thought Processes

The examiner then considers the patient's thought process. Is it rational, logical, and oriented toward a goal? Does the patient attempt to answer questions in a reasonably concise manner? Is the patient able to express thoughts clearly, or is there evidence of receptive and/or expressive aphasia? Deficiencies of thought include paucity of thought, which is a relative lack of expressed thought. Perseveration occurs when the same thought is expressed over and over again regardless of its relevance to the question asked. Other disorders of thought process include a loss of the normal logical pathways of human thought. When mild, this is called tangentiality, in which the person seems to constantly digress from the topic, or circumstantiality, in which the person "beats around the bush" but eventually answers the question. More severe loss of logical aspects of thought is called loose association or derailment. When severe, the person's speech may be almost impossible to understand. This situation is called a word salad. In addition, the patient may use neologisms, invented words that may have idiosyncratic meanings known only to the patient.

Thought Content

Next, one examines the content of the patient's thought. What is the patient specifically thinking, and is it relevant to the business at hand? Disturbances of thought content are several. One is vagueness of thought. Other disturbances of thought include compulsive repetition or obsessive intrusion of a thought alien to the patient's ego. The person may demonstrate *idées fixes,* which are unshakable and encapsulated ideas that may or may not be delusional. The patient may also be preoccupied with phobic ideas or fantasies. The patient may demonstrate delusions, which may be reasonably logical beliefs that are not based in reality. Delusions are frequently paranoid in the elderly. They may be encapsulated or limited to only a small part of the patient's life and may not affect the patient's functioning in other ways, or they may be unencapsulated, global, and severely disruptive. They may be organized into a delusional system, or they may be disorganized. The patient may also demonstrate confabulation or may create "factual" information to cover up memory deficits; this must be differentiated from willful lying. Depressive thought content, including self-deprecation, statements of irrational guilt, and feelings of helplessness, hopelessness, worthlessness, and uselessness, may also be demonstrated.

Finally, certain specific Schneiderian first-rank symptoms of schizophrenia are included as disturbances of thought. These include thought insertion (the belief that an outside force or person is putting thoughts in a person's head), thought control (the belief that an outside force is controlling a person's thoughts), behavioral control (a similar belief associated with behavior), thought withdrawal (the belief that an outside force is taking thoughts out of a person's head), and thought broadcasting (the belief that people are able to hear the individual's thoughts out loud). Schneiderian first-rank symptoms are believed to be pathognomonic of schizophrenia in younger people[35] but have no specific pathognomonic consequence in the elderly.

Perception

In examining perception one is examining the person's ability to understand the spoken and written word as well as looking for unusual perceptual experiences. Many major disorders of perception are pathophysiologic in nature, including receptive aphasias and the results of major sensory deficits.

Another common disorder of perception is the illusion in which things may be perceived in a manner different from a measurable reality. The optical illusion is one example with which most people are familiar. Misperceptions are another form of perceptual disorder, one in which something is misidentified as something that it is not. The most severe perceptual disorders are hallucinations, in which the person creates sensory inputs not based in the external environment; they may be auditory, visual, olfactory, gustatory, tactile, or kinesthetic. Specific Schneiderian perceptual symptoms include hallucination of two voices communicating with each other or hallucination of a voice keeping up a running commentary on the person's behavior.

Memory

Memory is examined, in part, during the process of obtaining a history, a process that allows the examiner to ascertain the accuracy of the patient's recent and remote memory. Questions about the patient's activities over the few days before the examination also tests recent memory. To test for immediate recall, one can give the patient three items to remember and check back several minutes later to see if they are recalled (but see also Ch. 5). Memory disturbances include specific amnesias and hypomnesias, as well as more global disturbances of immediate recall, recent memory, and remote memory and the part processes of registration, retention, recognition, and recall.

Orientation

One next tests for orientation. Does the patient know the day of the week, date, month, year, and season? Does the patient know the name of the place he or she is in, the address, the floor, the room number? Can the patient give a reasonable account of herself or himself? Is the patient aware of the present situation? (In other words, does the patient understand the environmental parameters surrounding him or her?) Difficulty with orientation is called disorientation; it is the person's inability to identify the time, the place, or basic information about herself or himself.

Intelligence

One assesses the patient's level of intelligence by examining ability to perform higher cortical functions. Can the patient serially subtract seven from a hundred? Can the patient follow simple instructions? Can he or she read and write a simple sentence? How well does she interpret proverbial statements? Are the proverbs interpreted abstractly or concretely? The adages I usually use are "you can lead a horse to water but you can't make it drink" and "people in glass houses shouldn't throw stones." Can the patient identify similarities and differences between items such as an apple and an orange? Disorders of intelligence may include lifelong intellectual deficits, as in mentally retarded persons, or acquired intellectual deficits. The latter may be specific, as dyslexia, or global, as in dementia, and may include difficulties following simple instructions, reading, calculating, and writing sentences. The deficit may also include loss of the ability to abstract proverbs, which is partially dependent on both the educational level and cultural background of the patient.

Judgment

One tests judgment by assessing what the patient would do in hypothetical situations. The situations I use are the following: "What would you do if you found a letter lying on the ground in front of a mailbox?" "What would you do if you smelled smoke while at the movies?" Responses give the examiner information about the patient's ability to integrate environmental cues and choose between alternative behaviors. Difficulties of judgment include impulsivity, failure to take the consequences of one's behavior into account before action.

Insight

The final part of the mental status examination is the assessment of the patient's level of insight. One asks the patient why she or he feels that the specific emotional, behavioral, or cognitive difficulty has developed. Levels of insight range from a complete denial of all symptoms, through the ability to identify symptoms but not consequences or etiology, through the identification of symptoms and consequences but not their etiology, to insight into the nature and cause of one's psychosocial difficulties. The level of insight will often dictate the type of intervention planned with the patient.

Laboratory Examination

The specific laboratory examination is dependent on the nature of the psychologic difficulty considered. All geriatric patients who develop psychopathology should have a complete blood count, renal, liver, and thyroid function studies, electrolytes, fasting blood sugar, electrocardiogram, chest x-ray, serology for syphilis, urinalysis, urine drug and alcohol screen, and serum concentrations of drugs that the patient is taking. In addition, if a diagnosis of brain failure is being considered, the patient should also have vitamin B_{12} and folate blood levels assessed, along with computerized axial tomography of the head, with and without contrast. Other specific laboratory evaluations, especially magnetic resonance imagery of the head, an electroencephalogram, or HIV (AIDS) virus titers, may also be necessary.

Social Examination

The social examination is the final part of the psychogeriatric evaluation. One includes information gathered from review of the patient's chart and discussions with social service staff, nursing staff, family members, neighbors, and other important persons in the patient's life. It will corroborate the history the patient gives the examiner and also gives the examiner insight into other symptoms that the patient may be unwilling or unable to discuss with the examiner. It will also help assess and enlist the interpersonal resources available to the patient. If feasible, the social examination includes a tour of the patient's home to assess resources, stresses, and barriers in the environment.

INTERVIEWING TECHNIQUES

The psychogeriatric evaluation is not necessarily done in a rigid sequence such as that listed above. A specific rhythm develops in a good interview: First, one starts with very broad questions that avoid "yes" and "no" answers; gradually, more specific questions are asked. Then one returns to broad questions as new areas are explored. The entire evaluation takes 1 to 2 hours.

I usually start by first introducing myself to the patient, asking if I can sit on the bed or chair, and then asking the patient how he or she feels and also what it is that bothers her or him. The patient should always be given the opportunity to discuss the immediate problem and what is of utmost concern to him or her. The patient is allowed to discuss this at her or his own pace and rhythm. Specific questions are geared to clarifying particular points and filling in some gaps as they develop.

Once the history of the present episode is elicited, I then seek answers to specific items of the psychogeriatric examination, again beginning with broad questions. For example, I might ask something about what it was like growing up as a child. From there, I can ask more specific questions about parents, siblings, and other childhood experiences; gradually the entire evaluation is completed.

The interview should be private and confidential and conducted without the presence of friends, relatives, or other staff. As part of the social examination, however, these collateral individuals should be interviewed with the patient present, as keeping secrets from the patient is likely to cause strain in the therapist–patient relationship.

The examiner should strive for a friendly, frank, and outspoken relationship, because his or her own insecurity and anxiety will become apparent to the patient and interfere with the examination. In part this anxiety can be overcome by being clear in one's own mind about what facts are to be elucidated and how to approach the patient. As noted above, it is usually best to discuss some aspect of the present difficulty or primary complaint first and then proceed as naturally as possible to other parts of the examination. "Yes/no" questions and leading questions must be avoided at all times. Tact, gentleness, and respect for the patient's sensitivities are most essential. If the patient should suffer from a catastrophic reaction or become severely agitated, it is usually wise to terminate the interview and return at a future time. Note-taking interferes with observation and also is frequently objected to by many patients; therefore I suggest that any notes needed should be written immediately after the interview, when the therapist is alone.

One way of assessing many aspects of the patient's mental status, especially memory, orientation, and higher cortical functioning, is to use the Mini-Mental State Examination[36] (Table 4-1). The Mini-Mental State Examination has the advantage of being reproducible, quantitative, and quick (it takes less than 4 minutes to complete with the average patient). It gives important clues to possible deficits of higher cortical functioning.

Following completion of the interview, I always ask the patient if there is anything important that has not been touched on that the patient wishes to share. I also tell the patient what I think about the patient's condition and what my plans are, even if my plans at that point are only to discuss the situation with the other members of the treatment team. I always give the patient the opportunity to question me, though I tactfully refuse to answer personal questions; instead, I limit questions to the clinical task. My interview is terminated with a request to see the patient again, with the patient's permission.

Table 4-1. Mini-Mental State Examination

BEGIN HERE: Now I would like to ask you some questions to check your concentration and memory. Most of them will be easy.

What is the ... *(RECORD ANSWERS AND CIRCLE APPROPRIATE CODE)*

		Correct	Error	Refusal Can't Do	Refusal Other Refusal
1.	...year?	1	2	6	7
2.	...season?	1	2	6	7
3.	...date?	1	2	6	7
4.	...day of week?	1	2	6	9
5.	...month?	1	2	6	7
6.	...Can you tell me where we are right now? For instance, what state are we in?	1	2	6	7
7.	...What city are we in?	1	2	6	9
8.	...What hospital are we in?	1	2	6	7
9.	...What building are we in?	1	2	6	7
10.	...What floor of the building are we on?	1	2	6	7

11-13. I am going to name three things. After I have said them, I want you to repeat them. Remember what they are because I am going to ask you to to name them again in a few minutes.

	Correct	Error	Can't Do	Other Refusal
Apple:	1	2	6	7
Table:	1	2	6	7
Penny:	1	2	6	7

Please repeat the three items for me.
"Apple" ...
"Table" ...
"Penny" ...

SCORE FIRST TRY. REPEAT OBJECTS UNTIL ALL ARE LEARNED.

14-18. Can you subtract (take away) 7 from 100, and then subtract 7 from the answer you get and keep subtracting 7 until I tell you to stop?

Record   ___ ___ ___ ___ ___
                 (93) (86) (79) (72) (65)

Number of Errors: 0   1   2   3   4   5

Refusal: Can't do   6
             Other refusal   7

19-23. *ALTERNATIVE TO Q. 14-18.*
Now I am going to spell a word forward and I want you to spell it backward. The word is W-O-R-L-D. Spell "world" backward.

REPEAT IF NECESSARY, BUT NOT AFTER SPELLING STARTS.

Print Letter: ___ ___ ___ ___ ___

Number of Errors: 0   1   2   3   4   5

Refusal: Can't Do   6
             Other Refusal   7

(continued)

Table 4-1. Mini-Mental State Examination

		Correct	Error	Can't Do	Other Refusal
				Refusal	
24–26.	Now what were the three objects I asked you to remember? Apple:	1	2	6	7
	Table:	1	2	6	7
	Penny:	1	2	6	7
27.	*SHOW WRISTWATCH.* What is this called?	1	2	6	7
28.	*SHOW PENCIL.* What is this called?	1	2	6	7
29.	I'd like you to repeat a phrase after me: "No ifs, ands, or buts." *ALLOW ONLY ONE TRIAL.*	1	2	6	7
30.	Read the words on this page and then do what it says. *CODE 1 IF PATIENT CLOSES EYES.*	1	2	6	7

CLOSE YOUR EYES

31–33.	*READ FULL STATEMENT AND THEN HAND OVER PAPER.* I'm going to give you a piece of paper. When I do, take the piece of paper in your right hand, fold the paper in half with both hands, and put the paper down on your lap. Right hand:	1	2	6	7
	Folds:	1	2	6	7
	In lap:	1	2	6	7
34.	Write a complete sentence on this paper for me.				
35.	Here is a drawing. Please copy the drawing on this page.				

SCORING FOR 34/35.

34.	*SENTENCE SHOULD HAVE A SUBJECT AND VERB AND MAKE SENSE. SPELLING AND GRAMMAR ERRORS ARE OKAY.*	1	2	6	7
35.	*CORRECT IF THE TWO FIVE-SIDED FORMS INTERSECT TO FORM A FOUR-SIDED FIGURE AND IF ALL ANGLES IN THE FIVE-SIDED FIGURE ARE PRESERVED.*	1	2	6	7

BLOCKS TO ADEQUATE ASSESSMENT

Several factors lead to an inadequate psychogeriatric assessment of elderly patients. Some of these blocks are based in the physical therapist's acceptance of societal attitudes toward and stereotyping of the elderly; others are an integral part of the structure of the delivery of health care services. Still others may be personal issues for the therapist, and others derive from the personality of the patient.

It is well known that health workers, regardless of specific profession, stereotype the elderly in exactly the same manner that the general population does (see various references cited in Refs. 22, 23, 25, and 37–41). Although there are no data specifically assessing the adherence of physical therapists to the stereotype, the consistency of data from other health professionals makes it reasonable to extrapolate such data to physical therapists.

Stereotyping has been defined by Solomon and Vickers[42] as "the holding in common of a standardized mental picture representing an oversimplified and uncritical judgment of another group." Stereotyping has been hypothesized to lead to the delivery of inadequate or inappropriate services to the elderly[43] (disputed by O'Dowd and Zofnass[44]) and is a factor in the development of learned helplessness in older people.[38,45,46] The stereotype of the elderly is as follows:[47]

1. They are conservative and old-fashioned.
2. They have limited activities and interests.
3. Physical deterioration is inevitable.
4. They are poor.
5. They have only negative or only positive personality traits.
6. They are dirty.
7. Mental deterioration is inevitable.
8. They interfere in the lives of others.
9. They are repudiated by their families.
10. They are asexual.
11. They are either in the best or the worst period of life.
12. They are pessimistic.
13. They are insecure and helpless.

As with all stereotypes, each of those statements is untrue for the elderly as a group, although some may be true for some older persons.

By believing in this stereotype of older people, the health professional is likely to prelabel behaviors and feelings of the older patient, which may then lead to an inadequate and inappropriate diagnosis of "senility" or a belief that psychotherapeutic and sociotherapeutic modalities are not efficacious in older people. In addition, the health worker who believes in the stereotype is likely to design an environment and therapeutic culture that further reinforces the stereotype. These beliefs will also lead to an independence of response outcome in interactions between the elderly patient and the therapist, thus leading to the development of learned helplessness.[38,45,46]

The second block to adequate assessment is ageism. Ageism is more than just discrimination on the basis of age; rather, it is an entire melange of negative societal attitudes and behaviors toward older people.[43] It encompasses the behavioral results of the stereotype described above but also includes four types of victimization (physical, economic, role, and attitudinal)[41,48] and resultant prejudice and misconceptions.

One type of medical model, the diagnosis-treatment model,[49] can be another factor that interferes with adequate assessment of older people. Negative attitudes and stereotypes will prevent even the use of this model, as they will preclude the accurate diagnosis of older people because of labeling. In addition, the medical problems of the elderly are almost always multiproblematic and not purely biological. The use of this rigid model is in conflict with a systems model more appropriate to the medical care of the elderly, and its use is further complicated by the fact that common diseases may present in uncommon ways in older people.[50]

There is a second medical model, the organizational model, in which the physician is atop a pyramid of other health workers, giving orders and making all major decisions.[49] This model frequently leads to a narrow view of the older person and inadequate examination of factors that influence rehabilitation. It also leads to rigid role definitions, which have consequences for the functioning of the different team members.[19-20]

Besides stereotyping and ageism, there may exist unresolved personality issues for the therapist that may cause problems for assessment.[25,51] The therapist may either infantilize or parentify the older patient and be blind to these specific intergenerational issues that may affect therapy. The therapist may also avoid certain specific issues, especially sexuality, chronicity, and mortality, during the assessment or intervention process.

The patient may have difficulty responding to the assessment process. Patients with dysarthria and aphasias present particular problems, as do those with severe cognitive impairment and those demonstrating catastrophic reactions. Severely depressed people may also be difficult to evaluate, as are those who are actively psychotic. It is virtually impossible accurately to assess an older person who is addicted to alcohol or drugs, or who is in a state of alcohol or drug intoxication or withdrawal. Yet it is imperative to do as complete an assessment of these patients as possible. For example, severe depression may mimic dementia or aphasia; however, because depression is much more treatable than these other conditions, an accurate assessment is essential. Other psychological issues in the patient may lead to blocks in assessment. The patient may infantilize or parentify the therapists[25,51] or refuse to deal with issues that are emotionally charged and laden with conflict, perhaps for an entire lifetime.

ASSESSMENT OF NEEDS

When the assessment data are collected, there is a need to organize them into a clinically useful paradigm. One such paradigm, developed by Vickers[52] and based on the work of Maslow,[8] allows for the development of a hierarchy of needs. The following discussion includes my minor modifications of Vickers' paradigm.

Maslow hypothesized that basic needs must be satisfied before one can successfully work toward the satisfaction of needs higher up the hierarchy.

Blocks in satisfaction of these basic needs thus have implications for all needs of the hierarchic pyramid.

At the base of the pyramid are biological needs. These are needs for physiologic homeostasis and absence of disease, including thirst, hunger, warmth, and other physical comforts. Problems that arise in this area are most commonly defined as medical problems. Problems may also include such biologically autonomous behaviors as panic and vegetative symptoms of depression. Biologically autonomous behaviors have physiologic concomitants and are self-perpetuating. Problems in this realm are treated by biological methods, especially medication and surgery.

The next level of the pyramid includes activities of daily living. These are the skills that allow daily survival, including ability to find an adequate diet, pay one's bills, get adequate income, dress oneself appropriately for the weather, and self-advocacy. It is at this level that the physical therapist is most active, as much of rehabilitation involves the correction of or adaptation to blocks to a person's ability to manage activities of daily living. For example, physical therapists do not work with cerebrovascular accidents per se; rather, they deal with the functional sequelae of this biological disorder. All blocks in activities of daily living, either physical or emotional, are treated with various rehabilitative and reeducative techniques.

On the third level of the hierarchy are social needs. These are needs to interact with others, to maintain meaningful social roles, and to avoid loneliness.[53] Problems in this realm may come from the individual because of inadequate social skills, social anxieties, or maladaptive interpersonal behaviors, or from society, including rigidly defined social and gender roles. Intervention at this level includes all therapies that involve the patient, the therapist, and at least one other person. Examples would include marriage counseling, group psychotherapy, and consciousness-raising groups.

These first three levels of needs are roughly equivalent to Maslow's basic needs. The next level of the hierarchy corresponds to Maslow's concept of esteem needs. This is the psychological realm and includes such constructs as mood, affect, identity, self-esteem, and body image, as well as the need for love, validation, and security. These psychological needs are primarily internal to the individual, although they may have interpersonal ramifications. Problems in the psychological realm are handled through a variety of individual psychotherapies involving only the patient and the therapist, including psychoanalysis, psychoanalytic psychotherapy, supportive psychotherapy, transactional analysis, and Gestalt psychotherapy.

The peak of the pyramid corresponds to Maslow's metaneeds. These are creative and self-actualization needs, including the need to express oneself in a meaningful way along with various existential issues, such as the meaning of life, mortality, life goals, and one's *Weltanschauung*. The problems meeting metaneeds are corrected through the various modalities developed from the human potential movement.

STRESS AND COPING IN THE ELDERLY:
A CLINICAL PARADIGM

A second way to organize the data gathered during the psychogeriatric evaluation is the psychodynamic paradigm, based on the pioneering work of Goldfarb[54,55] and expanded on by me.[25,41,48,56–58] The elderly experience a variety of stresses triggering a characteristic sequence of coping events (Fig. 4-1). Some of these stresses are rather sudden and unpredictable. These are stresses that may happen to individuals at any age but are more likely to occur in the elderly. They are also more likely to be clustered in the elderly. A common denominator of these stresses is that they all involve loss, including losses in the social support system—loss of friends, spouse, parents, children, neighbors, workmates. These losses may occur through death, illness, institutionalization, or relocation. Other losses occur in social role, including the shift from institutionalized roles at first to tenuous and informal roles, as described by Rosow,[59] and finally to a lapse into rolelessness.[56] In addition, the inability of men to perform traditional gender role behaviors is another significant loss that has important ramifications for rehabilitation; men faced with severe physical illness or functional disability are more likely to become severely depressed than women.[51,60,61] There are also other losses, including loss of health, mobility, income, adequate housing, and adequate opportunities for leisure-time activities.

Another set of stresses result from the daily victimization that the elderly face,[25,41,48,56] including economic, physical, attitudinal, and role victimization. Included here are ageism and stereotyping, as well as inadequate pensions and health insurance, high food prices, the effects of inflation, crimes against person and property, and inadequate medical evaluation and intervention. These stresses have been discussed in more depth elsewhere.[25,41,48,56,62,63]

When faced with these stresses, the elderly must cope with the feelings engendered. At first, the older person experiences a diminished sense of mastery over the environment. This decreasing mastery is associated with feelings of loss of control of one's destiny and over one's internal and/or external environment. These feelings then stimulate feelings of increased helplessness and ambivalent feelings about dependency. This sense of helpless-

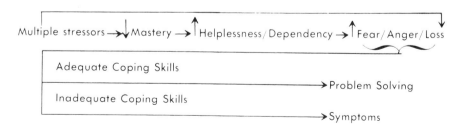

Fig. 4-1.   Stress and coping in the elderly. (From Goldfarb,[54] with permission.)

ness is often reinforced by health care workers because of stereotyping and ageism, the inappropriate adoption of the "sick" role[64,65] (which is antithetical to adequate intervention in a rehabilitation setting), and the power differential inherent in the interpersonal relationship between patient and therapist.[38,45,46] These feelings then stimulate the two underlying stress affects mediated by the general adaptation syndrome.[66] These affects (fight and flight) are experienced as feelings of anger or fear. The amount of anger and fear experienced by the older patient is largely determined by previous life experiences as well as the specific nature of the stress. In addition, anger and fear become separate affects as people age, so that the older patient experiences a third stress affect, loss.

The older person must then diminish the discomfort of these dysphoric feelings. The older person who has adequate coping skills will be able to regain a sense of mastery, avoid lapsing into a state of helplessness, ventilate feelings appropriately, and bring cognitive, problem-solving, and adaptative skills and psychogenic defense mechanisms into play. The dysphoric feelings are then minimized and the person alloplastically manipulates the environment.

However, if the person is unable to bring adequate coping skills into play, psychological symptoms will develop. These symptoms (Fig. 4-2) are largely dependent on the underlying affective experience. For example, the behavioral manifestation of anger is rage and physical assault; the behavioral manifestation of fear is panic. Various mixtures of these two affects lead to other psychopathological symptoms. The more loss the person experiences, the less manifest anxiety will be evident. In addition, if the person has always been narcissitic and oriented toward the body, somatization will be a concomitant symptom, regardless of the nature of the specific symptoms.

Three groups of older people have difficulty coping and are likely to develop psychological symptoms. The major group includes those elderly who have previously been able to cope well with stress; however, because of the severity of this stress and/or the clustering of stress, their coping mechanisms have become overwhelmed, and their coping abilities have broken down. A second group also previously coped well with stress; however, because of brain failure they have become unable to bring previously acquired coping skills into play and thus develop symptoms. These symptoms are usually an exaggeration of either the underlying affects or the individual's premorbid personality and coping mechanisms. The third group is the smallest but causes the most

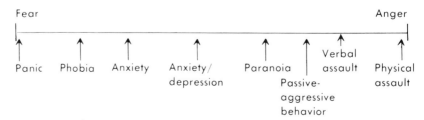

Fig. 4-2. Psychopathological symptoms in the elderly and their place on the fear–anger continuum. (From Solomon,[48] with permission.)

difficulty, and its members are the most difficult to treat. These are older people who have never been able to cope with stress, including older people with a history of personality disorders[25] or other major psychopathology.

This paradigm has many important implications for physical therapists. Most obvious is that loss of function is a very great stress at any age. There is a real loss of mastery, not only because the individual is no longer able to manage activities of daily living, but also because the stressful events themselves are not under the control of the individual in any way. Dependency on others is a reality issue, as is true helplessness, thus leading to conflict between real dependency and clinical goals that emphasize autonomy, independence, and minimization of disability. The sense of vulnerability engenders feelings of fear of recurrence of the underlying trauma or illness. Some patients feel anger at themselves for slow progression in therapy or for getting sick, or anger at God or at health care personnel for not being able to reverse problems and return the patient to the premorbid state. Loss of functioning requires that the individual grieve as he or she would grieve over any other loss. In addition, the older person must cope with the continuous stresses of ageism manifested in the health care system that reinforce learned helplessness and depressive symptomatology.[38,45,46,56]

COMMON PSYCHOPATHOLOGIC SYNDROMES IN THE ELDERLY

Adjustment Disorders

Adjustment disorders are virtually ubiquitous in the elderly. Such disorders are a response to any stress, and they are especially common following a major physical illness that requires rehabilitation. An adjustment disorder is a time-limited and mildly exaggerated form of the individual's usual coping mechanisms as the person experiences a wide variety of mood changes, including euphoria and elation, sadness, anger, self-blame, irritability, anxiety, hostility, and a variety of somatic complaints. The person's mood remains quite labile, and shifts within this range of feelings occur with minimal external or internal provocation. However, as the person begins to cope with the stress, these symptoms begin to improve, usually within days or weeks, which differentiates this disorder from other pathologic symptoms that tend to remain stable or get worse. The adjustment disorder differs from normative coping in that the individual acknowledges difficulty coping or the process of coping seems to become stalled for several weeks. The treatment of the adjustment disorder is psychotherapeutic and sociotherapeutic.

Affective Disorders

Affective disorders (depression and mania) are the most common major psychopathologic syndromes in the elderly. Estimates of the after-age-65 incidence of depression usually are approximately 30 percent, and depression accounts for 68 percent of psychiatric hospitalizations in the elderly.[67] Approximately 14 percent of the elderly suffer from depression at some time.[68] Depression is manifested by sad mood (or its equivalent) and various vegetative disturbances. There is a change in appetite (usually loss but occasionally increase) and a change in the sleep cycle (usually difficulty falling asleep, difficulty remaining asleep, and early morning awakening, but occasionally hypersomnia). The person demonstrates either psychomotor agitation or retardation and may complain of anxiety, weakness, or feeling slowed up, but not of sadness. The patient feels fatigued, even after adequate sleep, and feels lacking in the energy or the motivation for rehabilitation and other tasks. The patient feels guilty and blames himself or herself for these problems. The patient has difficulty concentrating and demonstrates a cognitive disturbance manifested by a disturbance of recent memory and immediate recall, concrete thinking, pervasive doubt, and what I have described as "viewing the world through gray-colored glasses." In addition, the depressed individual manipulates self and others into situations that will guarantee failure[69,70] and then internalizes the guilt and anger at others who do not respond to these failure-invoking manipulations.

The severely depressed person may verbalize suicidal feelings, ideation, or plans. As suicide is one of the leading causes of death in the elderly, the examiner must always ask the patient about suicidal ideation. Some severely depressed persons will also demonstrate a variety of psychotic symptoms, including delusions and hallucinations.

It is important to differentiate depression from an adjustment disorder, a relatively easy task except early in the course of the disorder. People with adjustment disorders with sad mood will gradually improve over time; those with depression will get worse. In addition, the depression may mimic a dementia (pseudodementia)[71] and must be differentiated from other causes of brain failure. Drug and alcohol withdrawal syndromes are frequently characterized by symptoms that are identical to depression, especially in patients addicted to short-acting benzodiazepines. Depressive symptoms are also common after detoxification and remit spontaneously over time. Thus, an addicted patient must usually be "clean" for at least 1 month before a diagnosis of depression can be made and treatment instituted. The treatment of depression is psychopharmacologic, psychotherapeutic, and sociotherapeutic.

Mania is much less common in the elderly than it is in younger patients and may have either an organic or psychological foundation. In some ways it is the extreme opposite of depression, as the manic individual's mood is elated or euphoric. The patient demonstrates extreme impulsivity, diminished need for sleep, increased energy, psychomotor agitation, and rapid speech. Many manic individuals are quite hostile and may be overtly paranoid. Some also demonstrate hallucinations and delusions. The treatment of mania also is psychopharmacologic, psychotherapeutic, and sociotherapeutic.

Alcoholism and Chemical Dependence

Approximately 25 percent of people over the age of 65 are at risk for developing alcoholism or chemical dependency. A major problem at this time is the addiction to short-acting benzodiazepines (Table 4-2), especially alprazolam, lorazepam, and triazolam. Indeed, this is a virtual epidemic in the United States at this time. Many of these persons have a long history of drug and alcohol abuse, with the short-acting benzodiazepines being the latest of a long line of abused medications. But many other patients were placed on these drugs after complaining to their physician about anxiety, depression, insomnia, or vague somatic complaints. Because of their short half-life in the body, tolerance to these medications develops rapidly, with withdrawal the consequence. Anxiety, agitation, and sleeplessness (withdrawal) are followed by either an increased dose of medication or increased frequency of dosage. Tolerance and withdrawal are the inevitable result, and a cycle of increased drug and increased withdrawal develops. Although this pattern occurs with all addictive drugs, it may take months to years to develop with alcohol or longer-acting medications. With the short-acting medications, however, a full-blown withdrawal syndrome, characterized by severe agitation, anxiety, panic attacks, depression, delirium, poor attention span, and even seizures may occur in the patient who has been taking these drugs for only 2 to 3 weeks, at very low dosage, *while the patient is still taking the drug.* Even when detoxification is complete, these symptoms may recur as long as 6 months after the last dose of drug has been taken. These medications should never be abruptly discontinued, as a full-fledged withdrawal syndrome can be fatal. For example, 20 percent of untreated delirium tremens (alcohol withdrawal) is fatal.

Another large group of these individuals are reactive alcoholics or chemically dependent patients who also suffer from severe depression. The drinking or abuse of drugs almost always begins after a major stress with loss. The use of alcohol or other drugs is clearly for self-medication of dysphoric affects. The pattern of drinking, in particular, is frequently different from that of other alcoholics or chemically dependent persons, as older reactive alcoholic/drug using men tend to drink alone to ward off feelings of depression, loneliness, and

Table 4-2. Benzodiazepines

Chlordiazepoxide (Librium, Libritabs)
Diazepam (Valium)
Oxazepam (Serax)
Clorazepate (Tranxene, Azene)
Prazepam (Vestran, Centrax)
Lorazepam (Ativan)
Halazepam (Paxipam)
Alprazolam (Xanax)
Flurazepam (Dalmane)
Temazepam (Restoril)
Triazolam (Halcion)

dependency. Older reactive alcoholic/drug using women often drink in the company of others and use alcohol to allow them to express feelings of anger and hostility. The treatment of alcoholism and chemical dependency first involves confrontation of denial and rationalization, education about the effects of addictive drugs and alcohol for the patient and family, confrontation of the family's enabling behaviors, and attendance at Alcoholics Anonymous, as well as supportive psychotherapy and appropriate detoxification. Once the patient is "clean" for at least 1 month, and preferably longer, then treatment of the underlying depression by appropriate psychotherapy, sociotherapy, and psychopharmocology is indicated.

Brain Failure

Approximately 6.2 percent of the elderly develop symptoms of brain failure.[72] As one-fourth of these individuals have a reversible condition, it is necessary that health workers not label the older patient with cognitive impairment as having an irreversible dementia. Depressive pseudodementia is only one of the common causes of reversible brain failure;[71] others are drug toxicity/withdrawal, malnutrition, infection, cerebral edema, and cardiovascular disease. The major cause of irreversible dementia is Alzheimer's disease, but other major causes are multi-infarct dementia, alcoholic dementia, tertiary neurosyphilis, head trauma, and cerebrovascular accidents. The symptoms of brain failure are either primary (based on the neurologic dysfunction itself) or secondary (symptoms that include the individual's attempt to cope with and adapt to the primary symptoms, using the coping mechanisms described above). Brain failure is discussed in more detail in Chapter 5.

Paraphrenia

Paraphrenia is a paranoid psychosis that develops for the first time in old age in the absence of an organic cause of brain failure. It affects approximately 1 to 2 percent of the elderly and is manifested by paranoid delusions usually limited to only small segments of the patient's life and allowing the patient to function in his/her usual way. Treatment is a combination of pharmacotherapy and psychosocial interventions.

Other Psychopathology

Personality disorders affect approximately 5 percent of the elderly[25] and are lifelong maladaptive interpersonal behavior patterns that may become evident for the first time or intensified in old age. The importance of personality disorders is that they often serve as the psychodynamic substrate for the development of more major psychiatric syndromes. Neuroses, phobias, and anxiety disorders are syndromes that are rare in the elderly. When they do occur, they are frequently indicative of an underlying depression or organic problem. The treatment of these disorders is psychotherapeutic. Sexual dysfunctions may also occur for the first time in old age; besides demythologization and education, treatment follows the techniques developed by Masters and Johnson.[73] And of course, schizophrenia, a disorder that begins in younger people, is chronic and continues into old age.

PRINCIPLES OF INTERVENTION

The goal of intervention is to change symptoms into adequate coping and adaptation by reversing the psychodynamic schema noted above. Most of this reversal can be accomplished by members of the rehabilitation team, using generalist skills. As Rogers[74] has pointed out, the major hallmarks of a good psychophysical therapist are not technical skills but rather empathy (the ability to psychologically put oneself in the other person's place), unconditional positive regard (the ability to accept the patient as she or he is; this is not the same as liking the patient), and genuineness (accepting yourself as you are).

The first step in therapy is a direct attack on the symptoms. If the person has psychotic symptoms (mania, delusions, hallucinations), catastrophic reactions, or organically based agitation that is not controlled by nonpharmacologic measures, antipsychotic medication (Table 4-3) is indicated. Antipsychotic medications should not be used to treat symptoms of anxiety, as there is no evidence that these medications are efficacious for such problems.[75] Nor should they be used in the treatment of organically based symptoms until the underlying cause of the symptoms are elucidated. If the patient meets the criteria for a diagnosis of major depressive disorder, antidepressant medication (Table 4-4) is indicated. Antidepressants should not be used in the treatment of anxiety nor for adjustment disorders, sadness, or grief reactions. If the patient is manic, lithium is the treatment of choice.

If the older person demonstrates phobic, compulsive, or obsessive symptoms, the use of behavior modification techniques is indicated.[76,77] Sexual dysfunctions may be treated by sexual therapies developed by Masters and Johnson.[73] Hypnosis may also be used for specific neurotic symptoms. A variety of nonpharmacologic techniques may be used in the treatment of anxiety. For episodic anxiety, the breathing exercises developed for use in Lamaze childbirth[78] are of help. For more continuous anxiety or tension, relaxation exercises, such as used in behavior modification or Lamaze childbirth, may be of help. For some patients regular strenuous physical exercise, transcendental meditation, yoga, massage, sex, or biofeedback may also be of benefit in mastering anxiety. Because of the unproven efficacy of benzodiazepines[75,79] (Table 4-2) and other antianxiety agents such as hydroxyzine or meprobamate,[75,80] as well as the dangerousness of these drugs, these drugs probably have no place in the treatment of the elderly.

Table 4-3. Antipsychotic Drugs

Phenothiazines
  Aliphatic
    Chlorpromazine (Thorazine)
    Promazine (Sparine)
    Triflupromazine (Vesprin)
  Piperidine
    Thioridazine (Mellaril)
    Mesoridazine (Serentil)
    Piperacetazine (Quide)
  Piperazine
    Prochlorperazine (Compazine)
    Trifluoperazine (Stelazine)
    Butaperazine (Repoise)
    Perphenazine (Trilafon)
    Fluphenazine (Prolixin, Permitil)
    Acetophenazine (Tindal)

Thioxanthienes
  Chlorprothixene (Taractan)
  Thiothixene (Navane)

Butyrophenones
  Haloperidol (Haldol)

Dihydroindolones
  Molindone (Moban)

Dibenzoxazepines
  Loxapine (Loxitane)
  Pimozide (Orap)
Diphenylbutylpiperidine
  Pimozide (Orap)

Table 4-4. Antidepressant Drugs

Tricyclics
  Iminobenzyls
    Imipramine (Tofranil)
    Trimipramine (Surmontil)
    Desipramine (Norpramin, Pertofrane)
  Dibenzoheptadienes
    Amitriptyline (Elavil, Endep)
    Nortriptyline (Aventyl, Pamelor)
    Protriptyline (Vivactyl)
  Dibenzoxepins
    Doxepin (Sinequan, Adapin)
  Dibenzoxazepines
    Amoxapine (Asendin)

Tetracyclics
  Maprotiline (Ludiomil)
  Trazodone (Desyrel)

Monoamine oxidase inhibitors
  Isocarboxazid (Marplan)
  Tranylcypromine (Parnate)
  Phenelzine (Nardil)

Bicyclics
  Fluoxitene (Prozac)

Following the direct attack on symptoms, the therapist next helps the patient ventilate the underlying affect. This involves giving the patient permission to feel fear, anger, or loss and to verbalize these feelings. Permission must be especially given to dependent patients who are afraid of antagonizing the therapist if they get angry at the therapist. It should be made clear that it is "okay" to be angry at members of the rehabilitation team and to direct this anger at them rather than toward oneself. Patients who are particularly labile in expressing affect must learn how to channel affect into verbal communication. Those who do not express affect must be pushed to do so.

The next step in therapy is to diminish helplessness and dependency. In part, this process uses the techniques of rehabilitation. The patient must internalize feelings that counter helplessness and dependency. Aside from the work of the rehabilitation team, one way of accomplishing this is to give the patient graded behavioral tasks with guaranteed success to build up a hierarchy of behaviors.

Regaining mastery requires that the patient have control over his or life. That requires choice and options. The patient must be made to understand that she or he is responsible for his or her own behavior; at first, this may be the patient's only expectation. The patient should be allowed to make all decisions for herself or himself, including decisions regarding clothing, menu, visitors, activities, and therapeutic goals. The patient should not be cut off from his or her network, but must use this network to help maintain autonomy and mastery. The older person must be encouraged to take risks and to try out new options, including options that may not be comfortable for the therapist yet are comfortable for the patient.

Whenever possible, the specific stresses must be reversed. It is important to realize that the specific physical stress may have ramifications involving the entire spectrum of stresses felt by the older person. For example, the stress of hemiparesis also involves the stresses of involuntary retirement, changed relationship with spouse and children, loss of ability to perform leisure activities, and financial problems.

For the older person who has previously functioned well, rehabilitation and psychosocial support are frequently all the therapy that is necessary. For the older person with a lifelong history of inadequate coping or who wishes to grow, long-term psychiatric intervention is indicated. If the problems are primarily intrapsychic, a form of individual psychotherapy is the treatment of choice. For those who are psychologically minded, an insight-oriented psychotherapy (psychoanalysis, psychoanalytically oriented psychotherapy, Gestalt therapy, transactional analysis, client-centered psychotherapy, or existential therapy) is the treatment of choice, augmented with a movement therapy, such as Feldenkrais or dance therapy, massage therapy, neurolinguistic programming, or art therapy. If the problems are primarily interpersonal, group psychotherapy or marital therapy is indicated. For those persons unable to work within an insight-oriented mode, the same techniques modified for supportive psychotherapy are helpful. These various therapies require appropriate members of the treatment team to adopt specialist roles.

CONCLUSION

Adequate treatment of the elderly begins with adequate evaluation. Adequate evaluation and intervention have cognitive, skill, and affective components.[22,23] The cognitive component is the knowledge of what it is that one needs to do; the affective components are the awareness of the therapist's attitude toward older people and working with them and how this relates to the stereotype of the elderly, all translated into daily interactions.

This chapter has examined these various issues and has offered therapists an outline of a comprehensive psychosocial assessment of the elderly and a general guideline for assessment and intervention in the hope that physical therapists will use these tools in their work with older people who require physical therapy.

REFERENCES

1. Solomon K: An objection to the use of the term "acting-out." Hosp Community Psychiatry 27:733, 1976
2. MacKenzie TB, Rosenberg SD, Bergen BJ, et al: The manipulative patient: an interactional approach. Psychiatry 41:264, 1978
3. Offer D, Sabshin M: Normality: Theoretical and Clinical Concepts of Mental Health. Basic Books, New York, 1966
4. Goffman E: Encounters. Bobbs-Merrill, Indianapolis, 1961, p. 84
5. Scheff TJ: Schizophrenia as ideology. Schizophr Bull No 2:15, 1970
6. Goffman E: Asylums. Doubleday, New York, 1961
7. Rosenhan DL: On being sane in insane places. Science 179:250, 1973
8. Maslow AH: The Farther Reaches of Human Nature. Viking, New York, 1971
9. American Psychiatric Association: Diagnostic and Statistical Manual of Mental Disorders, 3rd Ed., Revised. American Psychiatric Association, Washington, DC, 1987
10. Graham DT: Health, disease, and the mind-body problem: linguistic parallelism. Psychosom Med 29:52, 1967
11. Cohen RE: The collaborative co-professional: developing a new mental health role. Hosp Community Psychiatry 24:242, 1973
12. Harris M, Solomon K: Roles of the community mental health nurse. J Psychiatr Nurs 15:35, 1977
13. Howard M: The community mental health nurse and geropsychiatry. Presented at the 32nd Annual Meeting of the Gerontological Society, Washington, DC, 26 Nov 1979
14. Gottesman LE, Ishizaki B, MacBride SM: Service management—Plan and concept in Pennsylvania. Gerontologist 19:379, 1979
15. Ishizaki B, Gottesman LE, MacBride SM: Determinants of model choice for service management systems. Gerontologist 19:385, 1979
16. Pons SL: Roles of the community geropsychiatric social worker. Presented at the 32nd Annual Meeting of the Gerontological Society, Washington, DC, 26 Nov 1979
17. Romaniuk M: A look at the psychologist's role on a community geropsychiatry team. Presented at the 32nd Annual Meeting of the Gerontological Society, Washington, DC, 26 Nov 1979

18. Smith FS: Definition of a generalist. Albany, Capital District Psychiatric Center, Mimeo, 1972

19. Solomon K: The geropsychiatrist and the delivery of mental health services in the community. Presented at the 32nd Annual Meeting of the Gerontological Society, Washington, DC, 26 Nov 1979

20. Solomon K: The roles of the psychiatric resident on a community psychiatry team. Psychiatr Q 54:67, 1982

21. Rapoport M, Cahn B: The geriatric AHEC at the University of Maryland: a model for geriatric education. In Steel K (ed): Geriatric Education, Collamore Press, Lexington, MA, 1981

22. Grabowski BL, Kappelman MM, Cahn B, Solomon K: Geropsychiatric education in an interdisciplinary setting. Presented at the 33rd Annual Meeting of the Gerontological Society of America, San Diego, 22 Nov 1980

23. Grabowski BL, Kappelman MM, Cahn B, Solomon K: Geropsychiatric education in an interdisciplinary setting. Gerontol Geriatr Educ 3:29, 1982

24. Ayd FJ Jr: Treatment-resistant patients: a moral, legal and therapeutic challenge. In Ayd FJ Jr (ed): Rational Psychopharmacotherapy and the Right of Treatment. Ayd Medical Communications, Baltimore, 1975

25. Solomon K: Personality disorders in the elderly. In Lion JR (ed): Personality Disorders: Diagnosis and Management, 2nd Ed. Williams & Wilkins, Baltimore, 1981

26. Cicero: On old age (44 B.C.). In Selected Works, Grant M (transl.). Penguin, Baltimore, 1960

27. Weiss JAM: The natural history of antisocial attitudes. What happens to psychopaths? J Geriatr Psychiatry 6:236, 1973

28. Adams FD: Physical Diagnosis. Williams & Wilkins, Baltimore, 1958

29. Delp MH: Study of the patient. In Delp MH, Manning RT (eds): Major's Physical Diagnosis. WB Saunders, Philadelphia, 1968

30. Friedland E: Clinical Clerk Case Study Outline. State University of New York at Buffalo, 1967

31. Judge RD, Zuidema GD: Physical Diagnosis. A Physiologic Approach. Little, Brown, Boston, 1963

32. Menninger KA: A Manual for Psychiatric Case Study, 2nd Ed. Grune & Stratton, New York, 1962

33. Stevenson I, Sheppe WM Jr: The psychiatric examination. In Arieti S (ed): American Handbook of Psychiatry, Vol. I, 2nd Ed. Basic Books, New York, 1974

34. MacKinnon RA: Psychiatric history and mental status examination. Kaplan HI, Freeman AM, Sadock BJ (eds): In Comprehensive Textbook of Psychiatry, Vol. I, 3rd Ed. Williams & Wilkins, Baltimore, 1980

35. Kendell RE, Brockington IF, Leff JP: Prognostic implications of six alternative definitions of schizophrenia. Arch Gen Psychiatry 36:25, 1979

36. Folstein MD, Folstein SE, McHugh PR: Mini-Mental State: a practical method for grading the cognitive state of patients for the clinician. J Psychiatr Res 12:189, 1975

37. McTavish DG: Perceptions of old people. a review of research methodologies and findings. Gerontologist 11 (Part II):90, 1971

38. Solomon K: Social antecedents of learned helplessness in the health care setting. Gerontologist 22:282, 1982

39. Solomon K, Vickers R: Stereotyping the elderly: changing the attitudes of clinicians. Presented at the 33rd Annual Meeting of the Gerontological Society of America, San Diego, 25 Nov 1980

40. Solomon K, Vickers R: Stereotyping the elderly: further research on changing the attitudes of clinicians. Presented at the 34th Annual Meeting of the Gerontological Society of America and 10th Annual Meeting of the Canadian Association on Gerontology, Toronto, 10 Nov 1981

41. Solomon K: Victimization by health professionals and the psychologic response of the elderly. In Kosberg JI (ed): The Abuse and Maltreatment of the Elderly. Wright-PSG, Littleton, MA, 1983

42. Solomon K, Vickers R: Attitudes of health workers toward old people. J Am Geriatr Soc 27:186, 1979

43. Butler RN: Why Survive: Being Old in America. Harper & Row, New York, 1975 pp. 174

44. O'Dowd M, Zofnass J: Behavioral implications of attitudes toward the elderly. Presented at a regional meeting of the World Psychiatric Association, New York, 31 Oct 1981

45. Solomon K: Social antecedents of learned helplessness in the health care setting. Presented at the 31st Annual Meeting of the Gerontological Society, Dallas, 19 Nov 1978

46. Solomon K: Social antecedents of learned helplessness of the elderly in the health care setting. In Lewis EP, Nelson LD, Scully DH, et al, (eds): Sociological Research Symposium Proceedings (IX). Virginia Commonwealth University, Richmond, 1979

47. Tuckman J, Lorge I: Attitudes toward old people. J Soc Psychol 37:249, 1953

48. Solomon K: The elderly patient. In Spittell JA Jr (ed): Clinical Medicine, Vol. 12. Psychiatry. Harper & Row, Hagerstown, MD, 1982

49. Shagass C: The medical model in psychiatry. In Sachar EJ (ed): Hormones, Behavior, and Psychopathology. Raven Press, New York, 1976

50. Exton-Smith AN, Overstall PW: Geriatrics. University Park Press, Baltimore, 1979

51. Solomon K: The older man. In Solomon K, Levy NB (eds): Men in Transition: Theory and Therapy. Plenum, New York, 1982

52. Vickers R: Needs assessment of the elderly and community geropsychiatry. Presented at the 32nd Annual Meeting of the Gerontological Society, Washington, DC, 26 Nov 1979

53. Mijuskovic B: Loneliness: an interdisciplinary approach. Psychiatry 40:113, 1977

54. Goldfarb AI: Clinical perspectives. In Simon A, Epstein LJ (eds): Aging in Modern Society. Psychiatric Research Report No. 23. American Psychiatric Association, Washington, DC, 1968

55. Goldfarb AI: Minor maladjustments of the aged. In Arieti S, Brody EB (eds): American Handbook of Psychiatry, Vol. 3, 2nd Ed. Basic Books, New York, 1974

56. Solomon K: The depressed patient: social antecedents of psychopathology in the elderly. J Am Geriatr Soc 29:14, 1981

57. Solomon K, Zinke MR: Group psychotherapy with the depressed elderly. Presented at the 58th Annual Meeting of the American Orthopsychiatric Association, New York, 31 Mar 1981

58. Solomon K: Alzheimer's disease: the subjective experience of the patient. Presented at a regional meeting of the World Psychiatric Association, New York, 31 Oct 1981

59. Rosow I: Status and role change through the life span. In Binstock RH, Shanas E (eds): Handbook of Aging and the Social Sciences. Van Nostrand Reinhold, New York, 1976

60. Solomon K: Psychosocial crises of older men. Presented at the 133rd Annual Meeting of the American Psychiatric Association, San Francisco, 7 May 1980

61. Solomon K: The masculine gender role and its implications for the life expectancy of older men. J Am Geriatr Soc 29:297, 1981

62. Block M, Sinnott JD: The Battered Elder Syndrome: An Exploratory Study. University of Maryland, College Park, 1979

63. Kosberg JI (ed): The Abuse and Maltreatment of the Elderly. Wright-PSG, Littleton, MA, 1983

64. Parsons T: The Social System. Free Press, New York, 1951

65. Wilson RN: The Sociology of Health: An Introduction. Random House, New York, 1970

66. Selye H: The Physiology and Pathology of Exposure to Stress. Acta, Montreal, 1950

67. Ban TA: The treatment of depressed geriatric patients. Am J Psychother 32:93, 1978

68. Blazer D, Williams CD: Epidemiology of dysphoria and depression in an elderly population. Am J Psychiatry 137:439, 1980

69. Kovacs M, Beck AT: Maladaptive cognitive structures in depression. Am J Psychiatry 135:525, 1978

70. Bonime W: The psychodynamics of neurotic depression. In Arieti S (ed): American Handbook of Psychiatry, Vol. 3, 1st Ed. Basic Books, New York, 1966

71. Libow LS: Pseudo-senility: acute and reversible organic brain syndromes. J Am Geriatr Soc 21:112, 1973

72. Kay DWK: The epidemiology and identification of brain deficit in the elderly. In Eisdorfer C, Freidel RO (eds): Cognitive and Emotional Disturbance in the Elderly. Year Book Medical Publishers, Chicago, 1977

73. Masters WH, Johnson VE: Human Sexual Inadequacy. Little, Brown, Boston, 1970

74. Rogers CR: A theory of therapy, personality and interpersonal relationships as developed in client-centered framework. In Koch S (ed): Psychology: A Study of a Science. McGraw-Hill, New York, 1959

75. Solomon K: Benzodiazepines and neurotic anxiety. Critique. NY State J Med 76:2156, 1976

76. Wolpe J: The Practice of Behavior Therapy. Pergamon Press, New York, 1969

77. Shaefer HH, Martin PL: Behavioral Therapy. McGraw-Hill, New York, 1969

78. Bing E: Six Practical Lessons for an Easier Childbirth. Bantam, New York, 1969

79. Solomon K, Hart R: Pitfalls and prospects in clinical research on antianxiety drugs: benzodiazepines and placebo. A research review. J Clin Psychiatry 39:823, 1978

80. Greenblatt DJ, Shader RI: Meprobamate: a study of irrational drug use. Am J Psychiatry 127:1297, 1971

5 | Alzheimer's Disease and the Confused Patient

Nancy L. Mace
Sue R. Hardy
Peter V. Rabins

The rehabilitation therapist (physical or occupational therapist) is often called on to care for elderly persons with symptoms of impaired thinking or personality change associated with cognitive decline. We believe that the rehabilitation therapist's role in the care of such persons is important both in assessment of the person's function and in assisting the person to remain as independent as possible. This chapter briefly describes dementing illnesses and their diagnosis. We also discuss specific issues that commonly arise in the care of persons with dementing illnesses.

Although it had long been recognized that some individuals develop significant intellectual decline in later life, in the past there had been disagreement over the nature and the inevitability of this decline. More recently, however, significant advances have been made in distinguishing normal intellectual age changes from diseases causing cognitive decline and in understanding the prevalence and etiology of the dementing illnesses. It is now well recognized that a significant decline in cognitive function in later life is not normal, but is associated with a disease process.

Approximately 80 percent of those who live into very late life remain cognitively intact. However, in 1986 an estimated 2 million Americans had developed a senile dementia.[1] Approximately one-third (usually those most seriously ill and without family support) were institutionalized. A few nursing homes and day centers have established separate programs specializing in the care of people with dementia. Another 11 percent may reside in boarding homes and similar settings. More than half the impaired persons were cared for at home, usually by a spouse or adult child.[2] In 1983 the annual net cost per Alzheimer's disease patient was $18,517.[3] Nursing-home care for patients with these illnesses exceeded $2.5 billion.[4,5]

Significant disagreement still exists about specific cognitive changes in normal aging. However, it is generally agreed that slower response time and slight memory deterioration (what has been termed "benign senescent forgetfulness") occur. These changes interfere minimally with function. Such normal changes may be difficult to distinguish from the earliest symptoms of a disease process, but the differences become clinically obvious as the patient's level of function significantly declines.

DEMENTIA

A variety of terms have been used to describe the intellectual decline in late life. They include acute or chronic organic brain syndrome, senility, and Alzheimer's disease. Confusion over definitions of terms has led to misinformation about prognosis and treatment, and it is therefore important to review the generally accepted terminology.

Dementia is a global decline in intellectual function from a previous level occurring in clear consciousness. This decline from previous levels must affect several areas of mental function, for example, memory, language, praxis (motor abilities), and judgment. These patients are awake, alert, and aware of their surroundings.[6]

Delirium is defined as a decline in level of intellectual function in clouded consciousness. Although they may be either drowsy or agitated, delirious patients are not alert or fully aware of their surroundings and have difficulty shifting and maintaining a focus of attention. Clinically, delirium is often seen as having a more abrupt or more recent onset than dementia, and function often fluctuates over hours or days; thus the term "acute organic brain syndrome" was used to refer to delirium. Both delirium and dementia are syndromes, sets of symptoms that may be caused by a variety of diseases.

Alzheimer's disease accounts for about 50 percent of the cases of dementia. Another 20 percent of cases are diagnosed as multiinfarct dementia, and 20 percent of patients are believed to have both diseases.[7] The remaining 10 percent of cases are caused by a variety of rare conditions, including metabolic disorders (e.g., thyroid dysfunction), structural problems of the brain (e.g., normal pressure hydrocephalus, brain tumors, subdural hematoma), infectious disease (e.g., tuberculosis, tertiary syphilis), toxins (e.g., metal poisoning or alcoholism), degenerative diseases (e.g., Huntington's disease, Parkinson's disease, Pick's disease), autoimmune diseases, and psychiatric disorders (notably depression). About 10 percent of the patients seen[8] have reversible or treatable dementing illnesses.

Although the majority of the patients have a nonreversible dementia, many can be helped. The rehabilitation therapist can play a significant role in the care of such persons and their families by devising practical interventions that improve the quality of life for the patient and family or caregiver.

Alzheimer's disease is an irreversible, slowly progressive illness ending in death 4 to 15 (average 7) years after onset. The illness may be described as having three stages,[9] although the course is gradual, and many patients follow different courses. Symptoms of memory loss and sometimes personality change predominate in the first stage. These patients are usually still able to provide their own personal care, to socialize, and to function normally in many areas. They may be aware of their plight, and supportive psychotherapy may help them to adjust to the illness.

In the second stage memory loss worsens and aphasia, apraxias, and agnosia are increasingly evident. Aphasia is a disorder of language that often first appears as a difficulty in naming objects (anomia) but later is characterized by a misuse of words (e.g., "spool" for "spoon" or "fork" for "pen"). Apraxia, the inability to perform a learned motor movement although strength is intact, may first show up as difficulty in writing, in dressing, or in complex actions such as setting a table or knitting. Agnosia is the inability to know or recognize. There are many specific agnosias—for example, of faces or places, the inability to recognize objects, or seeing two objects at once. The patient in this second stage may have a lower tolerance for stress, may change eating patterns, may have difficulty walking, and may suffer disruption of sleep–wake cycles, and may be unable to communicate effectively.

In the third and final stage, the patient becomes incontinent, confined to bed, and severely aphasic. Strange sounds or single words may be produced. Alzheimer's disease patients have a shortened life expectancy. Death is often from a secondary condition such as pneumonia or a urinary tract infection, although this does not explain all early deaths.

The diagnosis of Alzeheimer's disease is based on the history of a gradually progressive dementia and on the elimination of other possible causes. Evidence from a CT scan, although supportive, is not definitive. Based on autopsy studies of clinical course, it is now believed that Alzheimer's disease of both early-onset (presenile) and late-onset (senile dementia) type are the same or very similar diseases.

Multiinfarct dementia is the cumulative result of a number of cerebral infarcts that may be individually too small to be clinically observed. Multiinfarct dementia usually presents a history of a stepwise progression (abrupt, intermittent worsening of symptoms), in contrast to the gradual progression of Alzheimer's disease. A history of diabetes, hypertension, and heart disease is often present. Multiinfarct dementia is a potentially preventable or treatable disease. However, in clinical practice a number of patients are seen who continue to deteriorate. Research into the treatment and prevention of stroke should reduce the number of such patients.

Depression is a cause of dementia in a significant number of elderly people and should never be overlooked as the primary cause of dementia. Although an "understandable" depression at the onset of the dementing illness is seen in some patients, in others the depression is primary. A depressive illness usually includes vegetative symptoms of weight loss, disturbance of sleep patterns, and depressive delusions. When the depressive illness is treated, the dementia will resolve or improve.[10]

A dementia often develops in patients with Parkinson's disease, particularly in the late stages of the disease. Korsakoff's syndrome is seen most commonly in patients with a history of alcoholism. It is characterized by an inability to form new memories, although other intellectual functions remain intact.

In the past, funding policies, the individual attitudes of some professionals, and the long-term patients course of the dementing illnesses led to a reluctance to commit resources to long-term patients with dementia. Because resources are finite and value judgments must be made regarding their distribution, the individual therapist who is interested in the care of these patients may be discouraged from helping such persons. There are other problems the therapist may encounter as well. The rehabilitation specialist in an acute care facility may be pressured to help patients in a limited period of time. Therapists may be faced with unrealistic requests for a cure from the medical team or the family. Despite such factors, the continuing care of these patients is a rewarding field for the therapist and can improve the quality of daily life for the patient.

THE FAMILY

The myth that the American family abandons its old and ill has been clearly disproven by Shanas.[11] Families do care for their elderly, often at great cost to themselves. The therapist may find the strength and resilience of family members to be one of the most rewarding aspects of caring for these patients (See Ch. 7).

Dementing illnesses create enormous burdens for families. Caregivers need to be monitored for stress-related problems such as alcohol abuse, medication misuse, and depression. Families in conflict often benefit from education about the disease and short-term counseling to help them accept and manage it. Caregiver *perception of burden* is a significant factor in caregiver stress. Caregiver characteristics are at least as important as patient characteristics in decisions to place patients.[12]

DIAGNOSIS

The first step in intervention with the patient with an impairment in thinking is a thorough evaluation to determine its type (dementia or delirium).[13] A search for its cause should be undertaken and other medical conditions treated (as much as possible). A complete assessment should yield the following information:

1. Nature and cause of illness or illnesses and their potential for treatment
2. Nature and extent of the disability and the areas of spared function
3. Social and psychological resources and limitations
4. Prognosis
5. Excess disability

A patient with confusion and declining intellectual function should be given a complete physical and neurologic examination. A detailed history should be taken and a mental status examination done. We have found the Mini-Mental State Examination[14] (MMSE) to be a reliable instrument that reveals memory impairment, aphasia, and apraxia (see also Ch. 4).

Persons suffering from difficulty in thinking are often able to function more independently when specific areas of spared function are identified and their environment modified to make best use of these areas. An Activities of Daily Living (ADL) evaluation will identify specific areas in which the patient needs assistance in order to make the most use of remaining abilities. An analysis of both cognitive function and task, which is designed to directly translate into supporting remaining abilities, is proposed by Weaverdyck.[15]

It has been our experience that family members and caregiving staff benefit from a careful explanation of the findings of the evaluation. For example, such findings show family members that the patient forgets an item as soon as a second item to be remembered is presented, or that a patient's slow gait is an apraxia rather than "laziness." The physical and/or the occupational therapist should participate in family conferences, because the therapist has observed the patient attempting such activities during the ADL assessment and because the therapist possesses the expertise needed to devise ways to maximize patient function.

ASSESSMENT AND INTERVENTION

Deficits may be more widespread with dementia than in other illnesses, such as brain trauma or stroke, but it may be difficult to determine the nature of the impairment. For example, a patient being treated for an apraxia may not be able to *remember* instructions or may not *understand* instructions, thereby failing a task that he or she is in fact able to do if the difficulties in comprehension are eliminated. An understanding of the nature of the impairment is essential for effective intervention. Because of this apparent uneven loss of cognitive functions, an assessment identifies both those functions that are lost or impaired and those that remain. Ways are sought to support these less-impaired functions. It is more successful to alter the environment to limit demands on impaired areas than to attempt to achieve relearning of lost skills.

An assessment must be based on a knowledge of the patient's environment. The therapist will find that change is most successfully effected in the environment rather than in the patient; it is helpful to keep this focus in mind as interventions are devised.

The ADL evaluation should describe the extent of self-care in terms of cognitive ability as well as physical impairment. For example, in bathing, is the patient cognitively able to learn to use a grab bar? In toileting, is a raised toilet seat confusing? Can the patient use a familiar toilet but not a public rest room? An ADL evaluation may indicate that the patient can feed himself when the plate is anchored or when weighted utensils give improved sensory clues. (Plastic, paper, or translucent utensils can increase confusion.)

The ADL evaluation can help the caregiver recognize that the patient can dress himself or herself but not select clothes or sequence the task or operate zippers but not buttons. It will examine home-making skills and identify impairments of judgment or sensation (e.g., ability to mix hot and cold water). It will determine whether or not the patient is able to use a telephone, make change, or tell time.

Tests of memory, praxis, and language help to define limitations and resources (Does the patient understand instructions? Can the patient remember enough to follow a three-stage command?). The ADL evaluation will clarify the patient's ability to read and comprehend. Some patients can read aloud but are unable to act on the information they read.

It may fall to the therapist to determine if prescribed interventions for a physical disability may cause more problems for the patient who cannot remember or learn, or if alternative interventions can be devised. For example, a confused patient may perceive splints as a restraint and become upset or tear them off.

An important function of the ADL evaluation is the identification of hazards to the patient (discussed at length elsewhere).[16] When skills have been lost, the environment can often be adjusted to compensate for the loss: the temperature of a water heater can be adjusted, throw rugs removed, and stairs blocked off. Families often need specific instructions, such as: the patient cannot be left unsupervised, must be prevented from driving, or must wear an ID bracelet. As the environment becomes more supportive and makes fewer demands on lost skills, the patient's anxiety will often decline, enabling her to function as well as possible and improving her overall quality of life.

EXCESS DISABILITY

Excess disability is described by Kahn[17] as more disability than can be explained by the disease alone. Persons with an existing dementing illness are especially vulnerable to developing delirium; this should be considered whenever an impaired patient worsens suddenly. The delirious patient may misinterpret reality, have false ideas or hallucinations, have incoherent speech, either sleepiness in the daytime or wakefulness at night, and either increased or decreased physical or motor activity. Delirium may be caused by a range of illnesses, such as pneumonia, urinary tract infection, congestive heart failure, malnutrition, dehydration, or even constipation. Medication is also a common cause of delirium (see Ch. 6). Thus when a patient displays intermittent intellectual impairment or memory or behavior disturbance of sudden onset, a delirium should be suspected and the underlying cause identified and treated. Pain may also increase patient confusion.

Psychiatric symptoms (depression, hallucinations, delusions, anxiety, and severe agitation) may contribute to disability and are generally responsive to treatment, reducing the patient's distress and enabling the patient to focus on therapeutic activities. Sensory impairments and stress also contribute to excess disability (see the next section).

SENSORY DEFICITS

Sensory deficits must not be overlooked as a cause of dysfunction in a person who presents with confusion. Sensory deficits are common in the elderly, and sensory deprivation may present as depression or disorientation. The person with a dementia is not aware of the impairment and is unable to compensate for sensory decline and may misinterpret sensory information. This person may also be unable to learn to adjust to compensatory devices such as hearing aids, which amplify irrelevant sounds, or contact lenses following cataract surgery.

The assessment must differentiate between sensory loss and loss of comprehension (does the patient not hear you or not understand you?), agnosia (can the patient not see you or not assess what is seen?), loss of sensation, and loss of judgment.

One should ask the patient's family or nurse whether the patient has glasses or a hearing aid. They are often aware of sensory deficits that may otherwise be overlooked. Sensory impairments may become evident during an ADL evaluation or therapeutic intervention. One can ask patients directly if they can hear or if they can see specific objects. Tests should be requested if sensory loss is suspected. The rehabilitation therapist can assist in devising ways to help a demented person adjust to glasses or hearing aids. Sometimes the problem is as simple as informing the family that they (not the patient) must be responsible for checking the batteries in a hearing aid or keeping eyeglasses clean. In other cases large print, less background noise, and bright colors may be environmental modifications that help the patient to function more effectively.

Changes in the physical environment are helpful. Glare and background noise should be eliminated. Light levels should be high enough to accommodate the aging eye. High contrasts should be tried (white plates on a blue placemat or a white toilet against a green rug). Large print and high contrast signs will help some patients. The physical environment should be examined to identify distractors and negative cues. Way finding, sense of place, and comfort can be enhanced.[18] Patient response to the physical environment will vary. It is helpful to experiment with low-cost changes to identify those that are most helpful to an individual.

MEMORY AND LEARNING

Memory impairment and the inability to learn new material are predominant features of dementia. Rehabilitation interventions can be more effective when the specific characteristics of the individual's forgetfulness are clearly defined. Some patients can retain certain types of information or can respond to memory cues in the environment. Many patients can respond to a one-stage command or single units of information but cannot handle more complex communications. This situation is easily evaluated and should be explained to everyone who will work with the patient. A patient who appears unable to follow instructions or complete a multistep task may in fact be able to do so if tasks are broken down into individual steps. For example, to help a patient transfer from wheelchair to toilet, give one-step instructions: "Put your hands on the rail." "Lean forward," "Push with your feet." Instructions should always be repeated exactly.

Patients may be better able to function if clues are given in several sensory modalities (e.g., putting a toothbrush in a patient's hand and touching the limb that should be moved as the patient is instructed to brush his teeth).

Often a patient can perform a task at one time but not at another. Function frequently worsens in the evening. Therefore, tests of function should be done at different times of day, with difficult or newly learned tasks scheduled for the patient's best times. The family or nursing staff may be able to chart the patient's daily variations. Testing in an unfamiliar setting may give inaccurately negative results. Confused patients often have difficulty orienting themselves in unfamiliar settings, which may distract them and cause them to function poorly. Tests of function and efforts to teach new skills should be carried out, if possible, in the setting in which the patient will need to function, because information learned in one setting, such as a hospital, may not carry over to another setting, such as the home.

Patients (especially those seen in an acute-care hospital) may have a delirium superimposed on the dementia that additionally limits learning ability. This should be watched for and evaluated, because the patient may be more functional when the delirium clears. Some patients are able to learn certain kinds of new information, such as the location of the bathroom in a new residence or the use of a prosthetic device, grab bar, cane, or walker; others will not be able to learn at all, and repeated efforts to teach them will frustrate both staff and patient. We have found that a 2-week trial is usually sufficient to determine whether or not a patient has the potential to learn new material.

Some patients can learn partially; for example, with consistant gentle reminders, they will use a grab bar. Many patients who never learn their way around a new environment do learn that a certain place is where they belong, so that wandering and complaints decrease. Benefits of reality orientation are limited. While it may be beneficial to frequently repeat to the patient information that is needed, little learning occurs or is retained. We tell the patients who we are, where they are, and what we are doing to them, and we repeat this information frequently, reassuring the patients that the therapist knows what is happening and will take care of them.

Everyone involved with a patient who has limited ability to learn must support the learning of new behaviors. Therefore, staff and family involvement is essential. If family and nursing staff are not able to continue the teaching process at home, newly learned tasks are likely to be forgotten. Everyone should use the same simplified one-step instructional phrases and give the same praise and encouragement. Families need to be told this explicitly.

Intermittent learning often confuses demented patients. For example, a patient learning to use a walker must be required to use it all the time. Positive reinforcement, the elimination of negative reinforcement, and the elimination of as much criticism as possible is important in working with a brain-injured person. It is not helpful to tell such patients that they are doing a task wrong because they lack the intellectual ability to remember how to do it correctly. The basic teaching approach would be to tell the patient what is being done right; suggest that the task be tried again; repeat instructions; give the patient the opportunity to rest between attempts; demonstrate the task; move the appropriate limbs; and give as many sensory clues as possible.

APRAXIA

Apraxias of dementia, particularly in Alzheimer's disease, are frequently more generalized than the apraxias seen in other conditions, such as a single stroke. Memory disorder or aphasia may interfere with the evaluation of specific apraxias. For example, patients may be able to feed themselves but be unable to understand or remember verbal instructions and therefore be unable to perform the same task in the evaluation setting. Direct observation in a familiar setting should replace verbal instruction. Asking the patient to copy a simple diagram is a reliable test for even subtle apraxias and is helpful in separating symptoms of apraxia from other symptoms.

Apraxias often present as the inability to do a complex task. Breaking down such tasks into individual steps can help a patient remain independent. For example, step-by-step instructions will help a patient bathe. Often one part of a task, such as undoing a zipper, proves to be the stumbling block to independence in an area such as self-toileting. Explaining to family members that they must assist at this one point can prevent accidents and reduce the patient's frustration (an alternative is to try Velcro in place of the zipper). In some cases a task can be simplified. For example, patients who have difficulty using eating utensils may be able to use one eating utensil but become confused by the presence of several.

When an apraxia interferes with a specific function, patients may be unable to learn new skills to compensate. For example, patients may be unable to learn to use a walker. They may carry the walker, creating a hazard to themselves and others. It may be necessary to accept only limited improvement in such situations. The object should be to improve the quality of life for the patients. They may be safer and more mobile in a wheelchair than with a walker they cannot learn to use. However, patient health and continence are associated with ambulation. Patients who are confined to bed during a concurrent illness should be helped to resume walking as soon as possible. Some frail persons may permanently lose the ability to walk if confined to bed. Falls present serious problems in this population. The physical therapist should assess risk to the individual patient and modify the environment to reduce the risk of falls.

Often, ingenious ways can be devised to use old skills to partially improve a patient's mobility or independence. A knowledge of the patient's past can help. Use familiar activities to initiate movements—for example, instruct a patient to "rock it like a baby," or "shake hands."

Apraxias can cause difficulty in swallowing. An ear, nose, and throat consultation should be obtained if choking, drooling of food, or dribbling occurs.

APHASIA

As with apraxia, other cognitive problems can complicate the assessment of aphasia. Some patients successfully conceal language problems so that an untrained observer or family member may not realize that the patient is aphasic. Failure to follow instructions can sometimes be misinterpreted as stubbornness. Confabulation, perseveration (repetition of a sound, word, or phrase), and other abnormalities of language are sometimes blamed on "old age," "living in the past," or an unpleasant personality. Thus aphasia should be specifically tested for. Most aphasic patients cannot repeat a phrase (e.g., "This is a nice day in October") and often misname familiar objects (Point to a watch, pen, or ring and ask the patient, "What do you call this?").

Communication is often possible even with severely aphasic patients.[19] Most patients communicate more successfully when they are relaxed; thus it is necessary to create a familiar, nonstressful atmosphere.

Words can be "filled in." We encourage family members to do so, as this seems to be less upsetting than forcing a patient to struggle to communicate. However, it is important to confirm that you are correctly understanding the patient. It is often possible to understand the meaning from the emotional content rather than the literal content. "I want to go home" may mean "I don't know where I am." Again, it is important to confirm with the patient the accuracy of your interpretation.

Watch the patient's nonverbal communications. If the patient is not listening to or understanding you, this may be clear from actions or facial expression. When working with a patient, watch his or her face: the patient may not be able to verbalize feelings of pain or fright.

When talking to a patient with a receptive aphasia or a dementia, first ascertain that you have the patient's attention and that she or he can hear you. Watch to see if the patient is paying attention to you. The patient who is distracted by activities in the room or who is upset may have difficulty focusing on what is being said.

Simplify information given to the confused person, and supplement verbal information with other environmental cues: give simple, one-stage instructions;

repeat them; *wait* for the patient to respond. Confused people often take longer to respond, and it is important that neither therapist nor patient feel rushed. Confirm that the patient comprehends your instructions before continuing. Patients may reply ''yes'' when in fact they do not understand. Ask questions in a way that requires an answer that demonstrates comprehension. (Say, e.g., ''Point to where it hurts.'')

Demonstrate a physical activity or assist the patient in moving through an exercise. Give information in ways familiar to the patient. For example, instead of teaching exercises as such, ask the patient to do a familiar task that will exercise the target muscle group. Instead of saying, ''Extend your arms,'' you may be more successful saying ''Reach for my hand.''

AGNOSIA

Agnosia is frustrating both to professional staff and to family members. Patients may be unable to recognize family members or friends or to recognize their own room or own home. Agnosias can be confused with sensory disorders, memory loss, or aphasia. Often other sensory clues will help to orient the patient. For example, the patient who does not recognize a face may be able to recognize the person's voice. Familiar odors or possessions may help patients orient themselves. Environmental cues, such as the smell of food cooking, familiar furniture, or the texture of one's own blanket, should be gently called to the patient's attention. Urinating in inappropriate places is usually caused by an agnosia—the person does not recognize that the wastebasket is not a toilet. Moving or covering the object often helps.

CATASTROPHIC REACTIONS

Patients with cognitive impairment may become emotionally distraught in the face of relatively minor stresses. Goldstein[20] has termed this behavior a ''catastrophic reaction,'' and it is one of the most common problems that families report to us.[21] The patient may refuse to cooperate, argue, cry, resist assistance, or ignore the therapist. Some patients, when severely upset, may yell, scream, throw things, or strike those who attempt to intervene. In some cases such reactions are almost continuous.

A key principle in working with a confused patient is to avoid catastrophic reactions or to defuse them as early as possible when they occur. Teaching the family or staff how to recognize them early and how to react is important. Our clinical experience has shown that an understanding of catastrophic reactions is often the most important single factor in helping an impaired person remain at home. Those involved in caring for and relating to the patient must understand that much of the unpleasant behavior is a factor of brain injury and not willful behavior. Understanding is the first step in learning to respond to the patient's behavior constructively rather than in anger. These reactions not only cause significant burden to the staff or caregiver, but are evidence of the patient's distress as well.

Catastrophic reactions are precipitated by

1. Misinterpretation of a request
2. Misinterpretation of sensory information
3. Cognitive overload (receiving too many sensory inputs simultaneously
4. The inability to perform a task
5. Fatigue
6. Inability to communicate needs, being misunderstood
7. Frustration
8. Response to demoralizing, punitive, or infantilizing treatment

Restructuring of the patient's environment to avoid or limit these factors is an important part of maximizing patient function.

Give patients clear, simple information, one step at a time. Tell them where they are and what is being done for them. For example, say, "I am going to lift your arm for you," or "I am helping you unbutton your blouse." Avoid complex explanations, such as, "You have to go downstairs to the therapy room to practice with your walker so you will get better and go home." Reassure the patient that she or he is all right. Whenever possible, give information both verbally and visually. You may have to repeat the same information frequently.

Stand where a patient can see you. Avoid approaching and touching a patient from behind or allowing others to remain out of sight. Provide adequate lighting. If patients have sensory losses, remind them gently that they might have misinterpreted what they thought they saw or heard. Avoid arguing with the patients; instead, respond with empathy to their distress.

Reduce the amount of noise and activity going on around a confused, disoriented person. Whenever possible allow the patient to be in a familiar place when doing a difficult task. Reduce the number of places where the patient has to look for things, and reduce the number of choices the patient must make. (For example, limit the number of items of food on a plate.)

Recognize that what may once have been a simple task may now be impossible (such as tying shoes). Gently helping patients may be better than coaxing them to do such a task themselves. In a chronic condition, efforts to teach or encourage the patient will not bring back lost abilities; they will only humiliate the patient.

Schedule stressful tasks, such as learning of new skills, bathing, visiting, or other activities that you have observed to upset the patient, at times of day when a patient is at his or her best and is least fatigued. Reconsider your approach: Avoid rushing the patient or ignoring her protests.

Occasionally medications are used to help control catastrophic reactions, but only as a supplement to environmental modifications. Medication should not be used as a substitute for efforts to make the environment comprehensible to a confused person.

Catastrophic reactions are sometimes misinterpreted as characteristics of personality, particularly when a patient's premorbid personality included elements resembling the catastrophic behavior and when a patient's social functioning remains superficially intact. An important part of the training of staff and family members is to overcome this tendency to interpret catastrophic behavior as a controllable aspect of personality.

Prevention is the most effective intervention. Encourage the caregiver to keep a log of the person's outbursts, noting especially those things that occurred just before the reaction. Caregivers should learn to recognize—and respect—the person's signals of increasing stress.

SUSPICIOUSNESS

Several factors contribute to the common phenomenon of excessive suspiciousness or suspicious uncooperativeness. Confused patients may easily misinterpret information or misinterpret procedures. For example, moving a patient's limbs for her or him may be misinterpreted as an attack or as sexual behavior. Forgetful patients mislay possessions, forget where items are, and misinterpret their absence as theft. The inability to make sense out of the environment and to remember can exacerbate and heighten normal behaviors of cautiousness.

However, some suspiciousness goes beyond misinterpretation and involves fixed delusions. When this situation occurs, it should be regarded as a factor of the brain disorder; it is usually not responsive to reason. Arguing with the patients or denying their feelings may precipitate a catastrophic reaction. Medication, judiciously used, may help with delusional ideas. Often it is equally important to reassure staff and family that the patient "cannot help" the behavior.

The therapist must take the time to establish rapport with the patient. This can be difficult for the therapist working in an acute-care hospital, where time with the patient is limited. However, gaining of the patient's trust is necessary to the success of interventions. Often a suspicious patient will cooperate with a person she or he trusts even when clearly confused or disoriented. One can empathize with the distress of persons who do not understand where they are or what is being done to them and who cannot remember what they are told. Respect for patients communicates itself no matter how ill the patients are. Taking time to listen to patients even when their speech is rambling and confused, visiting with patients about times past, and confirming that patients understand what the therapist is saying indicate that the therapist understands the patients' fears and anxieties and help to establish trust.

APATHY

There are many reasons why a patient is apathetic or refuses to cooperate in treatment. The brain damage itself may cause apathy. Failure to understand instructions or frequent catastrophic reactions are often contributing factors. Older people are often afraid of falling, particularly when they are unsteady or have already experienced a fall. Patients often refuse to do something because they do not understand the request or perhaps as a way of avoiding making mistakes. Gentle support and encouragement is helpful for patients who find even slight involvement too demanding.

Depression and delirium are frequently overlooked as causes of apathetic or even resistant behavior. Depression and delirium should be treated when identified. Confused, apathetic patients may have catastrophic reactions if they are addressed briskly or given firm orders. A good rapport, patience, and elimination of causes of catastrophic reactions is more effective.

SUPPORTING QUALITY OF LIFE

Caring for the person with a dementing illness is challenging. Families and staff may be stressed by the demands of managing behaviors and providing safety. However, a few congregate programs[22] are demonstrating that it is possible to improve patient quality of life. Some of the necessary interventions have been discussed above: Treat excess disability, reduce patient stress, and create a supportive environment. To make changes, the caregiver, whether staff or family, must be well supported, well trained, and given relief from the demands of caregiving.

People with dementia often lack the cognitive skills necessary to provide themselves with interesting or stimulating things to do. While the caregiver is engaged in necessary tasks, the patient may spend long hours in a mental "vacuum." Providing meaningful activities (including ADLs), appropriately paced, and with frequent rests, for more of the patient's day often reduces undesirable behaviors. Such activities must have meaning for the person, and the person must know what that meaning is.

Activities that reestablish old roles, support family relationships, and offer positive messages about one's identity are important. The dementing illness denies the person dignity, autonomy, and opportunities for small successes. Well-designed interventions that to some extent restore these support appropriate behavior as well as improve patient quality of life.[23,24]

All interventions must reduce anxiety and experiences of inadequacy. To do this, capitalize on remaining abilities, avoid demands on lost skills, and break tasks down into manageable steps. Because of the wide variation among patients, interventions must be individualized and flexible. For much of their illness, people with dementia are capable of experiencing pleasure. As patient anxiety is reduced, enjoyment often reappears spontaneously.

To make a significant change in the quality of life for these patients is difficult. Moreover, little is known about how frequently, or in which patients, behaviors, anxiety, and distress can be reduced or momentary enjoyment restored. In many cases the costs, the capacities of caregivers, and the resources of the therapist will limit what can be accomplished. The rehabilitation therapist plays a critical role in attaining these goals.

SUMMARY

The rehabilitation team and physical therapy can play a valuable role in the care of chronically ill demented persons. As with any other condition, the first step in such care is an accurate diagnosis and ongoing medical supervision of the illness and other health problems. When this has been accomplished, the rehabilitation specialist can contribute significantly to improvement of function, to reduction of risk or hazard to the person, and to enabling the person to remain as long as possible in their own familiar environment.

An understanding of the nature of the cognitive changes and their effect on the persons behavior, both in general and in terms of the individual, is essential for interventions to be successful. The rehabilitation specialist is in a unique position to define areas of spared and impaired function, to interpret them to other members of the health team and to the family, and to modify the environment to maximize the person's remaining abilities.

REFERENCES

1. Katzman R: Alzheimer's Disease. N Eng J Med 314:964, 1986
2. Brody EM: The formal support network: congregate treatment settings for residents with senescent brain dysfunction. Aging 15:301, 1981
3. Hay JW, Ernst RL: The economic costs of Alzheimer's disease. Am J Public Health 77:1169, 1987
4. Arbnett RH, McKusick DR, Sonnefeld ST, et al: Projections of health care spending to 1990. Health Care Financing Review 7:1, Spring 1986
5. Stone R, Cafferata GL, Sangl J: Caregivers of the frail elderly: a national profile. Gerontologist 27:616, 1987
6. McHugh PR: Dementia. In Beeson PB, McDermott W, Wyngaarden JB eds: Textbook of Medicine, 15th Ed., Saunders, Philadelphia, WB 1976
7. Blessed G, Tomlinson BE, Roth M: The association between quantitative measures of dementia and of senile changes in the cerebral gray matter of elderly subjects. Br J Psychiatry 114:797, 1968
8. Rabins PV: The prevalence of reversible dementia in a psychiatric hospital. Hosp Community Psychiatry, 32:490, 1981
9. Sjorgren T, Sjorgren H, Lindgren AGH: Clinical analysis of morbus Alzheimer and morbus Pick. Acta Psychiatr Neurol Scand (Suppl) 82:1, 1952
10. Folstein MF, McHugh PR: Dementia syndrome of depression. Aging 7:87, 1978
11. Shanas E: The family as a social support system in old age. Gerontologist 19(2):169, 1979

12. George LK: The Dynamics of Caregiver Burden. Report Submitted to the American Association of Retired Persons, Andrus Foundation, 1984

13. Folstein M, Rabins P: Psychiatric evaluation of the elderly patient. Primary Care 6:609, 1979

14. Folstein M, Folstein SE, McHugh PR: Mini-mental state: a practical method for grading the cognitive state of patients for the clinician. J Psychiatr Res 12(3):189, 1975

15. Weaverdyck SE: A Cognitive Intervention Protocol for Dementia: Its Derivation from and Application to a Neuropsychological Case Study of Alzheimer's Disease. PhD dissertation, University of Michigan, Ann Arbor, 1987

16. Mace N, Rabins P: The Thirty Six Hour Day: A Family Guide to Caring For Persons with Alzheimer's Disease, Related Dementing Illnesses and Memory Loss in Later Life. Johns Hopkins University Press, Baltimore, 1981

17. Kahn RL: The Mental Health System and the Future Aged. Gerontologist 15:24, 1975

18. Hiatt LG: Environmental design and mentally impaired people. in Altman HJ, ed: Alzheimer's Disease and Dementia: Problems, Prospects and Perspectives, Plenum, New York, 1987

19. Bartol MA: Nonverbal communication in patients with Alzheimer's disease. J Geriatric Nurs 5(4):21, 1979

20. Goldstein K: The effect of brain damage on the personality. Psychiatry 15:245, 1952

21. Rabins PR, Mace NL, Lucas MJ: The impact of dementia on the family. JAMA 248:333, 1982

22. U.S. Congress, Office of Technology Assessment: Losing a Million Minds, Government Printing Office, Washington, DC, OTA-Ba-323, April 1987

23. Zgola Y: Doing Things, A Guide to Programs and Organized Activities for Persons with Alzheimer's Disease and Related Disorders Johns Hopkins University Press, Baltimore 1987

24. Mace NL: Principles of activities for persons with dementia, physical and occupational therapy in geriatrics. 5(3): 13, 1987

6 | Clinical Pharmacology in the Elderly: Recognizing and Preventing Adverse Drug Effects During Rehabilitation

Dennis J. Chapron

The safe and effective administration of medications to the elderly can be a complex task. The combination of old age, multiple coexisting morbidities, and polypharmacy provides a setting with a high potential for serious adverse drug effects. The physical therapist who frequently works with the elderly is often confronted by patients who cannot realize their full potential for rehabilitation because of other disabling problems, some of which, in fact, may be drug-induced, (i.e., iatrogenic). To achieve the intended goals of rehabilitation optimally and effectively (i.e., to restore or arrest further decline in functional capacity), potential impediments to these goals must be identified, evaluated, and attenuated or removed if necessary. Adverse drug effects must be recognized as common and potentially serious impediments to rehabilitation in the elderly.

Elderly patients seen by the therapist are often receiving a large number of medications, some of which are being used to improve disabilities that the therapist is treating (e.g., L-dopa for Parkinson's disease). Many other drugs are prescribed for conditions that are not of direct concern to the therapist yet may affect the patient's response to rehabilitation. Regardless of a drug's indication or a therapist's professional orientation, anyone who makes an important contribution to the care and well-being of the patient must recognize that drugs can create new problems or exacerbate preexisting ones.

This chapter focuses on factors that influence drug response, with particular emphasis on the aging process, followed by a comprehensive discussion of several common side effects of drug therapy that may present as obstacles to successful rehabilitation of the elderly patient.

FACTORS INFLUENCING DRUG RESPONSE

The response of an individual to a medication is dependent on both pharmacokinetic and pharmacodynamic factors. Pharmacokinetic factors involve how the body handles a drug, that is, it deals with the movement of the drug into, around, and out of the body. Its focus is on quantitative information, such as (1) the rate and extent to which drugs are absorbed from sites of administration (e.g., gastrointestinal tract, muscle, or skin), (2) how rapidly and extensively drugs distribute from the circulating blood to various sites in the body, and (3) the overall efficiency of the body's ability to eliminate drugs via renal excretion and/or hepatic metabolism. The pharmacokinetic factors—absorption, distribution, and elimination—act in concert with the administered drug dose to govern the time course of drug levels in the circulating blood and, with long-term therapy, the degree to which drugs accumulate in the body.

Pharmacodynamics is the study of what a drug does to bodily processes. It identifies the specific actions of a medication (e.g., lower blood pressure, relieve pain, reduce spasticity) and examines the relationship between the magnitude of drug action and the concentration of drug in a biological fluid such as blood or urine that is in contact with the responding organ system. Thus pharmacokinetics and pharmacodynamics are closely interrelated. Because the relationship between drug concentrations in blood and response has been well established for numerous medications (see Table 6-1), the science of pharmacokinetics allows one to make good predictions of dosage requirements for a patient based on age, body weight, and estimates of their capacity to eliminate medications via the kidney or liver. Determination of blood concentrations of administered drugs may then be used to confirm or modify initial dosage estimates.

The determinants of drug responsiveness can be illustrated by a simple diagram (see Fig. 6-1). Only drug in plasma water is able to diffuse to its site of action to interact with tissue receptors and elicit a response. The concentration of a drug in plasma water is determined by the administered dose, the reversible binding of drug to plasma proteins and tissue constituents unrelated to the site of action, and the efficiency by which the drug is cleared from the plasma water by liver metabolism or renal excretion.

Table 6-1. Examples of Medications for Which a Therapeutic Range of Plasma Concentrations Have been Defined

Medication	Brand Name	Therapeutic Range
Carbamazepine	Tegretol	4–12 μg/ml
Digoxin	Lanoxin	1–2.0 ng/ml
Lithium	(Numerous)	0.3–1.2 mEq/L
Nortriptyline	Aventyl	50–160 ng/ml
Phenobarbital	(Numerous)	10–30 μg/ml
Phenytoin	Dilantin	10–20 μg/ml
Procainamide	Pronestyl	4–8 μg/ml
Quinidine	(Numerous)	2–5 μg/ml
Salicylate	(Numerous)	100–300 μg/ml
Theophylline	(Numerous)	10–20 μg/ml

The observed pharmacologic effect of a drug is initiated by its binding to a specific tissue receptor. This drug–receptor complex mediates a series of coupled biological events that culminates in an observable pharmacologic response. The magnitude of drug response is determined by the number of drug–receptor complexes formed and the efficiency by which postreceptor events are coupled. The former is determined largely by the concentration of drug surrounding its receptors, and the latter may be modified by homeostatic control mechanisms in the body that are often activated by drugs and can partly counteract their pharmacologic effects.

Thus aging may influence drug response by altering any of the loci—pharmacokinetic and/or pharmacodynamic—as shown in Figure 6-1. The majority of drug research in the elderly, however, has been in the area of pharmacokinetics. Numerous studies have shown that aging per se has no clinically significant effect on the rate or extent of drug absorption. Advanced age is associated with a significant reduction in renal blood flow, glomerular filtration, and kidney size. These changes translate into a reduced capacity of the elderly for renal drug elimination. For medications that have a narrow margin of safety and are predominately eliminated from the body by renal excretion, the daily dose must be scaled down to match the degree of existing renal function appropriately (Table 6-2). Amantadine (Symmetrel) and digoxin (Lanoxin) are common examples of renally eliminated drugs that are administered to the elderly in daily doses that are about one-half the doses given younger patients.

The metabolism of drugs by the liver to inactive products is another important means by which medications are eliminated from the body. Numerous studies have shown a differential effect of old age on the various enzymes in the liver that inactivate drugs. Generally, the enzymes that oxidize medications (see Table 6-3) appear to be impaired with advanced age whereas those enzymes that mediate conjugative reactions are not affected by aging.

The influence of advanced age on the pharmacodynamics aspects of drug response has not been extensively investigated. Several studies have shown

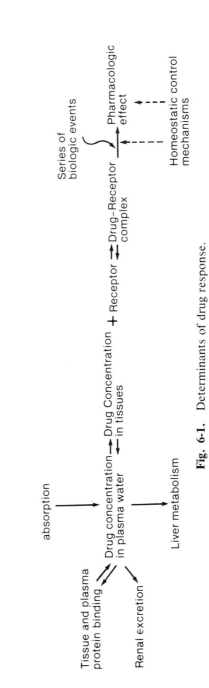

Fig. 6-1. Determinants of drug response.

Table 6-2. Selected Drugs Removed from the Body Primarily by Renal Excretion and for Which Dosage Adjustments Must be Considered in the Elderly

Generic Name	Brand Name
Acetohexamide	Dymelor
Allopurinol	Zyloprim
Amantadine	Symmetrel
Amiloride	Midamor
Atenolol	Tenormin
Captopril	Capoten
Cephalosporins	(Numerous)
Chlorpropamide	Diabinese
Cimetidine	Tagamet
Clonidine	Catapres
Digoxin	Lanoxin
Disopyramide	Norpace
Ethambutol	Myambutol
Fluorocytosine	Ancobon
Gentamicin	Garamycin
Kanamycin	Kantrex
Lithium	(Numerous)
Methotrexate	(Numerous)
Naldolol	Corgard
Procainamide	Pronestyl
Streptomycin	(Numerous)
Sulfonamides	(Numerous)
Tetracycline	(Numerous)
Tobramycin	Nebcin
Vancomycin	Vancocin

that the central nervous system depressant effects of benzodiazepines (e.g., Valium, Librium, Dalmane) are exaggerated in the elderly independent of potential age-related pharmacokinetic changes. Other drugs that have a high incidence of side effects in the elderly that cannot be solely explained by altered pharmacokinetics include antihypertensive, anticoagulant, and antipsychotic medications.

Table 6-3. Selected Drugs Metabolized at a Slower Rate in the Elderly and for which Dosage Administration Should Be Considered

Generic Name	Brand Name
Alprazolam	Xanax
Chlordiazepoxide	Librium
Diazepam	Valium
Imipramine	Tofranil
Naproxen	Naprosyn
Nortriptyline	Aventyl
Phenylbutazone	Butazolidin
Propranolol	Inderal
Quinidine	(Numerous)
Theophylline	(Numerous)
Triazolam	Halcion
Valproic acid	Depakene

ADVERSE DRUG REACTIONS IN THE ELDERLY

Epidemiologic studies have shown that adverse drug reactions occur with a greater frequency in the elderly.[1,2] Previously discussed age-related changes in pharmacokinetics and pharmacodynamics are partly responsible for these observations. Other factors that help explain the increased propensity for adverse reactions in the elderly include the following:

1. The elderly receive more medications than any other age group. The risk of reacting adversely to a drug increases with the number of drugs prescribed.[3]

2. In the aged the presence of multiple pathologies is common. Certain disease states can influence the pharmacokinetics and pharmacodynamics of drugs. For example, an elderly patient with intrinsic kidney disease will have a further reduction, beyond that associated with advanced age, in the ability to renally excrete medications. Furthermore, drugs are often prescribed in a setting of multiple comorbidities; although a specific drug may exert a beneficial effect for the condition that initiated its prescription, it may also adversely influence another existing and unrelated pathology—for example, haloperidol (Haldol), which may be beneficial for a psychotic patient, may also severely exacerbate coexisting Parkinson's disease.

3. The potential for multiple medication use in the elderly is great. The incidence of deleterious drug–drug interactions can be expected to increase as additional medications are prescribed. Such interactions can result in the development of exaggerated or reduced pharmacologic responses.

Selected drug side effects of concern to the therapist include the following:

1. Symptomatic postural hypotension
2. Fatigue and weakness
3. Depression
4. Confusion
5. Involuntary movements
6. Dizziness and vertigo
7. Ataxia
8. Urinary incontinence

It should be noted that these untoward drug effects do not necessarily occur as isolated events, but in fact often occur in clusters (e.g., fatigue, depression, and confusion).

Postural Hypotension

Postural hypotension is more common in the elderly than in any other age group. It may cause dizziness, light-headedness, faintness, a feeling of weakness, or unsteadiness, or in some cases lead to syncope (a sudden but transient loss of consciousness). These symptoms appear when the patient assumes an erect posture after lying or sitting for some time, particularly in the morning on getting out of bed. Postural hypotension is a major cause of falls in the elderly. Falls can cause trauma, particularly bone fractures, and thus are a major cause of morbidity in this age group. In many elderly, fears of repeated falls may lead to self-imposed restrictions on mobility and life-style. Symptoms of postural hypotension can be directly related to the sudden drop in blood pressure, which leads to a decreased perfusion of the brain and a subsequent impairment of cerebral metabolism.

When a person assumes an upright position, gravitational forces produce a fall in blood pressure predominately via pooling of blood in the venous system of the the lower extremities. This initial drop in blood pressure is sensed by baroreceptors in the carotid sinus and aortic arch bodies. These sensors activate certain cardiovascular mechanisms that blunt or abolish potentially serious orthostatic drops in blood pressure. As a result of these compensatory mechanisms, a fall in systolic blood pressure of 10 mm Hg or less and a rise in diastolic pressure of up to 5 mm Hg is seen in normal persons assuming an upright position. These blood pressure changes are often accompanied by a 5 to 20 beats per minute increase in heart rate. These adaptive mechanisms are neurogenically mediated via increased sympathetic nervous system activity and include primarily reflex arteriolar and venous constriction and an increase in heart rate so as to maintain cardiac output. There is good evidence that baroreflex responsiveness is impaired in advanced age.[4,5] Hypertension per se is associated with impairment of baroreflex response, thus the hypertensive elderly are more susceptible to postural drops in blood pressure.

Figure 6-2 illustrates the many hemodynamic factors that contribute to controlling blood pressure and demonstrates their interrelatedness. Arterial blood pressure can be expressed as the product of cardiac output and total peripheral resistance. This latter component is dependent primarily on the caliber of small vessels (mainly arterioles and to a lesser extent capillaries) and blood viscosity. Symptomatic postural hypotension leading to a reduction in cerebral perfusion may result from a decrease in cardiac output or a decrease in total peripheral resistance, or both.

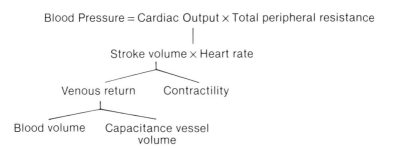

Fig. 6-2.   Factors controlling blood pressure.

Cardiac output may be reduced by a decrease in heart rate or stroke volume. Stroke volume is largely governed by the contractile force of the myocardium and the degree of cardiac filling. The venous system contains 70 to 80 percent of the blood volume, and rapid changes in its capacitance will markedly influence the amount of blood returning to the heart. Marked reductions in either venomotor tone (leading to increased vessel volume) or blood volume (hypovolemia) will decrease cardiac filling and subsequently reduce cardiac output. Arteriolar vasodilation is the primary mechanism by which total peripheral resistance is reduced.

To establish the diagnosis of clinical postural hypotension, blood pressure should be measured when the patient is lying down, immediately on standing, and frequently for 2 to 5 minutes thereafter. A recent study pointed out that orthostatic changes in blood pressure and heart rate can be detected as early as 30 seconds and reach a maximum at 2 minutes after a change in posture.[6] Symptoms synchronous with a fall in systolic blood pressure of 20 mm Hg or 10 mm Hg diastolic confirm the presence of clinical postural hypotension. For patients who already have low blood pressure while lying down, small postural drops may produce symptoms.

There is probably a multifactoral etiology to postural hypotension in the elderly, but often drugs may be the single most important contributing factor. Drugs can attentuate the normal physiologic compensatory mechanisms that accompany position changes and stabilize blood pressure. Furthermore, the effects of orthostatic drops in blood pressure may be accentuated by the presence of underlying pathology (e.g., diminished cerebral perfusion from postural hypotension superimposed on occlusive cerebrovascular disease). The risk of symptomatic postural hypotension increases with the prescription of multiple drugs, many of which may act at different or the same physiologic loci for orthostatic blood pressure regulation. Recent studies have shown that postprandial reductions in sitting blood pressure occur in many elderly institutionalized persons.[7] Systolic blood pressure fell an average of 25 mm Hg by 35 minutes after a meal in elderly subjects. In patients with documented postprandial hypotension, it seems reasonable to consider administering potentially hypotensive drugs at a time as distant from meals as possible.

Discussed next are the drugs that are particularly important causes of postural hypotension in the elderly.

Tricyclic Antidepressants

Tricyclic antidepressants (TCAs) (Table 6-4) presumably induce orthostatic changes in blood pressure by competitively blocking sympathetically mediated vasoconstriction. Imipramine is perhaps the best studied of the TCAs. Postural hypotension leading to ataxia, prolonged dizziness, and falls has been reported in approximately 20 percent of patients receiving imipramine.[8] Orthostatic blood pressure reactions can occur at any time during treatment and at plasma concentrations in the subtherapeutic or low therapeu-

Table 6-4. Tricyclic and Tricyclic-like Antidepressants

Generic Name	Brand Name
Amitriptyline	Elavil, Endep
Amoxapine	Asendin
Desipramine	Norpramin, Pertofrane
Doxepin	Adapin, Sinequan
Imipramine	Janimine, SK-Pramine, Tofranil
Maprotiline	Ludiomil
Nortriptyline	Aventyl, Pamelor
Protriptyline	Vivactyl
Trazadone	Deseryl
Trimipramine	Surmontil

tic range, suggesting that dosage reduction may not substantially alleviate symptoms. Tolerance does not appear to develop to this side effect. Advanced age, cardiac disease (especially congestive heart failure), elevated systolic blood pressure, and the presence of pretreatment postural hypotension may be important determinants of susceptibility to TCA-induced orthostatic drops in blood pressure. Studies have indicated that nortriptyline (Aventyl) may differ from other TCAs in that this drug does not appear to affect standing blood pressure significantly.[9] This property of nortriptyline probably contributed to its successful application in the treatment of poststroke depression.[10]

Antipsychotics

Antipsychotic agents presumably induce their orthostatic effects by a mechanism similar to that of the TCAs. There are marked differences among the specific agents regarding their propensity for inducing postural hypotension. Chlorpromazine, thioridazine, and mesoridazine have the greatest potential for inducing orthostatic changes in blood pressure. Although it is claimed that patients usually develop tolerance to the hypotensive effects of these agents, recent evidence suggests that in the elderly orthostatic effects may persist for a prolonged period.[11] Table 6-5 lists the available antipsychotic

Table 6-5. Selected Antipsychotic Drugs and Their Relative Incidence of Common Side Effects

Generic Name	Brand Name	Postural Hypotension	Parkinsonism	Sedation
Chlorpromazine	Thorazine	High	Moderate	High
Fluphenazine	Prolixin, Permitil	Minimal	High	Minimal
Haloperidol	Haldol	Minimal	High	Minimal
Loxapine	Loxitane	Minimal	High	Moderate
Mesoridazine	Serentil	Moderate	Minimal	High
Molindone	Moban	Minimal	High	Moderate
Perphenazine	Trilafon	Minimal	High	Minimal
Thioridazine	Mellaril	Moderate	Minimal	High
Trifluoperazine	Stelazine	Minimal	High	Minimal
Thiothixene	Navane	Minimal	High	Minimal

agents and ranks them according to their spectrum of common side effects. Because all these agents display similar efficacy, it seems prudent to use those with the least potential for orthostatic hypotension in patients who may already present with significant postural drops in blood pressure or who have important cardiovascular disease.

Antihypertensives

Many antihypertensive agents inhibit sympathetic neuronal function. It is via a nonselective effect on venous and/or arterial beds that they induce orthostatic changes in blood pressure. Postural hypotension is very common with guanethidine and is particularly troublesome with the initiation of prazosin therapy. Table 6-6 lists the commonly used antihypertensive drugs and rates them according to their likelihood for inducing postural hypotension. It must be emphasized that elderly patients are often very responsive to antihypertensive agents and that blunted baroreflex sensitivity makes this population especially prone to develop severe episodes of postural hypotension with any of these agents.

Diuretics

Diuretics (Table 6-7) act on the kidney to promote salt and water loss. Overzealous use of these drugs can produce an important reduction in circulating blood volume and result in decreased cardiac filling. There is no

Table 6-6. Commonly Used Antihypertensive Drugs and Their Relative Propensity for Causing Postural Hypotension

Generic Name	Brand Name	Postural Hypotension
Beta blockers	(See Table 6-9)	Rare
Captopril[a]	Capoten	Rare
Clonidine	Catapres	Occasional
Diuretics	(See Table 6-7)	Occasional
Enalapril[a]	Vasotec	Rare
Guanabenz	Wytensin	Occasional
Guanadrel	Hylorel	Common
Guanfacine	Tenex	Occasional
Guanethidine	Ismelin	Common
Hydralazine	Apresoline	Rare
Labetalol	Trandate, Normodyne	Occasional
Lisinopril[a]	Zestril	Rare
Methyldopa	Aldomet	Occasional
Minoxidil	Loniten	Occasional
Prazosin[b]	Minipress	Occasional
Reserpine	(Numerous)	Rare
Terazosin[b]	Hytrin	Occasional
Verapamil	Calan, Isoptin	Rare

[a] Pretreatment with a diuretic may greatly enhance the risk of postural hypotension.
[b] Severe postural hypotension has been noted with the initiation of therapy or with rapid and large increments in dose.

Table 6-7. Diuretics That Can Cause
Significant Volume Depletion and
Hypokalemia

Generic Name	Brand Name
Bendroflumethiazide	Naturetin
Benzthiazide	Exna
Bumetanide[a]	Bumex
Chlorthalidone	Hygroton
Chlorothiazide	Diuril
Cyclothiazide	Anhydron
Ethacrynic acid[a]	Edecrin
Furosemide[a]	Lasix
Hydrochlorothiazide	Hydrodiuril, Esidrex, Oretic
Hydroflumethiazide	Saluron
Methylclothiazide	Enduron
Metolazone	Zaroxolyn, Diulo
Polythiazide	Renese
Quinethazone	Hydromox
Trichlormethiazide	Naqua

[a] These are loop diuretics; all the remaining are thiazide or thiazide-like diuretics.

doubt that volume depletion is a major complication of diuretic treatment in the elderly. A recent study elegantly analyzed and demonstrated the enhanced propensity of the elderly to postural hypotension following moderate diuretic-induced sodium loss.[12]

Hypovolemia-induced orthostatic changes in blood pressure are particularly common in elderly patients taking diuretics who also have other conditions causing salt and water loss (e.g., diarrhea, vomiting, and fever). Reduced fluid intake as a result of impairment or loss of thirst sensation (a not uncommon finding in the elderly) or due to conditions associated with a clouded sensorium may also augment the potential for diuretic-related hypovolemia.

Nitrates

The administration of organic nitrates (Table 6-8) may sometimes lead to symptomatic postural hypotension. The sublingual route has been particularly associated with a hypotensive effect. Nitrate symptoms related to hypotension

Table 6-8. Nitrates

Generic Name	Brand Name
Erythrityl tetranitrate[a]	Cardilate
Isosorbide dinitrate[a]	Isordil, Sorbitrate
Nitroglycerin[a,b]	(Numerous)
Pentaerythritol tetranitrate	Peritrate, Duotrate

[a] Also available in sublingual form.
[b] Also available as a buccal tablet, ointment, spray, and transdermal patch.

are all increased when the patient is immobile and upright. These agents induce their orthostatic effects primarily via peripheral venodilation, causing substantial venous pooling, which leads to a decrease in venous return to the heart. Nitrate-induced postural hypotension normally leads to baroreflex stimulation of heart rate and increased vascular tone. These homeostatic mechanisms help to preserve blood pressure.

Certain drugs may augment the potential for nitrate-induced hypotension. These include the following:

1.   Beta-blocking agents (Table 6-9) depress sinus node function and thus can attenuate or prevent reflex increases in heart rate that often accompany nitrate-induced vasodilation.

2.   Diuretic agents (Table 6-7) can decrease the circulating blood volume (i.e., cause hypovolemia) and hence potentiate the "relative" hypovolemia caused by nitrate-induced venodilation.

3.   Intake of moderate amounts of alcohol, which by itself may cause postural hypotension but which probably has an additive vasodilating effect.

Narcotic Analgesics (Opiates)

Narcotic analgesics (Table 6-10) can cause peripheral arteriolar and venous dilation, thus decreasing the capacity of the cardiovascular system to respond to gravitational shifts and resulting in postural hypotension. Orthostatic changes are more prominent with parenteral (intravenous, intramuscular, or subcutaneous) than with oral administration.

Vasodilator Drugs

Numerous drugs (Table 6-11) are advertised as being useful in the treatment of obstructive arterial disease. These agents are vasodilators and act by relaxing vascular smooth muscle. Interestingly, there is little evidence to suggest that any of these drugs are effective for either peripheral or cerebral vascular disease. However, *these agents can cause postural or postexercise hypotension.*

Table 6-9. Beta-blocking Drugs

Generic Name	Brand Name
Acebutolol	Sectral
Atenolol	Tenormin
Metoprolol	Lopressor
Nadolol	Corgard
Pindolol	Viskin
Propranolol	Inderal
Timolol	Blocadren

Table 6-10. Narcotic Analgesics

Generic Name	Brand Name
Codeine[a]	(Numerous)
Hydrocodone	Hycodan
Hydromorphone	Dilaudid
Meperidine	Demerol
Methadone	Dolophine
Morphine	(Numerous)
Oxycodone[a]	(Numerous)
Oxymorphone	Numorphan
Pentazocine	Talwin

[a] Often marketed in combination with additional drugs.

Levodopa

Initial treatment with levodopa frequently causes postural hypotension. This effect is believed to be both centrally and peripherally mediated. Combining levodopa with carbidopa (Sinemet) does not seem to influence the incidence of this side effect.

Long-term treatment with levodopa or carbidopa is often associated with a decrease in the severity of postural hypotension. However, in many patients severe symptomatic postural hypotension may persist. This side effect may limit patients to a suboptimal dose of levodopa. Several methods have been tried to overcome persistent levodopa-induced hypotension, including elastic stockings, increased salt intake, or use of indomethacin or fludrocortisone. Bromocriptine (Parlodel), a relatively new antiparkinsonian agent, also elicits orthostatic drops in blood pressure with a frequency that rivals levodopa.

Fatigue and Weakness

Fatigue and weakness are common complaints from the elderly and may have either physiologic or emotional etiologies. Unfortunately these complaints are often ignored by caregivers and may even be equated with poor motivation. Prolonged bed rest, muscle disuse, certain acute and chronic illnesses, and primary depression can be obvious contributing factors. The role

Table 6-11. Vasodilating Drugs

Generic Name	Brand Name
Cyclandelate	Cyclospasmol
Ergoloid mesylates	Hydergine
Ethaverine	Ethaquin, Ethatab, Laverin
Isoxsuprine	Vasodilan
Nicotinic acid	Nicobid
Nicotinyl alcohol	Roniacol
Nylidrin	Arlidin
Papaverine	Pavabid, Cerespan

of drugs in producing fatigue and weakness is less well known and infrequently considered.

Beta-blocking Drugs

Beta-blocking drugs (Table 6-9) are a common source of fatigue. This side effect is probably due in part to their ability to reduce blood flow to muscle. With both short- and long-term treatment, heart rate is decreased at rest as well as during exercise. Stroke volume does not increase enough to compensate for the decrease in heart rate; hence cardiac output stays below pretreatment levels. During the first few weeks of treatment with beta-blockers complaints of muscle fatigue and heavy legs during and after exercise are particularly common. Although these side effects tend to disappear over time in young and middle-age patients, little is known about the development of tolerance to these effects in the aged.

Diuretics

Diuretics (Table 6-7) may produce weakness and fatigue via several different actions. Volume depletion from excessive diuresis can decrease ventricular filling, with a consequent decrease in cardiac output, leading to decreased perfusion of muscle and producing symptoms of tiredness. Hypovolemia may be particularly troublesome in patients with heart failure. Increased diastolic ventricular filling is one of the necessary compensatory mechanisms that increases the force of cardiac contraction and thus helps maintain cardiac output in the failing heart.

Hypokalemia (low serum potassium) is a common side effect of diuretic use in the elderly. The degree of hypokalemia induced by diuretic administration is dependent on the dose and type of diuretic. High doses are often associated with greater falls in serum potassium. In general, the incidence of hypokalemia is highest with chlorthalidone, intermediate with hydrochlorothiazide, and lowest with furosemide.[13] Skeletal muscle appears to be the major target organ that manifests the clinical impact of hypokalemia. When the serum potassium drops below 3.0 mEq/L (particularly below 2.5 mEq/L) some degree of muscle weakness is common. The weakness is most noticeable in the legs, particularly the quadriceps muscles. In addition, hypokalemia may produce muscle cramps and muscular pain, which tend to be more common during exercise, as well as serious cardiac arrhythmias.

Hyponatremia (low serum sodium) is another common side effect of diuretic treatment and may produce a feeling of overall fatigue. Localized feelings of fatigue or cramps in an exercising hand or limb may also be seen. Vulnerability to diuretic-induced hyponatremia seems greatest in a setting of liberal water intake and restricted sodium ingestion. Symptoms may be seen with a serum sodium of less than 130 mEq/L but are more common when sodium levels drop to 125 mEq/L or less.

Table 6-12. Selected Drugs Associated with Peripheral Neuropathies

Generic Name	Brand Name
Alcohol	(Numerous)
Chlorambucil	Leukeran
Chloramphenicol	Chloromycetin
Cisplatin	Platinol
Dapsone	Avlosulfon
Disulfiram	Antabuse
Ethambutol	Myambutol
Gold salts	(Numerous)
Hydralazine	Apresoline
Isoniazid	(Numerous)
Metronidazole	Flagyl
Nitrofurantoin	(Numerous)
Penicillamine	Cuprimine, Depen
Phenytoin	Dilantin
Procarbazine	Matulane
Vincristine	Oncovin
Vinblastine	Velban

Drug-induced Neuropathies and Myopathies

Drug-induced peripheral neuropathies and myopathies are important but uncommon causes of weakness. Tables 6-12 and 6-13 list drugs that have been implicated in these neuromuscular disorders. There are several excellent reviews on these topics.[14-16]

Drug-induced Sedation

Many drugs that have a major sedating action may produce a feeling of weakness and fatigue. These drugs include tricyclic antidepressants (Table 6-4), antipsychotics (Table 6-5), barbiturates, benzodiazepines (Table 6-14), antihistamines, and certain antihypertensives (methyldopa, clonidine, resperine). Their sedative effects usually disappear after several weeks of treatment.

Table 6-13. Selected Drugs Associated with Myopathies

Generic Name	Brand name
Alcohol	(Numerous)
Chloroquine	(Numerous)
Clofibrate	Atromid S
Corticosteroids	(Numerous)
Drug-induced hypokalemia[a]	(Numerous)
Lithium	(Numerous)
Lovostatin	Mevacor
Penicillamine	Cuprimine, Depen
Procainamide	Pronestyl
Vincristine	Oncovin

[a] Primarily seen with diuretics and laxative abuse.

Table 6-14. Benzodiazepines

Generic Name	Brand Name
Alprazolam	Xanax
Chlordiazepoxide	Librium
Clorazepate	Tranxene
Diazepam	Valium
Flurazepam	Dalmane
Halazepam	Paxipam
Lorazepam	Ativan
Oxazepam	Serax
Prazepam	Centrax
Triazolam	Halcion

To minimize the sedative potential of these drugs in the elderly, it is particularly important to begin treatment with a very low dose and increase it slowly if needed at 2- to 4-week intervals.

Finally, it needs to be noted that weakness and fatigue may be early signs of a depressive reaction to medication. These symptoms often coexist with other signs of depression and include early morning awakening, appetite disturbances, and multiple bodily complaints, especially gastrointestinal.

Depression and Confusion

As a group, the elderly are the most susceptible to mental illness. Depression and various degrees of impairment in cognitive function are the mental disorders most commonly noted in the aged. It is particularly noteworthy that depressive reactions in the elderly often have an important cognitive component that can easily mimic a progressive dementing process. This type of depression has been referred to in the psychiatric literature as pseudodementia.

Drugs acting on the central nervous system (CNS) are commonly prescribed in the elderly. Their use or sudden withdrawal may precipitate major depressive or confusional episodes in the elderly. Unfortunately, these drug reactions may not be easily recognized. Recognition of psychiatric symptoms related to drug toxicity is more difficult in the elderly than in younger patients because other or similar psychiatric problems more often may have been present before drug treatment. Furthermore, depression and confusion may be attributed to a prior history of poor physical and or mental health, the very factors predisposing a patient to the adverse CNS effects of drugs.

Many centrally acting drugs can have a very long duration of action and, with multiple dosing can accumulate slowly to high levels in the body. Their adverse CNS effects develop insidiously, and there may be no obvious improvement for several days or a week or more after the drug is stopped. A recent study has demonstrated a considerable excess risk for hip fracture in elderly patients prescribed long-acting (synonymous with a long half-life) sedative-hypnotic medications.[17]

Sedative and hypnotic medications can produce globally adverse depressive effects on brain function. Some centrally acting drugs, such as propranolol (Inderal) and methyldopa (Aldomet), appear to produce more selective deficits in cognitive function, imparing verbal but not visual memory.[18] Less obvious, however, are the effects of drugs whose primary and intended site of action is outside the CNS but because of their polypharmacologic spectrum have direct and important secondary effects on the CNS. For example, acetazolamide (Diamox) is a very effective, orally administered antiglaucoma drug, used most frequently by the elderly. Besides its direct action in the eye, this drug also partitions into the brain and can produce a disabling malaise syndrome consisting of depression, fatigue, anorexia, and weight loss in up to 50 percent of its recipients.[19]

Other drugs, via their peripheral effects, can create metabolic or cardiovascular disturbances that subsequently affect CNS function. Diuretic-induced hyponatremia and chronic hypoglycemia from oral antidiabetic agents are common examples of drugs indirectly disturbing CNS function and leading to confusional states. Hyponatremia from diuretics (almost exclusively owing to thiazide-type, see Table 6-7) usually occurs within several days following the initiation of therapy. Advanced age and being female has been implicated as important risk factors for this complication.[20,21] Confusion, drowsiness, disorientation, and lethargy are the common manifestations of hyponatremia provoked by diuretic use. Hypoglycemia from oral antidiabetic drugs (as well as insulin) produce what are described as neuroglycopenic symptoms, which may consist of confusion and inability to concentrate. Focal neurologic deficits may also occur with hypoglycemia and are probably more likely to be seen in elderly patients with underlying cerebrovascular disease and thus mimic a stroke-like state. The risk of hypoglycemia increases with aging and appears greatest with the oral agents chlorpropamide (Diabinese) and glyburide (Micronase/DiaBeta).[22]

A history of depression has been shown to predispose an individual to developing severe depressive reactions to certain drugs, particularly centrally acting antihypertensive agents (e.g., resperine, methyldopa, clonidine, and propranolol). It is reasonable to assume that preexisting brain damage will reduce a patient's tolerance to adverse CNS effects of drugs, confusional episodes being especially important. Finally, many metabolic, cardiovascular, and CNS disorders produce psychiatric symptoms, and great care must be taken to evaluate their contribution to the overall mental status of a patient.

In contrast to reactions related to the presence of drugs in the central nervous system, the sudden discontinuation of a drug may precipitate a withdrawal-type reaction. The onset of symptoms following sudden discontinuation of drugs is very much dependent on the individual agent involved, and onset may vary from as little as 6 hours to several days. Symptoms vary according to the drugs, but depression, confusion, and agitation are common with many withdawal reactions.

Prevention, recognition, and treatment of drug-induced depression or confusion are of obvious importance to the rehabilitation staff. Depressed

Table 6-15. Selected Drugs Associated with Depressive Reactions

Generic Name	Brand Name
Acetazolamide	Diamox
Alcohol	(Numerous)
Amantadine	Symmetrel
Antipsychotic agents	(See Table 6-5)
Barbiturates	(Numerous)
Benzodiazepines	(See Table 6-14)
Benztropine	Cogentin
Beta-blockers	(See Table 6-9)
Bromocriptine	Parlodel
Cimetidine	Tagamet
Clonidine	Catapres
Ethambutol	Myambutol
Glucocorticoids	(Numerous)
Guanfacine	Tenex
Guanabenz	Wytensin
Indomethacin	Indocin
Isoniazid	(Numerous)
Levodopa	(Numerous)
Levodopa-cabadopa	Sinemet
Methazolamide	Neptazane
Methyldopa	Aldomet
Naproxen	Naprosyn
Prazosin	Minipress
Prednisone	(Numerous)
Ranitidine	Zantac
Reserpine	(Numerous)

patients lack motivation, show disinterest, or refuse to cooperate in therapy. Even mildly confused patients may not be able to follow directions.

Because the number of drugs reported as a cause of depression or confusion is large, it is impossible to discuss each agent in this brief review. However, Tables 6-15 through 6-17 list those drugs most commonly associated with these types of reactions in the elderly.

Involuntary Movements

Parkinsonism

Drug-induced parkinsonism is a commonly encountered clinical problem following the administration of antipsychotic medications (see Table 6-5). Recent clinical studies have emphasized the importance of these drugs as a significant cause of parkinsonism in the elderly.[23,24] In some patients exquisite sensitivity to the offending medication has been attributed to the presence of an underlying subclinical form of idiopathic Parkinson's disease. Symptoms of parkinsonism usually appear during the first few weeks of antipsychotic drug therapy and are most often observed in elderly patients. Clinically, the effect appears identical to idiopathic Parkinson's disease.

Table 6-16. Drugs Associated with Confusional Reactions

Generic Name	Brand Name
Amantadine	Symmetrel
Aminophylline	(Numerous)
Antipsychotic agents	(See Table 6-5)
Barbiturates	(Numerous)
Benzodiazepines	(See Table 6-14)
Benztropine	Cogentin
Beta blockers	(See Table 6-9)
Biperidin	Akineton
Bromocriptine	Parlodel
Cimetidine	Tagamet
Codeine	(Numerous)
Cyclobenzaprine	Flexeril
Digitoxin	Crystodigin
Digoxin	Lanoxin
Glucocorticoids	(Numerous)
Indomethacin	Indocin
Isoniazid	(Numerous)
Levodopa	(Numerous)
Levodopa-carbadopa	Sinemet
Lithium	(Numerous)
Meperidine	Demerol
Methadone	Dolophine
Methyldopa	Aldomet
Morphine	(Numerous)
Mexiletine	Mexitil
Pentazocine	Talwin
Phenobarbital[a]	(Numerous)
Phenytoin[a]	Dilantin
Primidone[a]	Mysoline
Procyclidine	Kemadrin
Propoxyphene	Darvon
Ranitidine	Zantac
Theophylline[a]	(Numerous)
Tocainide	Tonocard
Tricyclic antidepressants	(See Table 6-4)
Trihexyphenidyl	Artane

[a] Confusional episodes are most often associated with large doses or high serum levels of these drugs.

Table 6-17. Drugs Associated with Withdrawal Reactions of which Depression or Confusion May Be an Important Component

Generic Name	Brand Name
Alcohol	(Numerous)
Amphetamine	(Numerous)
Anticholinergic agents[a]	(See Table 6-22)
Antipsychotic agents	(See Table 6-5)
Baclofen	Lioresal
Barbiturates	(Numerous)
Benzodiazepines	(See Table 6-14)
Clonidine	Catapres
Glucocorticoids	(Numerous)
Methylphenidate	Ritalin
Narcotic analgesics	(See Table 6-10)
Phenytoin	Dilantin
Tricyclic antidepressants	(See Table 6-4)

[a] This effect is limited to agents that partition into the brain.

Patients with drug-induced parkinsonism can show abnormalities of posture and gait, rigidity, bradykinesia, and resting tremors. Particularly noteworthy is the nearly always symmetrical distribution of symptomology in the case of drug-induced parkinsonism. There is a wide spectrum of disability associated with drug-induced parkinsonism, ranging from an annoying mild tremor to severe incapacitating bradykinesia and rigidity. Bradykinesia may be the earliest or even the only sign of parkinsonism in some patients and may be misinterpreted as depression. Certain antipsychotic drugs have a greater potential for producing parkinsonian-like symptoms than others (see Table 6-5). Thus, when an antipsychotic drug is needed, the selection of an agent least likely to produce parkinsonism seems particularly appropriate for those patients with preexisting disorders affecting ambulation, or activities of daily living, or who are already in an ongoing physical therapy/rehabilitation program.

Because drug-induced parkinsonism can be a serious threat to the independence and well being of the elderly, the indications for continued use of the offending medication must be thoroughly reevaluated and alternative therapies considered. When antipsychotic drug therapy is considered essential in the patient manifesting parkinsonian side effects, several measures can be taken to reduce the severity of this drug reaction. Symptoms, particularly when mild, may abate within several months despite continued drug administration. The dose of antipsychotic medications may be reduced with consequent reduction in the severity of symptoms, or one may choose to switch to another drug with a lower propensity for inducing parkinsonian reactions. Troublesome symptoms may be treated with centrally acting anticholinergic agents (typically benztropine or trihexyphenidyl). These drugs are remarkably effective for relieving symptoms of antipsychotic drug-induced parkinsonism. However, it is not wise to administer these anticholinergic agents with antipsychotic drugs indefinitely because of evidence suggesting that prolonged administration of this combination may substantially increase the likelihood of development of tardive dyskinesia (see below). Anticholinergic agents should be gradually withdrawn after 3 months of use in order to determine if relief from drug-induced parkinsonism has occurred spontaneously. Furthermore, the elderly are especially liable to confusional reactions to anticholinergic drugs as well as troublesome peripheral effects such as blurred vision, constipation, urinary retention, and reflux esophagitis.

Patients with Parkinson's disease often require rehabilitation intervention. It is important to be aware that certain medications may exacerbate this disorder and/or antagonize the beneficial effects of antiparkinsonism drugs. Medications that are potentially deleterious to the parkinsonian patient are listed in Table 6-18. Of particular note is the medication prochlorperazine (Compazine or in the combination product Combid), which has all the properties of an antipsychotic drug but is used almost exclusively as an antiemetic. This medication was responsible for more than 40 percent of all cases of drug-induced parkinsonism in the elderly according to a recent report.[24]

Table 6-18. Drugs That Can Aggravate Parkinsonism or Block the Beneficial Effects of Antiparkinsonism Drugs

Generic Name	Brand Name
Amoxepine	Asendin
Antipsychotic drugs	(See Table 6-5)
Benzodiazepines[a]	(See Table 6-14)
Methionine	Pedameth
Methyldopa	Aldomet
Metoclopramide	Reglan
Papaverine	Cerespan, Pavabid
Prochlorperazine	Compazine
Pyridoxine[b]	(Various vitamin preparations)
Resperine	(Numerous)

[a] Appear uncommon; further evidence for this potential adverse effect is needed.

[b] This potential adverse drug–drug interaction is seen only with levodopa and not in the combination preparation of carbidopa-levodopa (Sinemet).

Tardive Dyskinesia

One of the more serious adverse effects of long-term therapy with antipsychotic drugs is tardive dyskinesia. This manifests as a set of abnormal involuntary movements occurring most often in the oral region. They are typically localized movements of the tongue, lips, and jaws, consisting of mouthing, puckering, chewing, sucking, smacking, biting, and darting movements of the tongue. Less commonly seen are choreoathetoid movements of the fingers, head, body, and limbs. Diaphragmatic movements, although uncommon, may produce grunting, dyspnea, and hyperpnea.

Tardive dyskinesia is a late-appearing side effect of antipsychotic drug treatment. It has an insidious onset and becomes clinically evident months to years after initiation of treatment. Tardive dyskinesia may appear following a reduction or withdrawal of the medication or when centrally acting anticholinergic drugs are supplemented (e.g., trihexyphenidyl or benztropine). These movements can persist for long periods of time or for life even after the offending medication is discontinued. It is more commonly seen in the elderly, particularly females. Furthermore, in the aged symptoms are often more severe and less likely to remit following discontinuation of the antipsychotic medication. Patients with preexisting brain damage, including Alzheimer's dementia, are more likely to develop tardive dyskinesia.

Tardive dyskinesia is typically made worse by emotional distress and is diminished or absent during sleep. Many patients are aware of their abnormal movements and may be distressed by them, particularly when they experience functional impairment, usually when their arms and legs are affected. Severe cases of tardive dyskinesia may be complicated by difficulties of swallowing or speech, irregular respirations, and severely incapacitating movements of the axial musculature.

Although the most common cause of tardive dyskinesia is long-term treatment with antipsychotic drugs, this movement disorder is a recognized complication of therapy with metoclopramide (Reglan) and amoxapine (Asendin). Levodopa and any drug with central anticholinergic action may exacerbate this disorder.

Akathisia

Akathisia, a syndrome of motor restlessness, is a common extrapyramidal side effect of antipsychotic drugs. It is characterized by pacing, inability to sit or stand still, continuous agitation, and restless movement and intolerance to inactivity. Akathisia is sometimes mistaken for psychotic agitation and may (inappropriately) lead to an increase in antipsychotic drug dosage. Treatment of akathesia is difficult. This side effect usually does not respond as well to centrally acting anticholinergic agents as does drug-induced parkinsonism. Reduction of the dosage of the antipsychotic drug may be effective.

Essential Tremor

Essential tremor generally affects the distal parts of the upper extremities and sometimes involves the legs and head. It may be unilateral in onset, but almost invariably it becomes bilateral and symmetrical. It is most often seen in the elderly, and in this setting it is referred to as senile tremor. Typically the tremor is decreased or absent at rest and present when the limb is held extended in a sustained posture or in active movement. It is extremely troublesome when the limb is used for tasks that require precision or careful attention, such as writing or lifting a cup or glass. This latter situation may be socially embarrassing and is often attributed to manual clumsiness. Essential tremor may be exacerbated by certain drugs, including lithium carbonate, tricyclic antidepressants, and adrenergic drugs (e.g., albuterol, metaproterenol, terbutaline). Moreover, these drugs may produce an essential tremor-like syndrome in previously unaffected persons. If an adrenergic bronchodilator drug is prescribed for an asthmatic patient with essential tremor, an aerosol form that has less of a systemic action should be considered over the standard tablet or capsule formulation. Beta blockers (Table 6-9) and primidone (Mysoline) have a tremolytic action and may be beneficial in attenuating the severity of this disorder.

Dizziness and Vertigo

Dizziness and vertigo are important symptoms in the elderly and deserve thorough investigation. Falls secondary to these symptoms are particularly dangerous to the elderly because of their increased susceptibility to trauma, especially fractures. Furthermore, feelings of dizziness or vertigo may force individuals to severely limit their activities, leading to both social and geographic isolation.

A multitude of subjective symptoms may be interpreted as dizziness. Patients may complain of a sensation of giddiness or passing out, light-headedness, floating, postural unsteadiness, or faintness. Vertigo may be thought of as a more severe form of dizziness, with a definite feeling of spinning or whirling; it is often accompanied by sweating, nausea, and vomiting.

Drugs can easily produce these types of symptoms by (1) a direct action on those areas of the brain that control motor coordination and gait, (2) upsetting brain metabolism secondary to a reduction in brain blood flow or blood glucose, or (3) a direct toxic action on the vestibular system.

Studies in patients over the age of 60 years have shown drugs to be a major cause of dizziness.[25,26] Drug-induced dizziness or vertigo may occur alone or as part of a constellation of side effects.

Orthostatic hypotension leading to a decrease in blood flow to the brain is a common mechanism by which drugs cause dizziness. Every patient complaining of dizziness needs to be evaluated for orthostatic drops in blood pressure.

Drugs that cause dizziness and vertigo by a toxic action on the vestibular system are listed in Table 6-19. It is important to realize that certain drugs may produce irreversible injury to the vestibular apparatus (e.g., gentamicin, tobramycin), whereas with other medications, symptoms abate very quickly on their discontinuation. Many drugs that have a nonselective action on the central nervous system may cause dizziness. Such drugs commonly include sedatives, hypnotics, anticonvulsants, tricyclic antidepressants, and antipsychotics. Table 6-20 lists other medications that may cause symptoms of dizziness or vertigo.

Table 6-19. Drugs That May Cause Dizziness and Vertigo by a Toxic Effect on the Vestibular System

Generic Name	Brand Name
Alcohol	(Numerous)
Amikacin	Amikin
Fenoprofen	Nalfon
Gentamicin	Garamycin
Ibuprofen	Motrin
Indomethacin	Indocin
Meclofenamate	Meclomen
Minocycline	Minocin
Naproxen	Naprosyn
Oxyphenylbutazone	Tandearil, Oxalid
Phenylbutazone	Butazolidin, Azolid
Quinidine	Quiniglute, Quinidex, Quindra
Salicylate	(Numerous)
Streptomycin	(Numerous)
Sulindac	Clinoril
Tobramycin	Nebcin
Tolmetin	Tolectin

Table 6-20. Other Drugs That May Cause Dizziness or Vertigo[a]

Generic Name	Brand Name
Acetazolamide	Diamox
Alcohol	(Numerous)
Barbiturates	(Numerous)
Benzodiazepines	(See Table 6-14)
Beta-adrenergic blockers	(See Table 6-9)
Cimetidine	Tagamet
Diphenhydramine	Benadryl
Encainide	Enkaid
Flecainide	Tambocor
Hypoglycemic agents[b]	(Numerous)
Isoniazid	(Numerous)
Meprobamate	Equanil, Miltown
Metronidazole	Flagyl
Mexiletine	Mexitil
Naladixic acid	NegGram
Narcotic analgesics	(See Table 6-10)
Nifedipine	Procardia
Nitrates	(See Table 6-8)
Nitrofurantoin	Macrodantin, Furantin, Cyantin
Oxolinic acid	Utibid
Pentoxifylline	Trental
Phenytoin	Dilantin
Primidone	Mysoline
Tricyclic antidepressants	(See Table 6-4)
Tocainide	Tonocard
Verapamil	Isoptin, Calan

[a] Antihypertensive drugs or other drugs capable of causing postural hypotension can precipitate these symptoms.

[b] Symptoms related to excessive reduction of blood glucose.

Ataxia

Whereas drug-induced dizziness and vertigo create a feeling of disorientation in space, ataxic reactions to medications manifest as an impairment of upright stance and locomotion. These untoward effects are characteristic of drugs that have a diffuse action on the central nervous system, and they are particularly prevalent with anticonvulsants and hypnosedatives. Ataxia is a common sign of excessive blood concentrations of anticonvulsants. Of the hypnosedatives, benzodiazepines (Table 6-14), because of their widespread use and well-documented altered metabolism and or response in the aged, are probably the most common cause of drug-induced ataxia in the elderly. These and other drugs associated with ataxic reactions are listed in Table 6-21.

Urinary Incontinence

Lack of control of bladder function is a clinical problem that can have a devastating effect on rehabilitation efforts in the elderly. Urinary incontinence in the elderly often causes anxiety, severe distress, and depression, which can lead to social isolation and can undermine the confidence and motivation

Table 6-21. Drugs Associated with Ataxic Reactions

Generic Name	Brand Name
Alcohol	(Numerous)
Barbiturates	(Numerous)
Benzodiazepines	(See Table 6-14)
Carbamazepine	Tegretol
Carbidopa-levodopa	Sinemet
Levodopa	Dopar, Laradopa, Parda
Indomethacin	Indocin
Lithium	Eskalith, Lithane
Minocycline	Minocin
Nitrofurantoin	Macrodantin, Furadantin, Cyantin
Phenobarbital	(Numerous)
Phenytoin	Dilantin
Primidone	Mysoline
Valproic acid	Depakene

essential for successful rehabilitation. Incontinence is not a disease. It is a symptom that may reflect a serious underlying disorder and needs to be thoroughly investigated. Included in this investigation is the possibility of medication-induced incontinence. The normal or compromised bladder can be adversely affected by many drugs. These drugs and the complex means by which they exert their untoward effects on continence mechanisms have been well reviewed and will only briefly be addressed here.[27-29]

The most common cause of urinary incontinence in the elderly is the uninhibited bladder. This condition is usually caused by a decrease in cortical control of the micturition process. Simplistically viewed, bladder emptying involves a reflex arc with the spinal cord wherein sensory fibers in the bladder detect urinary filling pressures and relay this information to the spinal motor fibers that can activate the bladder musculature (detrusor muscle) to contract when a critical pressure is reached. Cortical function, however, strongly modulates the spinal relex arc, allowing an individual to suppress or follow through on the sense or desire to void. This reflex arc cannot be modulated well if the higher centers of the brain are damaged by disease (dementia, stroke) or suppressed by pharmacologic agents. Drugs that depress cerebral function (e.g., benzodiazepines, barbiturates) can decrease one's ability to inhibit bladder contractions, thus bringing on or exacerbating preexisting incontinence.

Sphincter weakness or insufficiency is another common cause of incontinence in the elderly and is often referred to as stress incontinence. In this condition intraurethral sphincter tone is not sufficiently strong enough to overcome the passive rise in intravesicular pressure that accompanies the rise in intraabdominal pressure from such activities as coughing or sudden move-

Table 6-22. Selected Drugs with Potent Anticholinergic Effects

Generic Name	Brand Name
Amitriptyline	Elavil, Endep
Amoxepine	Asendin
Benztropine	Cogentin
Biperiden	Akineton
Chlorpromazine	Thorazine
Dicyclomine	Bentyl
Diphenhydramine	Benedryl
Disopyramide	Norpace
Doxepin	Sinequan, Adapin
Glycopyrolate	Robinul
Imipramine	Tofranil
Loxapine	Loxitane
Maprotiline	Ludiomil
Mepenzolate	Cantil
Molindone	Moban
Nortriptyline	Aventyl
Procyclidine	Kemadrin
Propantheline	Probanthine
Protriptyline	Vivactil
Thioridazine	Mellaril
Trihexyphenidyl	Artane
Trimipramine	Surmontil

ments. The phenothiazine drugs, thioridazine (Mellaril) and chlorpromazine (Thorazine) have been found to exacerbate stress incontinence by compromising sphincter tone.

Overflow incontinence represents a third common cause of involuntary urine loss in the elderly. Mechanical (e.g., prostatic hypertrophy) or functional (e.g., drugs) obstruction to bladder outflow leads to retention of urine with eventual overflow incontinence as intravesicular pressure overcomes urethral sphincter pressure. Drugs with an anticholinergic action (see Table 6-22) relax the detrusor muscle of the bladder, causing urinary retention and potentially overflow incontinence. Furthermore, rapid inhibition of detrusor tone by drugs may produce acute urinary obstruction, particularly when given to patients with a history of prostatic hypertrophy.

The inappropriate timing of diuretic administration is a common and easily remediable cause of incontinence. Diuretic use is particularly likely to exacerbate the incontinence caused by the three disorders described above. Rapidly acting potent diuretics like furosemide and bumetanide induce a considerable diuresis over a period of several hours and careful attention needs to be paid to the scheduling of these agents relative to therapy sessions.

CONCLUSION

In this brief review an attempt has been made to point out to the therapist that certain drug effects can present as obstacles to successful rehabilitation. Although these deleterious drug effects can occur in any age group, the elderly are particularly vulnerable. Scheduled periodic reviews of medications used by the elderly patient need to be multidisciplinary and include input from the therapist.

REFERENCES

1. Hurwitz N: Predisposing factors in adverse reactions to drugs. Br Med J 1:536, 1969
2. Seidl LG, Thornton GF, Smith JW, Cluff L: Studies on the epidemiology of adverse drug reactions. III. Reactions in patients on a general medical service. Bull Johns Hopkins Hosp 119:299, 1966
3. Williamson J, Chopin MJ: Adverse reactions to prescribed drugs in the elderly: a multicenter investigation. Age Ageing 9:73, 1980
4. Gribbin B, Pickering TG, Sleight P, Peto R: Effect of age and high blood pressure on baroreflex sensitivity in man. Circ Res 29:424, 1971
5. Caird FI, Andrews GR, Kennedy RD: Effect of posture on blood pressure in the elderly. Br Heart J 35:527, 1973
6. Kennedy GT, Crawford MH: Optimal position and timing of blood pressure and heart rate measurements to detect orthostatic changes in patients with ischemic heart disease. J Cardiac Rehab 4:219, 1984
7. Lipsitz LA, Nyquist RP, Wei JY, Rowe JW: Postprandial reduction in blood pressure in the elderly. New Engl J Med 309:81, 1983
8. Glassman AH, Giardine EV, Perel JM, et al: Clinical characteristics of imipramine-induced orthostatic hypotension. Lancet 1:468, 1979
9. Thayssen P, Bjerre M, Kragh-Sorensen M, et al: Cardiovascular effects of imipramine and nortriptyline in elderly patients. Psychopharmacology 74:360, 1981
10. Lipsey JR, Robinson RG, Pearlson GD, et al: Nortriptyline treatment of post-stroke depression: a double blind study. Lancet 1:297: 1984
11. Branchey MH, Lee JH, Amin R, Simpson M: High and low-potency neuroleptics in elderly psychiatric patients. JAMA 239:1860, 1978
12. Shannon RP, Wei, JY, Rosa RM, et al: The effect of age and sodium depletion on cardiovascular response to orthostasis. Hypertension 8:438, 1986
13. Perez-Stable E, Caralis PV: Thiazide-induced disturbances in carbohydrate, lipid, and potassium metabolism. Am Heart J 106:245, 1983
14. Argov Z, Mastaglia FL: Drug-induced peripheral neuropathies. Br Med J 1:663, 1979
15. Lane RJM, Mastaglia FL: Drug-induced myopathies in man. Lancet 2:562, 1978
16. Sahenk Z: Toxic neuropathies. Semin Neurol 7:9, 1987
17. Ray WA, Griffin MR, Schaffner W, et al: Psychotropic drug use and the risk of hip fracture. N Engl J Med 316:363, 1987
18. Solomon S, Hotchkiss E, Saravay SM, et al: Impairment of memory function by antihypertensive medication. Arch Gen Psychiatry 40:1109, 1983
19. Epstein DL, Grant WM: Carbonic anhydrase inhibitor side effects. Serum chemical analysis. Arch Ophthalmol 95:1378, 1977
20. Ashouri OS: Severe diuretic-induced hyponatremia in the elderly. A series of eight patients. Arch Intern Med 146:1355, 1986
21. Sterns RH: Severe symptomatic hyponatremia: treatment and outcome. A study of 64 cases. Ann Intern Med 107:656, 1987
22. Ferner RE, Neil HAW: Sulphonylureas and hypoglycaemia. Br Med J 296:949, 1988

23. Murdoch PS, Williamson J: A danger in making the diagnosis of Parkinson's disease. Lancet 1:1212, 1982
24. Stephen PJ, Williamson J: Drug-induced parkinsonism in the elderly. Lancet 2:1082, 1984
25. Skiendzielewski JJ, Martyak G: The weak and dizzy patient. Ann Emerg Med 9:353, 1980
26. Blumenthal MD, Davie JW: Dizziness and falling in elderly psychiatric outpatients. Am J Psychiatry 137:203, 1980
27. Bissada NK, Finkbeiner AE: Lower Urinary Tract Function and Dysfunction. Diagnosis and Management. Appleton-Century-Crofts, East Norwalk, CT 1978
28. Williams ME, Fitzhugh PC: Urinary incontinence in the elderly. Ann Intern Med 97:895, 1982
29. Resnick NM, Yalla SV: Management of urinary incontinence in the elderly. New Engl J Med 313:800, 1985

7 | The Aging Client and the Family Network

Carl I. Brahce

The unprecedented aging of the American population and the equally dramatic demands that will be made on the health-care system present both challenges and opportunities for those who will service the elderly. Not only will the system need to establish policies for extending health-care benefits to the larger geriatric population, to find ways to train new cadres of well-trained professionals, or to fund the delivery of services equitably to all in need, but there will be a corresponding opportunity to design new concepts of care that can creatively use the new patterns of family interrelationships between older persons and their family members.

As a member of the geriatric health-care team, the physical therapist will need to be knowledgeable of critical relationships between geriatric patients, their meaningful others (family and/or friends), and professionals in meeting this future challenge. The central proposition of this chapter is that the physical therapist will assume a greater responsibility for improving health care of older persons through orientation and training of the informal support system, chiefly the family network or extended kinship or social structure.

A corollary of this premise is that geriatric patients and their family members will continue to seek and require assistance from health and medical personnel in the effort to gain improved functioning and health status. As the primary caregivers, middle-aged women will require understanding and skillful help from the physical therapist and the rehabilitation team. The past decade, notes Cantor,[1] has seen the emergence of considerable research that validates the role of family and other informal supports in caring for frail and chronically ill elderly. The informal support network for older persons goes much further than providing help and assistance; it speaks also to the affectional and social lives of the elderly, with strong implications for their emotional well-being.[2] Sociologists and others have shown that the family network is, in fact, superior

173

to the bureaucracy in performing nonuniform, nonexpert tasks like socialization and the exchange of affection in caring for older persons.[3,4] Several factors, however, are accounting for rapid and significant changes in the intergenerational relationships of family members.

Women are now an integral part of the labor force; women at work has nearly tripled since 1951, increasing from 18,181,000 to 45,915,000 in 1984.[5] This larger labor force participation, in turn, is influencing the relation of employment income to available medical services, to security in retirement, to differential relationships with spouses, and, most certainly, to the traditional kinship role of women. Surprisingly, as will be shown, working women still are retaining their responsibilities as nominal family-member caregivers. Still, the situation has become more stressful and complex and will be a future factor in the continuing role of the family in caring for the most vulnerable elderly. With the greater longevity of the old old (those age 75 and older), it is not uncommon to see new retirees delay their leisure plans in order to care for an aging parent or in-law. For many of the frail elderly, especially single women, but also for men, the extended life span can mean a fragile existence with multiple illnesses. American society has not yet accepted the fact that there is a rapidly increasing chronically ill aging population that will require more diversified supportive services and health care in the future.[6,7]

Researchers continue to find that contrary to prevailing stereotypes, the informal support system provides more assistance than do formal organizations in the care of frail and chronically ill elderly and that without such care institutional living would be inevitable.[1] The family is especially important as a resource in coping with impairment and disability.[7] Health-care professionals now recognize that quality of life is an important issue. To facilitate the individual's coping with disability and quality of life, a holistic approach to care includes patient/family systems treatment during the hospital stay and follow-up in the community in physical rehabilitation.[8] A major task of the rehabilitation team is to provide assistance to family caregivers to improve performance of the nurturant role to the elderly. The patients' well-being is directly related to the extent that they receive assistance from both formal and informal support systems.[9]

The services provided by the formal support system in conjunction with those provided by the informal are important for the physical, social, and psychological well-being of the elderly. The informal support system, composed of family, friends, and neighbors, is viewed as providing the more personal and idiosyncratic services. The formal system, through volunteer agencies and large-scale governmental organizations, provides basic entitlements of health, housing, education, safety, and transportation, as well as those that are mandated under law as the Older Americans Act, Social Security, Medicare, and Medicaid.[10]

In terms of providing quality care to the frail elderly, the relationship between the natural or preexisting helping network and the formal support system needs special attention. The family network may see the formal helping agency representative or medical-team professional (e.g., the physical therapist) as an intruder, and the professional may have difficulty in moving away from traditional service-delivery techniques to work in a peer relationship in an unstructured situation. For this reason, a high level of professional training and discipline is necessary to strengthen the natural system without disturbing its delicate balance.

In the following sections the preceding concepts and premises are discussed in detail. The roles and tasks of the physical therapist as a member of the rehabilitation team caring for the aged will be examined in light of (1) changes in demographics and sociologic patterns of the elderly and the family, (2) health needs and support for elderly, (3) the family's responsibility for care of the elderly, (4) intergenerational relationships and caregiving, (5) the importance of family education, and (6) model approaches to care and programs designed especially for the elderly.

THE PHYSICAL THERAPIST AND GERIATRICS

Why should the physical therapist be concerned about geriatrics? The first part of a rationale for studying geriatrics is to imply a professional requirement. As explained by Hawker in *Geriatrics for Physiotherapists*, geriatrics has finally been established as a branch of general medicine concerned with the clinical, preventive, remedial, and social aspects of health and disability in the elderly.[11] The purpose of geriatric medicine, states Nichols, in the foreword to Hawker's book, is to help restore elderly patients to activity and independence in the home setting or, if this is not practicable, to help patients gain maximum independence and live successfully in an institutional or hospital setting. As part of the total concept of reablement of elderly disabled people, physical therapy can have no meaning unless there is understanding of aging in all its implications, explains Hawker.[11]

> Without this understanding it is easy to believe that the problems of the elderly are unrewarding and insoluble—a matter for do-gooders and geriatricians. It can be more comfortable to think of people in this age group as non-people and so it follows that their needs and problems as individuals do not exist.

In a cross-cultural study of health-care policies and practices in Sweden compared to the United States, Purtilo[12] observes that perhaps the greatest strength of the Swedish approach is an interpretation of justice regarding the quality and extent of medical rehabilitation services as a standard for resource allocation. This leads to policies and practices that enhance the opportunity for a more independent existence for those chronically ill and disabled.

To study geriatric patients and their special needs means acknowledging that the important support usually provided the patient by the family network in the home must be assumed by the members of the rehabilitation team when the patient is institutionalized. Ideally, for any age group, but particularly the elderly, the only time that the family network should be removed or put in a position of secondary importance is in the emergency situation. As soon as the life-or-death crisis is stabilized, the family network should be invited and encouraged (through education programs and counseling as needed) to help the patient prepare for a return to the previous living environment whenever possible. If this step is not taken, the elderly patient will become dependent on the staff and make heavy emotional demands on them. Our goal is to help the family network to work with the rehabilitation team in order to meet the elderly patient's physical, psychological, and social needs and to avoid when possible disrupting the preexisting patterns of support.

The physical therapist needs to recognize that aging is an evolutionary process that affects individuals at different rates and degrees and is an inescapable aspect of life, until death. Old age is not a stage like adolescence that with proper intervention the individual "gets over." It is not a phase but a culmination. The later years of life need not be filled with empty hours or days or with uselessness, but can be especially meaningful and rewarding. The older person has needs that go beyond survival or coping with the problems and losses of life—needs that enable the person to be an expressive and contributing member of the community.[13] Older persons, if they are to achieve maturity, must respond to the needs for relatedness or association with others, for creativity, for security, for individuality, for recognition, and for an intellectual frame of reference.[14]

In terms of the quality of medical rehabilitation services, a weakness in the Swedish practice observed by Purtilo is that compassionate care does not automatically flow from policies and practices that meet the requirement of a needs-based interpretation of justice. She tells of being haunted by the words of a physical therapy student in Stockholm, who was amazed that every time she asked elderly persons about their homes they began to cry. The student did not understand why the older persons were still unhappy, when they had tried so hard, done so much.[12]

Quality of life, reminds Mock,[8] is an issue that rehabilitation always has to address. It means not only health maintenance and functional abilities, but also adjustment to disability, a meaningful life in the face of losses, and management of the reaction of others coping with barriers to full participation in society.

The community is a focal point for helping the elderly remain in or regain a state of well-being in the later years. Community-wide planning must strive to meet the exceedingly complex health needs of older persons and show as great variability as in planning for child services. Convalescent facilities and rehabilitation are special problems requiring combined operations of health, welfare, and educational groups in the community.[15] As members of their society, the elderly want to maintain their independence, they desire above all else to continue being active, contributing, and therefore useful members of the community in which they live.[11]

Growing old is not sudden, but physiologic and psychological changes that take place slowly. Few professionals are prepared for these changes. In addition, normality in an aging population has never been defined. Until recently, there seemed to be no need to distinguish between aging and illness.[10]

As the government and health-care workers look for ways to provide increasingly targeted services to the elderly, one of the foci for planning is the support of the family network that gives care and assistance to elderly members.[2]

THE ELDERLY—A POPULATION IN TRANSITION

It is now accepted that increased life expectancy, the social opportunity for retirement, and independent living for older couples affects the present generation of elderly. Today's seniors, with their "on-the-go" vigor and with their general mobility despite chronic illness and sensory loss in varying degrees, would hardly be recognized as aged persons a few decades ago. They are starting new after-retirement careers; going back to college; taking part in elderhostels; being useful in volunteer activities; helping other, less fortunate elderly; assisting classroom teachers in creative teaching of elementary school children; traveling around the country and beyond in senior travel groups; assuming important advocacy roles through membership in the Gray Panthers or local organizations; and otherwise enjoying their status as senior citizens.

Today's older citizens are contributing to a change in public attitudes or stereotypes on aging through their active roles in volunteer, advocacy, learning, and helping activities—a phenomenon never before seen in our nation, where values of youth and newness have dominated.[16] We are finally discarding the stereotype that the elderly are a homogeneous group and replacing it with a truer image of the enormous diversity among our elderly, observes Lennie-Marie Tolliver, U.S. Commissioner on Aging.[17] A recent issue of *Time* magazine featured today's mobile, energetic older Americans as individuals launching new and successful businesses after retirement, pursuing educational goals in colleges and universities, assuming community roles, and confounding the experts with their vitality and exuberance for life.[18] Such actions, however, do not alter the fact that many elderly, particularly those of minority populations, are still in need of medical and health-care services or will be as they reach their eighties and nineties. The changing demographic patterns are, in fact, indicative of future health-care needs of our oldest citizens, needs that will be of great economic consequence.

T. Franklin Williams, Director, National Institute on Aging, told conferees of the 1988 14th Annual Meeting of the Association for Gerontology in Higher Education that the projections show we are going to need from two to ten times as many health-care professionals—physicians, dentists, psychiatrists, psychologists, social workers, physical therapists, occupational therapists, and others to the level of aides and technicians—in order to prepare for the health-care needs of the older population,[19] and the need for funding to train health and medical-care professionals will increase dramatically. He estimated that Medicare reimbursements for the training of health-service providers for meeting the health needs of Medicare recipients will approach $3 billion, including residency fellowships to train physicians in geriatric medicine. At present, $47 million is being invested in gerontologic education and training, in addition to efforts by the Administration on Aging and the Health Resources and Services Administration. The Administration's $1.6 billion budget now provides funding for 31 Geriatric Education Centers, for geriatric traineeships and fellowships, and other training programs.

The negative consequences of the fact that life expectancy has increased from 49 at the turn of the century to 74.9 in 1986[15] are that the older population itself is getting older. In 1986 the 65 to 74 age group (17.3 million) was eight times larger than in 1900, but the 75 to 84 group (9.1 million) was 12 times larger, and the 85+ group (2.8 million) was 22 times larger.[20]

Medical-health professionals in the future, therefore, can expect to be caring for the most vulnerable elderly as a major part of their practice. Most elderly persons have at least one chronic condition, many have multiple illnesses. In 1984, about 6 million (23 percent) older persons in the community had health-related difficulties; one or more with personal-care activities (19 percent of men, 25 percent of women) and 7.1 million (27 percent) had problems with home-management activities (18 percent of men, 33 percent of women). For the health-care system, these changes pose tremendous challenges for decades ahead when the baby boomers will swell the ranks of the older population. In 1986, older persons accounted for 31 percent of all hospital stays and 42 percent of all days of care in hospital. The elderly also require a larger proportion of the nation's health-care expenditures. In 1984 the 65+ population represented 12 percent of the U.S. population, but was projected to account for 31 percent of total personal health-care expenditures. These expenditures are expected to total $120 billion and to average $4202 per year for each older person (more than three times the $1300 spent for each younger person).[20,21]

Two results of these demographic patterns are important for the practitioner serving the elderly. First, the period in a couple's life beyond child-rearing responsibility can now last for 30, 40, or more years. It is not uncommon for a retired couple to delay moving or travel after work ceases because they are caring for one or more parents.

The existence of four stages of postparental life, rather than one, have been suggested by Thompson and Streib.[22] In the first stage, family of late maturity, the couple's ages are generally between 45 and 54. The majority live in their own homes; 84 percent of the men and 75 percent of the women have been married. More than half these couples still have a child under age 18 at home. The second stage is preretirement; chronologic ages are 55 to 64, and most such persons are still living at home with a spouse. Sex differences in survival are apparent, with 80 percent of the men still married, compared with 62 percent of the women. One third of the still-married women continue to work. In the third stage, the family of early retirement, the ages are 65 to 74. Now the earlier mortality rate for men is noticeable; only 45 percent of women are married, compared to more than 70 percent of the men. During the final 5 years of this period this ratio drops to 36 percent for women, and less than 10 percent of wives are still working. In the fourth stage, late retirement, the ages of husband and wife are 75 and older. Of men aged 75 to 79, 61 percent are still married, 49 percent at age 80 to 84, and 34 percent over age 85. The number of women still married is considerably less: at age 75 to 79 it is 25 percent; at age 80 to 84 it is 14 percent, and over age 85 it is only 6 percent. It can be seen that the health-care needs of older women are related to their single status as widows or never-marrieds who often live alone. Many have outlived not only their spouses but their children as well.

A second result of demographic changes in the elderly for the health-care team has to do with grandparenting. Several trends regarding modern grandparenthood are suggested by Hagestad.[23] Because women are completing childbearing responsibilities early in adulthood, active parenting days are over by the time they become grandmothers. Gutmann[24] coined the term "emeritus parents" for these women who assume new roles as managers of the extended family. They are supporters (kinkeepers) for more generations, serving such vital functions as safety-valve relievers for family members or supporters of teenagers. The dynamic changes in family patterns, including divorce and mixed families, suggests new, potentially complex family networks. Hagestad observes that we now have four- and five-generation families, unprecedented duration of family relationships, as well as unique webs of experiences for individual members.[23]

In our society, notes Hagestad, the greater life expectancy of women and their younger age at marriage results in the world of the very old being a world of women.[23] Among the oldest old, there are 41 men for every 100 women; and for the younger old (65 to 74), there are only 75 to every 100 women.[20,21] Half of all older women were widows in 1986, and there were five times as many widows (8.1 million) as widowers (1.5 million). And yet, research findings continue to substantiate that family influence remains strong in caring for their elderly members. The majority (67 percent) of noninstitutionalized elderly persons lived in a family setting—83 percent of older men and 57 percent of older women. About 14 percent were not living with a spouse but were living with children, siblings, or other relatives. Another new trend is that of more congregate living arrangements participated in by older persons. An additional 3 percent of men and 2 percent of women, or 616,000 older persons were living with nonrelatives in 1986.[20,21]

As pointed out by Troll,[25] grandparenting has become a middle-age rather than an old-age event. Earlier marriages, earlier childbirth, and longer life expectancy result in grandparents who are only in their forties. Because these grandparents usually have only a few children, they are truly grandparents in identity and not also themselves parents of young children. In addition, owing to the increase in three- and four-generation families, the grandparent becomes a second- rather than a first-generation event (not the oldest generation). Therefore, the old rocking-chair image of grandmother sitting and idly knitting or crocheting is manifestly false today.

THE FAMILY IN TRANSITION

For the elderly, meaningful participation in a family group is a major source of important activity.[4] Institutionalization for the elderly, whether voluntary or involuntary, is often seen as a final surrender to the realization that they can no longer care for themselves. Fierce independence in old age is a mark of the elderly who combated depression, endured hard, long years of backbreaking work, and lived primarily for their children. Going to the hospital or nursing home or other long-term facility is still unthinkable for many. Salber, in a collection of rural elderly voices, reports this tradition:[26]

> "What do I want for myself, right now? I just want to be able to wait on myself. I don't want to put myself on my children. I don't want to be a bother to nobody."

> "Now if I got sick, I have the children to look after me. But I just hope and pray when I gets sick to die, I hope I'll just die. I don't want to be no trouble to nobody. . . . I don't know about nursing homes. As far as I'm concerned, I don't think I'd want to go to one. . . . I stayed in the sanitorium for three years (I had T.B. and I had to have my lung out) and I didn't like that too good, so I know I wouldn't like a nursing home. You don't get the treatment that you should get I don't think."

> "I was raised to work and I still enjoy it. I'll go on working as long as I'm able. When I'm not able, when I get to that, I hope I'll do a big day's work and lay down at night and go to sleep and not wake up. I tell people. Don't send me flowers when I'm dead. I want them now. It wouldn't do me two cents worth of good after I'm dead to put me in my grave and put a pile of flowers on me as high as this house. If you've got a flower you want me to have, give it to me while I'm living."

Such beliefs are an important factor in postponing as long as possible the entering of homes for the aged or hospitals for the chronically ill.[4] The multidisciplinary geriatric team is crucial to the evaluation and care of the complex and frail elderly patient.[27] Rehabilitation specialists such as the physical therapist often view independent living (or returning to work) as target outcomes of successful rehabilitation. They recognize, however, that these may be unrealistic goals for many elderly persons. It is the responsibility of the rehabilitation team to provide a setting where education, support, and the provision of alternatives are constantly in exchange.[8] The needs of rehabilitation patients defined by Towle[28] as basic to psychological survival are (1) self-respect, (2) social acceptance, (3) satisfying work, (4) adequate recreation, (5) freedom of choice, (6) an intimate love relationship with mutually satisfying exchange of human affection and an uncomplicated release of biological energies, and (7) a physically healthy body that can be taken for granted.

The important role of the patient's daughter or other primary family caregiver in giving the older person emotional support in view of fear of impending treatment as well as potential losses is evident. The physical therapist emphasizes with the patient and family member the importance of setting short-term goals or plans. In this process, that which is dreamed of or wished for (level of unreality) becomes separated from what is expected (level of reality) in the future.[8]

Anderson[27] notes that goal setting includes early identification of conflicts among combinations of patient–family goals and individual treatment programs; enhancing family–patient–staff interaction through negotiation; and the setting of treatment priorities, including the patient and family members as active and responsible team members. The family is taught how to develop longer lasting rehabilitation goals through compromise goals. The team aims at reducing sabotage of treatment goals by the patient or family.

The rehabilitation team includes besides the physical therapist, the physician (usually the team leader), rehabilitation nurse, psychologist, social service worker, occupational therapist, speech pathologist, vocational counselor, recreational therapist, dietician, prosthetist, orthotist, and others as needed.

Facilitating communication and understanding between the family and the interdisciplinary team is a significant task during the treatment phase.[8] The social worker in this effort is supportive to the patient's familial needs and problems. Continued educational information is provided as necessary in order to assist with gaining those community resources that the patient will need after discharge. The systematic process of problem identification and resolution usually depends on the interactions that various team members have with the patient and family members. This includes their interpretation of what will be required in continuing medical care, caregiving needs, obtaining supplies and equipment, safety factors, and community resources. In terms of the now current philosophy toward deinstitutionalization, the family is viewed as the most logical support and possible caregiver.

On rehabilitation, points out Mock,[8] the family systems approach is preferable to individual treatment. Advantages are (1) the treatment team receives more information and a clearer perspective about the family situation and is able to give feedback to the entire family system; (2) the treatment team can have the family do things they cannot do, such as small tasks like home measurement to the greater responsibility for providing continuing support and care—this process reinforces the family's sense of integrity and control; (3) problem solving together as a family system within the hospital prepares family members for doing this at home; and (4) the focus for concern is not only the patient; everyone's problems in coping are discussed.[8]

In this interaction, the family is defined as two or more persons with a mutually interactive support system. Members can be married (spousal) or related (children). They have strong emotional bonds and a method of communication, and share rules and values. In family-systems theory, as defined by Kramer,[29] the therapist looks on families as holistic functioning units that are composed of interdependent parts.

Patients, then, are not the only ones in this process to have problems; families also have problems. Symptoms of these may include very stressful reactions, communication barriers or secrets, scapegoating, or emotional alienation. Here, in the context of the older patient, it will be well to review the special relationships that can prevail.

The elderly and their family network need to be educated as to the importance of temporary, short-term (up to 3 months) institutional placements for rehabilitation that can lead to discharge to their homes.

The family network is important in helping the elderly to remain both active and independent. The well-being of the older person is directly related to the extent that assistance is received from both the informal support system (the family) and the formal support system (organized health and medical services).[4] The family network helping the elderly person who needs to deal with the bureaucracies in order to survive often serves as a mediating link between the older person and societal institutions and organizations.[4]

Just how important is the family to the old in terms of this linkage to formal systems? In a study of informal and formal supports to maintain older people in a community, clients and their primary informal caregivers were interviewed. The research, dealing specifically with those older persons who had turned to an agency in New York City, was funded by Title III of the Older Americans Act to provide homemaker services to the marginal poor in need of such services. These services included housekeeping, shopping, and escort, as well as hands-on assistance with bathing, dressing, toileting, and such. More than half of the respondents indicated the reason for requesting homemaker services was an accident or sudden illness; 42 percent felt they gradually needed more help in order to manage at home. Findings showed that even while formal services were being provided, the family caretakers, friends, and neighbors continued to play an active role in caring for the frail elderly.[10]

The hierarchic–compensatory model is generally viewed to be a function of the primary relationship of support given to the older person rather than by the nature of the task. Elderly persons, according to this concept, would prefer to receive assistance from their family. If family is not available, friends and neighbors are the next choice, followed by formal organizations.[30]

It needs to be emphasized that numerous studies have shown that the family remains the critical bulwark against personal and social loss for the elderly. As Sussman[4] reminds us:

> The immortal adage of "blood is thicker than water" seems to hold even in this postindustrialized period. In societies undergoing rapid changes from rural to an industrial based-economy, such as Egypt, Iran, and Pakistan, family bondings are the primary structures vis-a-vis mechanisms for making bureaucracies functional and tolerable.

Lebowitz[7] elaborates on two common misconceptions about the family. The first notion concerns the low level of functional utility of the family in contemporary industrial society:

It seems common sense to many that geographic mobility, industrialization, the rise of specialized organizations for education, child care, and work have all made the family a useless or vestigial manifestation of an earlier mode of social organization. After all, the argument goes, grandparents no longer live upstairs from their married children, family gatherings rarely take place, and people would rather be in some nuclear family unit of one or perhaps two generations. Contemporary scholarship has shown this to be an inadequate conceptualization in at least two ways. First, historical studies have shown that the idealized characterization of family life in the past is both inadequate and inaccurate. Things were not so good in those good old days, as the historical and comparative studies in family structure are beginning to show. Second, the loss of family based functions has only succeeded in re-defining the notion of family into such notions as the "modified extended family" [Shanas and Streib[31] cited]. Other studies have identified the fictive kin functioning of networks of friends, neighbors, and others within a person's social environment. It is therefore safe to say that notions concerning the death of the family are misplaced and of dubious validity.

The second misconception holds that if families still function, they do not do so for the elderly. This argument says that most old people are alone, without support, and therefore both physically and socially isolated. It is true that many elderly live alone—14 percent of the men and 36 percent of the women over age 65, but it does not necessarily follow that they are isolated.[7] It has been noted that despite the geographic mobility of the U.S. population, many older persons who have children live close to at least one of them. In addition, such parents do see their children often.[32]

HEALTH NEEDS AND SUPPORTS FOR THE ELDERLY

The older person's family network is significant in maintaining the well-being and supporting the independent status of that individual. This informal support system becomes especially important for the chronically ill person or someone who has suffered a debilitating impairment. Such impairments, particularly progressive neurologic diseases (e.g., parkinsonism), interfere with function. As such, they threaten to undermine personal independence and those older persons need much support.[11] In addition to these illnesses, persons in the later stage of life may suffer from skeletal disorders, respiratory diseases, and sensory losses, which can be equally disabling and which often contribute to psychological disorientation. Depression or mental impairment is especially demanding on the adult-child caretakers or others in the family kinship network providing support. The physical therapist, whether involved with the patient in the home, hospital, or nursing home, can benefit from an awareness of the family role in maintaining the older patient's independence and/or facilitating rehabilitation to an enhanced physical and mental capability.

To better understand the needs of older patients, let us look at normal dependencies of aging. Blenkner[33] points out that dependency for the old is a state of being, not a state of mind; a state of being in which to be old—as to be young—is to be dependent.

> Such dependency is not pathological, it is not wrong; in fact, a right of the old recognized by most if not all societies. It cannot be cured and the only way to forestall it is to die young.

These normal dependencies may be explained as follows:

1. Economic dependency stems from having crossed over from the productive to the consumer status in the economy. No longer a wage earner, or the spouse of a wage earner, and not having been able to accumulate sufficient savings to support oneself through 15 to 25 years of retirement, the older person typically finds himself or herself dependent on income transfer from the currently working generation, provided primarily through taxes but also by contributions from children and other younger relatives.[34]

2. Physical dependency arises from the simple fact that in the process of advanced aging muscle strength inevitably diminishes, sensory acuity decreases, reflexes are slower, coordination is poorer, and the general level of energy is lower. The ordinary chores of living—personal self-care and grooming, keeping up one's living quarters, preparing or securing food, transporting oneself from place to place, shopping, participating in social functions, etc.—become increasingly difficult, strenuous, and eventually impossible to perform entirely without aid.

3. Mental dependency arises from a decline in the power of mentation paralleling the decline in physical power, but occurring more slowly or not reaching such magnitude as to be seen as a source of dependency until quite advanced old age, and in some cases never. At that time, when deterioration or change in the central nervous system produces marked deficits in memory, orientation, comprehension, and judgment, old persons quite literally no longer can use their heads to solve their problems and direct their affairs; they must rely on the cognitive functions of others.[35]

4. Social dependency develops out of a matrix of factors and losses. As persons age, they lose others who are important objects and sources of affection, stimulation, and assistance. They lose roles that are the basis of status and power and avenues to social participation. They lose contemporaneity as their knowledge, values, and expectations become obsolete in a fast-changing society. They become without volition progressively isolated and disengaged nonparticipants in the surrounding social world, increasingly dependent on bureaucratized substitutes for missing kith, kin, and agents of former days, increasingly dependent on recognition by others of their rights rather than their power. They become dependent on the social conscience of the generation in positions of authority, dependent on those who currently have all that they have lost in the way of vitality and performance.[33]

Blenkner[33] suggests that there are three sources of help or types of solution for the normal dependencies of aging. The first is self-solution, whereby the older person seeks to modify her or his behavior or circumstances. Examples would be balancing one's budget by restricting consumption, conserving energy by restricting activities, bolstering failing memory by writing notes to oneself, countering social losses by social disengagement—a first line of defense. These methods are sensible and valid ways of coping, but they work only up to a point. The individual may increase such devices until they become pathologic and perhaps jeopardize survival of the individual.[36]

The second is the kinship solution, which requires the existence and proximity of children or other relatives. For those aged who are fortunate enough to have concerned and capable kin, most of their dependent needs can be and usually are met by family members providing caregiving services.

In this situation the typical old person remains in his or her own household as long as he or she is capable of personal self-care. Children or other relatives (traditionally a daughter or niece) increasingly take on or assist with the heavier tasks of housekeeping and home maintenance; provide transportation and escort; manage financial affairs; supervise health care; nurse the person in time of illness; and generally substitute their strength, mobility, and judgment for the older person's declining abilities. If or when the older person becomes too ill or frail, she or he may be taken into the caretaker's home. When the demand for intensive and skilled care rises beyond the capacity of the family network, the elderly person may be institutionalized.

These family kinship support roles are sensible and valid, up to a point. An excessive burden of care, however, can be too much for the caretakers and other family members.[33] (Difficulties with the intergenerational aspects of caretaking are described below.)

The third solution is the societal solution. In this arrangement society assists its members through established programs or policies that are beyond the resources of individuals and their primary group. Examples of these solutions are social insurance, public housing and rent supplementation, and Medicaid.

Some State Departments on Aging or Commissions on Aging recently have undertaken the development and funding of social support programs administered through Area Agencies of Aging to extend more health and home support services in the expectation that these efforts will delay institutionalization of elderly persons. For example, the Pre-Admission Screening System Providing Options and Resources Today (PASSPORT) is a partnership program between the Ohio Department of Human Services and the Ohio Department of Aging. This program is designed to slow the growth in Medicaid nursing-home spending by increasing the availability of lower-cost community-based care allowing clients in need of services to remain in their homes. In 1981 the federal Omnibus Budget Reconciliation Act was passed, allowing the states to apply for Home and Community-Based Service Waivers that opened the door for program like PASSPORT to be established around the country.

Ohio is one of the eight states accounting for about half of persons age 65 and older. Receiving its waiver in 1984, PASSPORT started in nine counties and added three more in 1986. State planners are aiming for statewide expansion of the program by 1991. Physical therapy is one of a number of in-home services (case management, registered nursing home-health aide, home-delivered meals, adaptive and assistive equipment, occupational and speech therapy, adult day care, and noninstitutional care) provided to the elderly.

Gerontologists and other social scientists continue to investigate health service needs of elderly persons in view of available supports and the increases in persons age 65 and older. Research-based national and regional surveys have demonstrated that the use of health services is highest among divorced and separated, widowed, and never-married persons than among those who are married.[37]

It should not be thought that societal measures are adequate for health maintenance and long-term care of the elderly. There is a tremendous need to develop and expand imaginative and inventive societal solutions to the normal dependencies of aging.[33] With the extension of life after retirement and the continuing rise of inflation, many elderly people are increasingly in need of a national policy of long-term care and a community care system available to all. In addition to Medicare and Medicaid, the elderly need a broad array of social and health-related services that are supportive of home-based care. The escalation of costs, coupled with a mounting public concern over the gross inadequacies of current programs, is resulting in public recognition that action is needed. An indication of this urgency is to be found in the 1981 White House Conference on Aging Act, accepting the findings by Congress that there is a great need for a more comprehensive long-term care policy (with a strong home-care component) responsive to the needs of older patients and their families.[38]

The need for a comprehensive long-term care program to offset the devastating cost of acute catastrophic illness is more evident than ever before with the increase in the oldest segment of the population to more than double their present number to 5.4 million. Legislative action to provide long-term care protection against the ravages of Alzheimer's disease or to protect against extended nursing-home stays that literally wipe out savings of elderly persons in less than a year remains an urgent priority for a Congress faced with a massive budget deficit and rising costs for present health assistance programs. A national strategy to attempt an answer to some of the problems occurred in October 1983 when Medicare introduced a prospective payment system (PPS) based on diagnosis-related groups (DRGs) in an effort to control the escalating cost of Medicare-funded hospitalizations. This new system has brought about a major change in the long-term health-care system.[39]

The following sections discuss the medical-health needs of the elderly and the family roles in responding to responsibilities for caregiving in conjunction with the community and professional systems.

FAMILY RESPONSIBILITY IN CARE OF THE ELDERLY

In a study that examined marital status and living arrangements as they affect the use of informal and formal health services by the elderly, Cafferata[37] found that both physician visits and the likelihood of a hospitalization are affected primarily by the need for care, particularly in the presence of a chronic condition, worry about health, and the total number of bed-disability days. Older persons who lived with others besides a spouse had significantly more bed-disability days than did those who lived alone. Disability days were found to be affected by age (positive); education (negative); employment (negative) and health status measures: perceived aging, poor health, the presence of a limitation; presence of a chronic condition, and worry.[37] The importance of this study is that the large number of persons who live alone in the United States and their relatively higher rates of use compared with those living with others has implications for the health-care economy (even more so, when one considers the present and projected numbers of frail elderly who will require health-care services in the future.)

In another study, Antonucci and Akiyama[40] investigated the extent of social support networks for older adults using a national sample. They borrowed the term convoy from anthropologist David Plath to convey the image of protective layers of family and friends that help the individual cope with life's challenges. They learned that it was the middle-aged group, not the oldest or youngest, who received support from the largest number of network members. This suggests that the older persons receive more various support from fewer network members. Also, respondents in the middle-age group reported that their network members received the most respect from them.[40]

Providers of health and social services to the elderly must realize that the idea of alienation of the old by the young has been found to be a groundless misconception. This social myth—that old people who live alone or apart from their children are neglected by their children—is perpetuated by aged persons themselves, especially childless old people, and by professional workers.[9,41] Elderly persons prefer to maintain their independence as long as possible, but when no longer able to manage they expect their children to assume that responsibility. Research of the past two decades shows that children give services involving physical care, shelter, and household and other related tasks, as well as sharing leisure time.[42] More significantly, as has already been shown with regard to linkage of formal services to family caregivers, without the care extended by their informal support networks, more elderly persons would very likely be forced to leave their homes and enter long-term care institutions. A recent study of the nature of the informal support system for older persons revealed that spouse and children were the cornerstone of the support system, followed by friends and neighbors.[1] The family is increasingly seen as the focus for treatment in clinical or social services for the elderly.[43] An earlier study showed that 87 percent of the elderly in Cleveland reported having a primary source of informal assistance available on a long-term basis, usually the family.[44] According to the National Center for Health Statistics,[45] family assistance to elderly family members comprises up to 80 percent of the care that elderly persons receive. The common forms of help are homemaker services, transportation, and personal care, including care in times of illness. As noted earlier, family members also serve as mediator and advisor to the elderly and as a linkage to formal or bureaucratic services, including health, financial, and social-recreational.[4]

The Cleveland study[44] revealed that family services are more extensive for assisting the severely impaired elderly, a fact noted by officials and gerontologists advocating policies to provide financial assistance to family caretakers. Califano stated that too often programs for the elderly have been designed with the individual but not the family network in mind: "We have failed to tap the strength of the family in caring for the elderly." It seems that family and kin, however defined, will continue to be the primary groups who will respond in service and kind when elderly family members call or are in need.[4]

The place of the elderly in family structures is shown by studies of living arrangements of persons 65 and older. Because women live longer than men and thus have less choice in partners for second marriages, they are more active in linkage activities within the family. Age and number of children seem to be the most important predictors of moving into a family member's household when living alone becomes untenable because of diminished health and mobility.[4]

Four kinds of relationships or dimensions have been suggested to assess family or kin structure:[25] (1) residential proximity—how close relatives live to each other; (2) interaction frequency—how often relatives visit, phone, or write each other; (3) economic interdependence or mutual aid; and (4) a variety of more subtle qualitative measures, such as the valuing of "familism," the transmission of values, and the strength of affectional bonds.

Researchers agree that the kinship ties are strongest between female members in the helping relationships. It is usually the daughter or daughter-in-law who acts as caretaker. The mother–daughter relationship tends to be stronger than the mother–son bond from adulthood on. Other researchers have found that the sister–sister tie is stronger than either the sister–brother or the brother–brother tie. Although most studies show a bias toward female-linked relationships in the family network (residence is closer to wife's parents; interaction is greater with wife's relatives, interaction is mutual and more frequent along female lines; and affection is said to be greater among women), Adams found little sex differentiation in his research on kinship interrelationships except for patterns of mutual aid. More men than women gave help in both money and services, such as work in the house, to their parents. Also, because women outlive men in the later years of life, more older men than women actually live in families. Widowers are much more likely to remarry than widows. On the other hand, older widows (closer to their daughters) are more likely to move in with children, usually daughters, when they no longer can manage to live alone than are older widowers.[25,47,48]

As pointed out earlier, the current generation of elderly are a hardy cohort, and research of the past several years shows that they prefer to live independently in their own household. Even after a spouse dies, and faced with the emotional difficulties associated with bereavement, older persons strive to maintain their independence. The important fact for physical therapists and others on the health-care team to recognize is that the family members do provide meaningful strength and support to the elderly across many dimensions. As Sussman states,[4]

> The continued psychological well-being of the aged, similar to the needs of persons at all stages of life, is largely dependent upon a high level of activity, involvement with other persons, and with interests beyond their own personal lives. Meaningful participation in a family group is a major source of such activity for the elderly.

As noted by Stone and coworkers, research of the past four decades has successfully shattered the myth of the lack of family involvement.[49] Litwak[50] theorized that helpers feel an even stronger extended family orientation than do the elderly themselves. Research has shown that older persons continue to play a role, often reciprocal, in family networks, maintaining close communication with relatives, friends, and neighbors; that the primary caregiver is usually a wife or daughter; and that a pattern of intergenerational reciprocity exists in most families. Rosenmayer[51] termed ''intimacy at a distance'' the findings that widowed, divorced, or never-married elderly prefer to live independently but near their relatives.

The nature of caregiving activities varies from family to family, but even working daughters provide considerable emotional support as well as performing a variety of tasks. Horowitz[52] conceptualized caregiving behavior as being in four primary areas: emotional support, direct support provision, linkage with the formal sector, and financial assistance. Family and friends do not necessarily specialize in particular support assistance, but increase it as the need arises.[1,49]

As a number of studies have consistently shown, it is usually the spouses, daughters, or daughters-in-law who provide the most help of all kinds. Men, other than spouses, are more likely to assist with financial and transportation, as well as home-repair assistance, to their parents and in-laws.

Probing the impact of caregiving, researchers have found that the most serious problem for caregivers is stress or emotional strain causing caregiver burden. Stress also is exacerbated by conflicting demands of time, especially for working women, in particular those who still care for dependent children as well as a spouse. Investigating caregiver burden, Pearson et al.[53] studied elderly psychiatric patients, patient depression, and caregiver stress. They found descrepancies between patient abilities and behaviors to be important contributors to caregiver stress and perceptions of burden. Their findings supported earlier research that patient confusion and physical dependency were associated with caregiver burden.

In a comprehensive study using a national data base, Stone et al.[49] examined major characteristics of caregivers. The findings are as follows: in 1982 approximately 2.2 million caregivers aged 24 or older were providing unpaid assistance to 1.6 million noninstitutionalized disabled elderly with one or more ADL limitations. About one-fifth of care recipients were 85 or older, with a mean age of 78 years. Of the total, 60 percent were women, 51 percent were married, and 41 percent were widowed. Approximately 40 percent lived with a spouse only, 36 percent resided with their spouse and children or children only, and 11 percent lived alone. Recent estimates from the National Center for Health Statistics indicated that one third of the overall noninstitutionalized elderly population live alone.[49]

Investigating attitudes of filial obligation, Finley and associates[52] learned that regardless of the personal motivation for caregiving, obligations to provide care to an older parent do not simply result from feelings of affection. It is role conflict, rather than employment status or number of children, that is suspected of influencing levels of filial obligation. For some persons, social and environmental factors like distance and role conflict do make it difficult to meet societal expectations.

INTERGENERATIONAL RELATIONSHIPS AND CAREGIVING

Research in intergenerational relations is a relatively recent phenomenon. As observed by Troll,[25] there is nearly a 30-year gap between parent–child relationships dealing in the launching stage, when the parents are in early middle age, and relationships involving aged parents and their adult children. Between these two points, both parental and child couples are growing older, but there are few data on life-cycle patterns of behavior in this period.

During the first phase, middle-aged parents are frequently visited by children, and parents provide help to children in the form of services or money. The American norm requires independence of the newly married couple. They are expected to establish a home separate from both sets of parents, raise their children, and be economically independent, by virtue primarily of their own efforts and successes. At the other end of the age scale, the stereotype of old parents is that they desire dependence on their adult children and demand services, moving in with children where possible; but generally they are neglected and unwanted.

Actually, most young couples in the United States seem to live reasonably close to both sets of parents, receive help in the form of either services (babysitting) or money, and visit often. Most old parents prefer to live alone and to see their children frequently. Blenkner[9] has described the concept of "filial maturity" seen for that stage as part of the developmental sequence representing the healthy transition from genital maturity to old age. This concept has its own sequence of stages. A filial crisis may be said to occur in most persons in their forties or fifties, when the individual's parents can no longer be looked to as a rock of support in times of emotional trouble or economic stress but may themselves need their children's comfort and support. Successful accomplishment of the filial task or performance of the filial role promotes filial maturity. This has its own gratification, leading into and preparing the middle-aged person for successful accomplishments of the developmental tasks of old age—the last of which is to die.[9]

In this concept Blenkner refutes the earlier concept of role reversal formerly held by many gerontologists—that as the parents age they take on the child's former dependent role while the child assumes the parents' supportive role. Blenkner postulates that the son or daughter does not assume the parental role toward the parents but rather grows into a mature filial role. This role is that of being depended on and therefore means being dependable. In achieving this filial maturity that occurs in middle age, the adult turns again to the parent, no longer as a child but as a mature adult with a new role and a different love. The adult child sees the parents for the first time as individuals with their own rights, needs, limitations, and life histories that to a large extent made them the people they are long before the child existed. As Blenkner explains, this is what parents want of their children; this is what society expects; this is what many Americans do accomplish, with varying degrees of success, in their late forties and fifties. It is also one of the ways in which the adult children prepare themselves for their own aging, through identification with the parent, just as in childhood they similarly prepared for adulthood.[9]

A major role of the therapeutic professions can be that of helping the middle-aged family member, client, or patient accomplish this task as best as possible. This is important because it will ultimately determine how successfully the challenge of growing old is met.[9]

The importance of reciprocity in relationship is suggested by Troll.[25] The significance of the parent–child relationship is that it continues throughout life. Parents who continue to mature throughout their lives, who accept their own development as meaningful and satisfying, are really assisting their children to mature in turn.

The situation of the caretaker as helper to elderly parent(s) or relatives—that is, one who carries out the concept of filial maturity and is responsible—can become critical for the middle-aged caretaker. Usually a woman whose children have just left the home may be in the process of adjusting to important changes in her own life cycle. These changes for the middle-aged woman may have to do with conflicting obligations to teenaged children or to spouse, the postponement of assuming a career again, or returning to school to learn new skills. Because members of the older generation are remaining independent longer, the adult caretaker may also be coping with retirement. There are many parent–child pairs in which the children themselves are at or near retirement.[55] In addition to these pressures, career obligations may conflict with the caregiving role, especially with the increase in numbers of women now in the labor force. The middle-age crunch of responsibility is a time of midlife crisis for the adult caretaker; who becomes a member of the sandwiched generation.[56]

As illustrated earlier, certain differences between the age cohorts of adult children and aged parents are a result of both social changes and personal expectations due to changes in the life cycle. In the matter of providing supports these two generations may experience difficulty or conflict. The first fact to be considered is that for middle-aged and older parents, or young-old and very old generations, parents and children are adults or social equals. The earlier socially sanctioned power imbalance based on the minority position of the child and the child's economic dependence is gone. Also gone, along with the public entitlements of social insurance, Social Security, and Medicare, is the reverse situation—complete economic dependence of an elderly parent on children. Along with this status, both older generations, if still married, retain primary emotional investments in and obligations to their marriage partners. (This becomes more complicated in the case of in-laws).[57]

Second, regardless of time or social context, members of different generations have vastly different life experiences and are products of different social influences. In this sense the middle-aged and old will continue to bring different motivations, aspirations, beliefs, and expectations, as well as different capacities, to their mutual relationships. Even when they may experience the same historical events, such as war or depression, their different age locations and cohort memberships mean the event will have varying impacts on their lives. Each has encountered unique life situations, and, consequently, the middle-aged and old have self-interests that are potentially productive of conflict in the societal arena—and of strain in the intergenerational relationship.[57]

The intergenerational difficulties may be of two orders: those arising from age structure alone, and those compounded by long-standing conflict within the family.[55] The first group is marked by the following[55]:

1. The problem of fatigue. Pressures on the caretaker may be too much, particularly in the case of illness or incapacitation.
2. The problem of competing demands. Particularly pressured are those sons or daughters caught between spouse, children, and the elderly parent.

Intergenerational difficulties created by old patterns of conflict within family include the following[55]:

1. The problem of anaclitic age and depression. Adults may be unable to accept a dominant parent's decline.
2. The problem of the wrong survivor. If the family script has called for the other parent to die first, it may be hard for members to relate to the real survivor.
3. The problem of sibling rivalry. Sibling rivalry may persist to the very deathbed of the courted parent. Generally, one sister or brother is doing most of the work; another appears to be getting most of the credit. Often the put-upon sibling is not giving the other a chance to do a fair share because the purpose is to show how unworthy the rival is. None of this is helped by a parent who instinctively grasps the benefits to be derived from the competition.

4. The problem of the unemancipated son or daughter. Most adolescents separate painfully from their childhood selves with all their dependence on parental approval and all their fantasies of parental omnipotence, but a few adults continue to behave as if governed by an ambivalent drive for independence. Sometimes the aging adolescent forgoes marriage and remains an uneasy son or daughter in the home. If the parent is unable to let go, the relationship may be marked by alternate periods of appeasement and explosion.

These problems can be synergistic, but generally several approaches can be useful. The following are applicable[55]:

1. Encouraging all parties to make reasonable demands before these take the form of confrontation improves the climate.
2. Emphasizing that now is not then improves reality testing, even without much insight or working through.
3. Accepting the negative part of the ambivalence and putting it in the context of the total behavior promotes better relations.
4. Redefining the old person as interactive reduces guilt and restores perspective. This is especially important if the parent is becoming confused or going into an institutional placement.

One common error of adult children is to exclude the parent from planning or decision-making on the grounds that they are too fierce to be faced, too impotent to be counted, or too vulnerable to be told. In so doing, the adult children reduce the older parent or relative to objects. Similarly, children caretakers need to understand that confusion is not constant and that even persons incapable of ultimate responsibility may contribute to a decision. Persons not fully oriented may still be aware of their own feelings and sensitive to the way others in the family are responding to them.

THE IMPERATIVE OF EDUCATION FOR FAMILY
CARETAKERS AND PROFESSIONALS

The beneficial aspects of caretaking within the family are strengthened with an educational intervention offering both knowledge and emotional support to caretakers.[58] Professionals and social workers providing health and medical services to elderly patients could similarly profit from an opportunity to learn about the realities of the aging process and the pitfalls or stress points in the vital function of family care of the elderly.[59] Lebowitz noted that most older persons are tied into a network of social support (primarily adult children) and that fictive kin (friends and neighbors) provide important supportive services. He identified certain gaps in research findings that need attention; one fundamental gap in knowledge concerns the manner in which portions of support systems are activated to provide assistance to the older person.[7]

We do not have the basic understanding of the decision (making) process whereby an older person reaches out for help or in which family members or friends offer support. Our studies have not captured the complexity of this dynamic situation.

Research also has failed to conceptualize adequately the dynamic processes of identification, conflict, evaluation, and decision that are characteristic of the relationship between family members. Too little is known about disagreements between older people and their family or friends, or the dimensions of depression. Someone who is depressed is unlikely to seek help and often is reluctant to accept it when offered. Consequently, supports may not be activated. This issue represents another gap in knowledge.[7]

Institutionalization of the elderly is not required for the majority of aged persons. As noted earlier, the current philosophy is toward deinstitutionalization and return to natural, nonrestrictive environments.[8] The family plays a critical role in maintaining the psychological well-being of the elderly family members.

The family group is seen as the most logical support of possible caregivers, especially if the program is for long-term disability. As pointed out earlier, present governmental efforts are directed to supporting home health-care services and extending home care. Research indicates that many families adjust well to caring for a disabled family member, changing in role flexibility, group cohesiveness, as well as evidence of more problem-solving and self-regulatory behavior.

Family involvement, education, and counseling are sensible strategies for the total rehabilitation management of patients. The outcome of rehabilitation is related to the specific environment, not only in terms of accessibility but in family understanding and ability to cope with ensuing exchanges.[6]

In maintaining the psychological well-being of the elderly family member, the family plays a critical role; the health-care professional can be a consultant in the helping pattern of services. To the aged, institutionalization, as suggested previously, may be seen as a final surrender of self-care and meaningful activity. One recommendation to improve hospital rehabilitation is to increase the flexibility of hospital rehabilitation programs sufficiently to allow the elderly person to return to the community as quickly as possible[4] (e.g., short home visits during the rehabilitation process).

Nothing is more unbearable to the older person than being alone and feeling unwanted. The family has the capacity to give the older person a sense of being accepted and being loved. When the family can give its love and understanding, the physical handicaps that older persons must live with become easier to bear.[6] It is therefore necessary to support the patient–family contact during institutional-based rehabilitation so as not to alienate the patient from the family network in the name of rehabilitation. In home-based rehabilitation programs or institutional-based programs with a strong family education and counseling component, both the patient and the family are more likely to be accepting of the final outcomes.

Butler and Lewis[60] have pointed out that countertransference in the classic sense occurs when mental-health personnel find themselves perceiving and reacting to older persons in ways that are inappropriate and reminiscent of earlier patterns of relating to parents, siblings, and such key childhood figures. Because the professional relationships are critical for physical therapists as well as professionals involved in psychotherapy, difficulties from ageist attitudes of staff are worth noting. Butler states that staff members have to deal with leftover feelings from their personal pasts that may interfere with their perceptions of an older person. They also must be aware of a multitude of negative cultural attitudes toward the elderly that pervade social institutions as well as individual psyches. The Committee on Aging of the Group for the Advancement of Psychiatry listed the following major reasons for negative attitudes of staff toward treating older persons.[60]

1. The aged stimulate the therapist's fears about his or her own age.
2. The aged arouse the therapist's conflicts about her or his relationship with parental figures.
3. The therapist believes that he or she has nothing useful to offer older people because she or he believes that they cannot change their behavior or that their problems are all due to untreatable organic brain diseases.
4. The therapist believes that psychodynamic skills will be wasted in working with the aged, since they are near death and not really deserving of attention.
5. The aged patient might die while in treatment, which could challenge the therapist's sense of importance.
6. The therapist's colleagues may be contemptuous of efforts on behalf of aged patients.

(One often hears the remark that gerontologists or geriatric specialists have a morbid preoccupation with death; their interest in the elderly is therefore "sick" or suspect.)

Another difficulty that may affect the health-care worker's treatment of the aged is what seems to be a human propensity for hostility toward handicapped persons, stemming from unconscious overidentification with older persons, especially those who are physically handicapped or thought to be crippled and powerless. What may result is oversympathetic concern, resulting in hostility.[60]

On the whole, we do not know much specifically about old age, as most clinical experience and research has been of the sick and institutionalized rather than the healthy, active elderly. One consequence of this limitation, observes Butler,[60] is the loss of the more enduring, intensive relationship of treatment for personnel and patients, which could be an important source of data about older persons as well as a check on therapist evaluation of them. Similarly, the physician rarely encounters a member of the older patient's family (except the spouse) until the patient's capability for living independently is challenged.[43]

There are definite reasons why the physical therapist and other members of the rehabilitation team now prefer the family system treatment approach to individual treatment.[8] Advantages are (1) the treatment team can receive more information and a clearer perspective of the family's needs as well as being able to give appropriate feedback to an entire family system; (2) the treatment team can have the family do things they cannot do, from small tasks to larger ones like providing ongoing care; (3) problem-solving together as a family system in the hospital is good preparation for doing it at home; (4) everyone's problems in coping are discussed—the focus for concerns goes beyond the patient to everyone in the system.[8] At the point where the elderly patient's functional independence is challenged, the physician must be aware of potential family problems and strengths that relate to the elderly patient's care.

As noted earlier, adult caretakers may be facing crises of their own when their parent becomes dependent or disabled. In review, these could include loneliness secondary to the children leaving home (the empty-nest syndrome); the necessity of reexamining personal relationships with spouse and children; conflict with other siblings over the caretaking responsibilities; a renewal of earlier communication or interrelationship conflicts between themselves and the parent; facing one's own middle-life adjustment problems, including one's own aging. In addition, a problem that is sure to be exacerbated in the future is that of the woman caretaker being forced to delay or interrupt her own activities and priorities (education or career).

The supportive role for the therapist is emphasized by Milloy.[61] In this perspective the worker's interest needs to be centered on helping the older person maintain external and internal depleting and restorative forces—the nature of the ego and its capacity to deal with both internal and external stress. The worker's proper concern, then, is not so much pathology and treatment as those ego and life forces that are still intact or capable of restoration. The worker needs to acquire a longitudinal view of the client in order to determine the strength of the patient's anchorages, how well they have served the client, and how adequate they are in the present. This perspective means viewing aging as a development stage in order to evaluate both the older person's success in mastering the tasks and crisis of previous stages as well as the residue of unsolved problems complicating the mastery of the current crisis.[61] The professional therefore requires a knowledge of the aging process from a psychological perspective, including the patient's history of ego functioning at various age levels. The worker also should be familiar with the degree of conflict that might exist between the client's and society's expectations with regard to patient role performance in various statuses, including spouse, parent, child, older person, unemployed person, and roles in relation to race, religion, education, and occupation.

It is important to realize that the transition from one set of roles to the other cannot be accomplished without great pain and anxiety, not only for the older person but also for those who are affected by role definition or participation in roles, such as adult children when they feel they should assume roles of parents to their own parents.[61]

The older person's losses may also stem from the painful loss of spouse; the necessity of giving up a lifelong occupation or career because of illness; or simply the loss of health. Coping with bereavement can be important in maintaining the older person's sense of purpose or value in living. Such adjustment may be expressed in depressive reaction. The older patient may seem to have lost an anchor, a habit pattern of daily living related to the lost person. Although the patient may appear not quite oriented, she or he will not have lost touch with reality. But reassurance is needed along with expressions of interest from intimate persons and help in making new connections and activities. The point is that the health-care therapist must make an unusually heavy emotional investment in the older client—not a personal one, but a professional one—through which the client learns that his or her own thoughts and feelings are truly important.[61]

An example of how a multidisciplinary treatment team can provide appropriate diagnosis and treatment for elderly patients is that of the Geriatric Evaluation and Treatment Team at the Methodist Hospital, Houston. Seven elderly patients without antecedent psychiatric histories presented hysterical behavior symptoms of pseudodementia. They were treated by a team that included managing physician, nurse, social worker, dietician, speech patholo-gist, pharmacist, psychiatrist, clinical psychologist, physical therapist, speech therapist, and physiatrist. One patient, age 91, had been living successfully at home until shortly before hospitalization. She became confused, vividly describing symptoms of dementia. Social investigations uncovered several recent losses, including the departure of a nephew and a neighbor. As the team gained the patient's confidence, her functional disabilities began to ameliorate. Primary treatment intervention consisted of environmental restructuring of the patient's eroded social system including the fact that the nephew was able to return to be closer to her again.[61]

As noted earlier, an overinvestment in the older client to satisfy the therapist's own needs is not beneficial. Rather, the therapist needs to have a controlled empathy with the client that is focused to help the client.

For the physical therapist it is important to assist the elderly patient to learn new ways to initiate and to respond behaviorally. The most helpful professional response is to demonstrate respect and to expect the best from patients.[8] Calling an elderly patient by her/his first names without permission, or assuming that a person's useful life is over, is not going to help the patient feel positive toward herself or the health professional.

A knowledge of available community resources can be useful for the health-care worker in assisting the family. The two most important criteria[61] for utilizing any services are as follows: (1) Will using the service increase or maintain the client's capacity for self-directed behavior? (2) Will it tend to lessen the client's sense of isolation and increase the feeling of being needed?

The physical therapist may find it necessary to assist the family in decisions about living arrangements or resorting to institutionalization as the condition of the patient worsens. In answering questions such as the need for institutional care, the physical therapist needs to be cognizant that each person is a product of unique life experiences. Plans for living arrangements should be based on the principle that as long as a person gains more gratification than pain from living in the community, it is better to help the patient remain there.[62]

In all patients, but especially the elderly person for whom relocation can be traumatic, there is a need to establish or reestablish oneself in a familiar environment or life space. The older person lives in a complex, modern society facing a variety of life challenges—physical, mental, psychological, social, economic, legal, and spiritual.[63]

Many needs call for the involvement and assistance of helping professionals. Although the elderly patient's needs may lie within the domain of one professional, many needs that older persons face require a particular degree of interprofessional, multidisciplinary skills, knowledge, and practices. In geriatric medicine, there are strong legal and ethical bases for achieving effective interprofessional and multidisciplinary cooperation.[63]

The adult child who seeks assistance in relation to caring for an aging parent or relative can be helped in several ways. One of the most important is in separating reality from the mass of feelings that color it.[61]

> The worker can be most supportive if he (sic) can help the client understand that his parent is not a child for whom he must assume complete responsibility: the parent is an adult, who, although suffering from serious limitations, has a right to make decisions and to take responsibility for the consequences of those decisions.

Specific programs that have been developed to assist the elderly in coping with losses and provide support for family members are discussed next.

FOUR CONCEPTS—EDUCATION STRATEGIES TO SUPPORT THE AGING CLIENTS AND THEIR FAMILY NETWORK

A perspective is emerging that the practicing physical therapist will ultimately be involved with families providing assistance to their elderly. In such involvement the professional can benefit from an understanding and knowledge that goes beyond the functions of technical competence and practical skills. To illuminate some new dimensions with regard to family caretaking, I will describe four programs that are considered to be innovative, relative, and timely. The descriptions cover the reason or rationale and purpose of the programs, clientele served and family relationships, program objectives, program content, and results, with implications discussed in subsequent sections. It is hoped that the physical therapist will gain a clearer understanding of the scope of the problem as well as the opportunities involved in approaches to care of the elderly that involve the family network as part of the rehabilitation team.

Peer Supports for Older Adults

A peer support system was started as part of the psychosocial component of the Turner Geriatric Clinic, an outpatient clinic at The University of Michigan Hospital, Ann Arbor. It began as a program of monthly health-education workshops planned and implemented by a group of peer counselors, that is, older persons.

The staff at Turner Clinic were struck by the patients' needs for information and attention. Frequently they would tell the staff of their frustration with doctors who only had a few minutes to give to each patient, "rushing me in and out," or the family doctor who said, "What can you expect, you're just getting older. Nothing can be done about it." Despite relatively good health, many of the older persons had generalized worries about the future and a set of specific concerns (e.g., treatment of chronic conditions, exercise, diet, and the effects of new drugs and their interaction with drugs already taken). Part of their worries, the staff noted, was a result of too much rather than too little information from the mass media. The staff realized that many of their patients' concerns were shared by many, for example, worries about cataract operations, memory lapses, hearing loss, stiffening joints, and general uncertainties about how all of these might threaten their independence. Once a program to address this need was decided on, the staff agreed that they needed input from the elderly before drafting the program.

The first step was to identify a nucleus of older adults (from patients) who had leadership potential and who might be willing to serve as peer counselors. Patients, colleagues, and social agency staff were asked to suggest candidates. Subsequently, 12 persons became the first peer counselors. It was subsequently decided by counselors and staff to organize a series of workshops.

Frequently, workshops served to introduce new ideas and to stimulate interest in pursuing a subject in more depth. As a result, the formation of small groups grew out of workshop presentations.

Although few peer counselors would have called themselves advocates, the fact that they were better informed about services and resources than the average person and had a number of channels through which to spread information placed them in this role. One peer counselor was particularly effective in convincing persons that they have the right to ask questions and receive answers from ophthalmologists and others who work with the visually impaired. Others have written letters to editors and taken part in community planning meetings and advisory groups. Most important, according to the Turner Clinic staff, they are models, by their behavior and attitudes, for older adults who are active participants in their community and able to take responsibility for issues affecting their interests and the needs of those less able. One visitor remarked to a group, "I just can't wait to get old."[64]

Older Women Caring for Disabled Spouses

A multiservice program directed toward women who are caregivers of their elderly spouses evolved into a respite project that incorporated several community based supportive services. The original impetus for the wives' support group started in Marin County, California, in 1977. The initiator was a woman who had cared for a stroke-disabled husband for 17 years and who also was a leading advocate for the development of a community day-care program.[65]

The project funding initially received came from the Senior Community Employment Program (Title V, Older Americans Act). Primary outreach efforts were directed toward the day-care population, where the number of women involved in caregiving was significant. Of the participants, 50 percent were men; 85 percent of them were cared for by their wives. This was comparable to research findings that men are more likely than women to be cared for by a spouse. Such women are identified in the literature as being "the hidden victims," a high-risk group of elderly women. For such caregivers the emotional strain and the physical demands of caregiving are superimposed on the stress they already are experiencing in attempting to cope with their own aging processes. Most of the women experience isolation, loneliness, and role overload.[65]

The primary purpose of the wives' group was to build mutual support. They began with monthly meetings, but these were expanded to twice monthly because the caregiving wives wanted more time for educational programs. For these sessions resource persons were invited to address issues of concern that ranged from preparing financially for a spouse's institutional care to the physiologic and psychological aftereffects of a stroke. All meetings took place at the day center, with arrangements made for the husband to attend the center that day if he was not a regular participant. Group meetings were facilitated by coleaders, the group's founder, and a social worker who also served as program director at the day center. Their role was to encourage each woman participant to express her feelings and to foster a nonjudgmental atmosphere where others refrained from giving advice.

As with similar groups, the participants were experiencing stress and a prevailing sense of isolation, both social and emotional. The majority of women were caring for husbands who were brain-injured to some degree. Because many of the spouses no longer had full capacity for empathy or interpersonal sensitivity, they could rarely satisfy their spouses' needs. The group's founder described this as a loss of closeness, of loving. The group experience gave the wives an opportunity to share common experiences as well as to explore alternative methods of coping and problem solving.

One general need surfaced—the need for adequate, affordable respite services in the community that would relieve the women of daily demands of caregiving. Most of the women could not afford the community's proprietary (for profit) home-care services. This issue led to the submission of a grant proposal to a local foundations to support a 2-year respite care service. One benefit was that the respite service provided both husband and wife the opportunity for periods away from the intense interaction and stresses inherent in their relationship. It had been 3 to 12 years since any of the wives had had a vacation. All commented on the peace, quiet, and rest they were able to enjoy. Comments on the benefits ranged from, "The nurse's visits raise his mood," to "One day away from me—he would have to enjoy the change." The reactions demonstrated the positive effects of the respite program for the husbands as well as the wives. Two special programs were generated in the project: (1) a community workshop was directed to both the public and health-care providers (the latter generally fail to understand the ongoing problems faced by wives once the husband is discharged from the acute care or rehabilitation facility); (2) a videotape was produced with the help of a nonprofit agency in the community—entitled "Women Who Care: Living with Disabled Husbands," the videotape focuses on one of the couples involved in the project. Personal interviews with other participants provided information on their personal experiences. The community workshop attracted many women and other family caregivers as well as health-care providers.

The Natural Supports Program

The purpose of Natural Supports Program (NSP) was to explore the nature and extent of care provided by families to the aging and to determine how services might be designed to enhance and prolong caregiving efforts.[67] NSP was initiated in October 1976 by the Community Service Society of New York based on the premise that a family's caregiving efforts on behalf of its elderly can be supported by the development of services designed specifically for its members. NSF has concentrated on the role of the family, both nuclear and extended. The project sought to supplement rather than substitute for the care provided by informal supports.

Two distinct service modalities were used: (1) family-centered social casework, and (2) community based group services. The objectives of NSP were as follows:

1. To promote and document the development and use of groups comprised of caring relatives of the aging in order to strengthen their caregiving capacity.

2. To develop a variety of community based group models and assess their replication potential across a diversity of family types and communities.

3. To provide training for group leadership and to attempt to mobilize or develop community organizational structures that will provide for local accountability and maintenance of these groups.

Four contrasting areas of New York City were chosen to assess the applicability of service models in relation to a variety of community and population characteristics. The areas varied in demographic characteristics, types of family constellations, extent and nature of services for the elderly, and geographic proximity of the older person to supports.

Community assessment meetings for caregivers that also involved professionals from related agencies were held. Information on the aging process, nature of the caregiving role, and services benefits for the elderly was provided by speakers, resource persons, demonstrations, and literature. Supportive services were offered in small discussion groups comprised of up to 12 caregivers, a leader, resource person, and a recorder. These provided an opportunity for ventilation of concerns, problem solving, and service requests. A social worker was present at each program to deal with crises and individual service requests.

Attendees reported disabilities of 187 older relatives of concern as follows: 59 percent had multiple disabilities, with 35 percent reported as confusion, 35 percent depression, 34 percent mobility, 26 percent vision, 19 percent hearing, 16 percent heart condition, 10 percent for each use of hand/arm and for speech, and 9 percent for bowel and bladder control. Attendees were asked to check the number of formal services received by their older relatives. Of 72 responses, 69 percent were not receiving any formal services and 30 percent were receiving one or more services. Of the attendees (200), 60 percent reported that they were the only caregiver for their older relative; 21 percent reported one other person involved, and 15 percent reported two or more other caregivers. Of 249 respondents, 77 percent reported no friends or neighbors in the caring network, and 23 percent reported one or more friends involved.

Caregivers using group services tended to be primarily white, middle-aged, middle-income women of diverse religions and ethnicity. They were primary caregivers for widowed parents over 70 years of age with mild multiple disabilities. There was a disproportionate representation of attendees who were single, given the predominance of married households in the four target areas. As evidenced by the data, they were primarily sole providers of care for their older relatives, and it appears that they lacked informal supports for their own caregiving roles. Therefore they may have been more likely to need peer support and mutual aid from a group.

As to use and value of the groups, both caregivers and professionals expressed the positive value of the group experiences. Some caregivers primarily sought information regarding resources (that proved helpful in finding and using services). Others gained a more realistic understanding of the aging process, enabling them to plan and cope with changes in the caregiving situation. Such understanding helped to assuage fears regarding anticipated physical and mental decline and potential increases in caregiving demands.

Greater toleration and decreased frustration, especially in relation to caring for the mentally impaired, was reported. Caregivers were able to begin addressing their feelings regarding their own aging. Members learned the importance of mutual communication of needs with their older relatives. They developed communications skills that assisted them in involving others in caregiving responsibilities as well as decision-making.

A high degree of interaction and group cohesion developed as a result of caregivers' participation in ongoing small discussion groups. Attendees considered the group programs to be as the first nonjudgmental, supportive environment in which they could express feelings of anger, frustration, and resentment regarding caregiving roles and responsibilities. Members provided each other with recognition and support for their caring roles. Caregivers were eventually able to recognize and define their limits in caregiving, to adjust better to new and changing responsibilities, as well as to develop coping strategies. Some evidenced skill and knowledge in the area of community resources and entitlements and in functioning as indigenous resources persons. Group sharing for some served as sanctioned opportunity for socialization as well as respite from the caring role.

As Parents Grow Older: An Intervention Model Program to Assist Family Caretakers of Elderly Members

The As Parents Grow Older (APGO) program model was implemented and evaluated in several Michigan community sites in an Administration of Aging (AoA) funded project entitled The Development and Evaluation of Community Based Support Groups for Families of Aged Persons.[59] The prototype in the Child and Family Service, Washtenaw County Branch, Child and Family Services of Michigan, Inc. developed from a recognition by social workers that adult children caring for aging parents had special needs. These needs, and those of their aging parents, often resulted in tensions and stress for the caretakers.[59,67]

To test the applicability of this program with various caretakers and families living in different communities as well as to develop a training strategy for agency personnel who would serve as program facilitators, a proposal was written by the Institute of Gerontology, The University of Michigan, in collaboration with Child and Family Services of Michigan, Inc. Objectives of the 2 1/2-year Model Project included the development and evaluation of a facilitator's manual. In addition, the project sought "to assess the ability of an existing community structure (Child and Family Services of Michigan, Inc.) to improve services to families with older members through staff development and training."[58]

Purpose and Objectives. The project model, a series of six group sessions, is designed both to help induce supportive behavior in adult children and to provide a link between the parents and community service resources. It is a blend of two traditional interventions and theories—education and learning theory and counseling and problem-solving models.

The content of the sessions cover sequentially (1) the psychological aspects of aging, (2) chronic illness and behavioral changes with age, (3) sensory deprivation and communication, (4) alternative living situations and shared decision-making, (5) the availability and utilization of community resources, and (6) dealing with situations and feelings.

The prevention and education functions of the APGO model support the premise that despite inherent difficulties families are and will continue to be responsible for supporting their aged members. Project data support the fact that educational and supportive services are needed to supplement family assistance and strengthen its capacity to care for its elderly members.

The information and concepts provided to the adult-child caretakers form a nucleus of educational content of value to physical therapists as well. As noted earlier, medical health service providers will be carrying out their professional duties on behalf of older patients more and more in conjunction with families.

Based on the subjective reactions of the participants to the APGO model, the program intervention was clearly successful. A total of 91 percent of the participants thought that they had gained in their understanding of the aging process; 78 percent believed they had improved understanding of their older person's needs and feeling; 71 percent reported that they had achieved a greater insight into their own aging. A total of 78 percent of the participants believed they were better prepared to cope with the current and the potential future needs of the elderly, and 81 percent believed that the group process approach, with its combination of information and interpersonal support, proved to be a helpful forum for meeting their needs.[58] Finally, 79 percent indicated that the information and group problem-solving capabilities of their groups seemed most useful.

Every participant experienced improvement in at least one problem area, and 44 percent experienced improvement across four or more of the nine problem areas. Personal feelings showed nearly a 60 percent improvement rate; living arrangements and health problems showed substantially smaller rates of improvement. It seems clear that problems that are more situational may be less amenable to the APGO type of intervention and that APGO is more able to alleviate situations dealing with interpersonal problems, personal adjustment, and problems in communications. When asked how they learned about community programs, 51 percent responded by indicating that it was a direct result of the APGO program.

Perhaps equally relevant for persons working in the medical health-care field was the result of the changes due to improved understanding of the aging process. The project staff developed a true–false test with matched pre–post schedules. Using this instrument, participants showed a decided increase in acquired knowledge.

THREE CARE PROGRAMS FOR ELDERLY PATIENTS

To better illustrate the importance of the physical therapist in the role bridging elderly patient needs, family assistance, and professional–community interventions, I describe three rehabilitation-respite programs selected for their creative approach to specific problems. Each program is summarized according to background need for the program, the methodology, implementation, and outcome.

A Community-Oriented Geriatric Rehabilitation Unit in a Nursing Home

The program recognized that elderly people past age 75 often develop a frailty that leads unnecessarily to a diminished quality of life and to placement in nursing homes and other institutions. If an age-specific rehabilitation program could be established for elderly persons with disabilities (stroke, lower limb amputations, hip fractures), elderly patients could achieve a level of independence that allowed them to be discharged back to their homes, families, communities. The Jewish Home and Hospital for Aged (JHHA) in New York City opened a special geriatric rehabilitation unit. It was the first community-oriented inpatient rehabilitation unit in Manhattan that was based in a nursing home. JHHA was one of the oldest, most advanced long-term facilities in the United States. In 1982 it became a teaching nursing home, in affiliation with the Ritter Department of Geriatrics and Adult Development, The Mount Sinai School of Medicine.[67]

The JHHA rehabilitation unit used two teams, one for admissions, the other for patient management. A physical therapist was assigned to each team. Criteria for admission to the rehabilitation unit included: minimum age of 60, cognitive function adequate to enable patients to comprehend and follow the rehabilitation program, stable medical status, and a potential for return to a suitable, safe home environment or capacity to attain independence for the rest of their institutionalized lives. Team efforts focused on diagnostic evaluation, patient management, and conferences with families. The rehabilitation program consisted primarily of individualized physical and occupational therapy. From July 18, 1983 through November 5, 1984, 47 patients were admitted to the rehabilitation unit and 27, or 57 percent, were discharged to home. In mid-December 1984, a follow-up survey was carried out through home visits by a social worker and a psychiatrist on all 27 patients discharged to the community. Of the 27 rehabilitation patients discharged to home, 23 patients remained in their homes.

A rehabilitation unit that is based in the nursing home, and is made available to older people in the community, is an innovative concept in health care for the elderly. Serving a group of elderly who have the possibility of returning home is a welcome and positive experience for staff members in the chronic care facility. The exposure of staff to the cohort of rehabilitation patients did much to dispel stereotypes about older people in general. A sense of triumph also occurred with each discharge; the high level of enthusiasm of the rehabilitation team had positive repercussions throughout the institution.

A Post-Hospital Nursing Home Rehabilitation Program

A critical consequence of the DRG prospective payment system for elderly patients is that where they used to remain hospitalized to regain functional ability, the present system requires some form of post-hospital care. Emphasis has shifted from hospital-based rehabilitation to that of less costly community care. The DRG prospective payment system has stimulated hospital involvement in providing short-term after-care services.

A collaborative arrangement was initiated as a service demonstration project of The Cleveland Clinic Foundation (CCF) and the Benjamin Rose Institute's Margaret Wagner House (MWH), a skilled nursing home. The overall project goal was to provide post-hospitalization, short-term rehabilitation care for CCF hospital patients. An innovative component of the arrangement, whereby six nursing-home beds were reserved for CCF patients, was that continuity of medical care was provided by the hospital—a psychiatrist continued to be responsible for the medical care of discharged hospital patients during their nursing-home rehabilitation. The emphasis was on the formalized linkage between CCF and MWH for ensuring continuity of care. One outcome of the innovative collaboration was the interinstitutional learning process resulting from the program's implementation. Both institutions were aware that each provided a distinct form of health care for elderly persons. The nursing home provided ongoing patient care with a focus on the social, health, and nursing needs of older persons. Problems tended to be of a chronic nature, often necessitating long-term care. This was in sharp contrast to the hospital environment, which was focused on medical research, diagnosis of disease entity, and treatment of the acutely ill.[69]

For patients, survey data revealed that 98 percent were satisfied with their rehabilitation experience. They were generally satisfied with physician communication, nursing care, physical and occupational therapy, social work involvement, and the quality of dining and recreational facilities. The participants showed a dramatic improvement in physical functioning during the rehabilitation period and a sharp leveling off, with slight improvement, subsequent to discharge from the rehabilitation facility. Interviews with staff participants showed that the affiliation was beneficial to both institutions, primarily because it served as a learning and teaching vehicle. Later problems of communication indicated a need for additional modes of communication among all participants. An important outcome of the affiliation was gaining a better understanding of the logistical and operational programs of maintaining continuity of care by two distinct facilities. Through negotiation, a key objective was achieved; patients were provided with consistent, comprehensive care from time of admission to the hospital until completion of rehabilitation.

Respite Care: A Partnership

Researchers over the years have documented the need for providing caregivers of the elderly with respite care—temporary supervision and care given to a disabled person in order to provide relief to the patient's primary caregiver. The Palo Alto Veterans Administration Medical Center (PAVAMC) supports caregivers of frail elderly veterans. In 1977, the PAVAMC developed a plan for a continuum of care for aging veterans based on the premise that inappropriate institutionalization could be limited if programs were developed that would support in-home caregivers of aging veterans. When a 150-bed nursing home was constructed at the VA's Menlo Park Division, beds were filled rapidly.[37] To prevent inappropriate institutionalization and to support caregivers needing short-term relief, five respite beds were opened. The program was expanded to 10 beds later. All respite patients were housed in one section of the nursing home to underscore the concept that respite patients lived in the community and not in the nursing home.[70]

The typical respite patient is a 69-year-old man with multiple medical problems in need of moderate to intensive skilled nursing care. The three most frequent diagnoses are cerebrovascular accident, dementia, and chronic obstructive pulmonary disease. While in the program, primary medical treatment responsibility stays with the family physician, again affirming that the patient lives in the community. The program's physician's role is to provide medical observation and to implement the care plan developed by the family physician. The patient also receives skilled 24-hour nursing care; physical and occupational therapy are offered to those with potential for more independence. An important goal is to help each veteran return home as independent as possible in bathing, feeding, walking, toileting, and dressing.

Psychosocial services are essential for respite patients. For many patients, the respite stay is the first time they have ever been in a nursing home. The adjustments they must make can be stressful. To ease this transition, staff learns the patients preferred routine and does as much as possible to maintain that routine. The staff encourages socialization within the unit. Emotional support and information are shared by patients and caregivers. Telephone numbers are exchanged, and many lasting friendships are made. Each caregiver receives assistance in organizing a home caregiving plan that addresses three basic questions: Who is assuming responsibility for the various aspects of the care plan? Is the care plan realistic? Have all potential sources of help been used (e.g., family, friends, neighbors, and community resources)? The location of the respite program in the nursing home has had a major impact on the facility. It has changed the reality of the nursing home. Since the program opened, the number of community persons coming into the nursing home has increased dramatically, because veterans in respite are temporary patients and not permanent residents. They have families, friends, and neighbors who enter the nursing home social system, causing it to expand and become more dynamic. Isolation from the outside world is reduced.

Respite also offers positive role models for permanent nursing-home residents because many respite patients are frail elderly who improve their health and self-care skills while in the nursing home. Additionally, the long-term residents gain emotional and intellectual stimulation from the presence of the relatives and friends of the respite patients. The nursing home is transformed from a single-purpose institution where isolated elderly reside until they die into a multipurpose geriatric facility providing services that help older families stay together in their own home. The respite program enables the nursing home to serve a larger number of families because of its emphasis on short-term stays. With health-care resources diminishing and an increasing number of aging persons in society requiring long-term care, inpatient respite programs will be increasingly in demand in the VA system and in the broader community.

IMPROVING PROFESSIONAL CARE IN THE FUTURE

In conclusion, the physical therapist's future role as a member of a geriatric team striving to provide quality of care to elderly patients in partnership with the family kinship and other support individuals or groups will continue to change. There could well be creative breakthroughs in this mutual effort using the new technology and in conjunction with a dramatically improved practice. Potential areas of research that could open new awareness and understanding for the elderly person and his/her family will be discussed.

One area that needs further illumination is that of the variable ethnicity. The future racial and cohort variations in family relationships and such areas as filial responsibility, especially for black and Hispanic families, could affect future populations of the elderly. When Hanson and associates[71] looked at racial and cohort variations in filial responsibility norms, they found little evidence that black families gave greater help and kinship assistance to their older members, in contrast to earlier findings. They concluded that the elderly of both races require alternative sources of support, and these must come from organizations and groups in the community. Few researchers have sought answers to intriguing questions in this area of inquiry, but such indicators as the recent rapid increase in Hispanic births and increased longevity for black elderly suggests that more knowledge will be useful for future cohorts of elderly.

Research is needed to evaluate model approaches to assist institutionalized elderly to resume independent living and community participation, using family support, the physical therapist, and other health-care professionals. A crisis situation can occur when the patient realized he or she will not change back to a former physical state. The physical therapist can help the individual adopt previously successful adaptive behaviors and provide information and assistance to family members to locate environmental resources.[8] One program used physical therapists and other team members to support in-home caregivers of frail elderly, working out a partnership between a Veterans Administration nursing home and family members. The families received program services, being taught health-care delivery skills needed to maintain the frail elders at home, as well as how to build community support systems.[70] Additional service programs could be designed and evaluated to assist families in conjunction with health-care professionals who are committed to extending quality of life after institutionalization. Similarly, research on short-term programs following hospitalization stays might investigate model instructional programs in which the health professionals teach family members, using videotape, computer technology, and other educational tools that could be adapted to the home environment.

As the patterns of family interaction evolve with different work–career–educational roles for women, particularly single parents, mixed-marriage families, research will be useful to study the effects of these changes on traditional family kinship roles. Researchers could explore the mechanism of interprofessional relationships as they also affect treatment and care of geriatric patients and potential approaches involving family members of elderly.

With the increasingly larger cohorts of elderly women living into their eighties and nineties and older, the traditional communications and assistance roles of reciprocity take on different dimensions. More longitudinal investigations could study the dynamics involved to seek out possible future directions for health professionals to assist other caregivers. As HMOs and other forms of health care become normalized, various delivery systems could be studied to provide health professionals with knowledge most applicable to policy changes in various forms and community settings.

With new systems of medical care being targeted to larger subpopulations of workers and retirees, researchers need to examine their effect on elderly groups of various makeup and socioeconomic status. It is especially critical to study health-care delivery approaches for the single elderly living alone, various ethnic populations, those who are surviving at or near the poverty level, those last independent persons who shy away from official programs and services, including the rural and city ghetto-bound residents. Their needs for assistance and know-how to negotiate an increasingly complex system, with assistance from family, friends, or others, in order to maintain some dignity and self-identity as individuals must be studied as more specialization in the delivery of health-care demands an extension of the knowledge base around the quality care issue for everyone, at any age.

The entire arena of professionalism and ethics as they involve not only the physician and nurse but also the physical therapist and other health professionals requires careful study in relationship to the health needs of the elderly geriatric patient and the family kinship network. The potential of technology and its creative and humane application to assist elderly persons must be tempered with careful regard for the rights of the individual older person as well as the younger patient who needs specific organs or other surgical techniques.

REFERENCES

1. Cantor M: Strain among caregivers: a study of experience in the United States. Gerontologist 23:597, 1983
2. Silverstone B: An overview of research on informal supports: implications for policy and practice. Presented at the Gerontological Society Meeting, Dallas, 1978
3. Litwak E: Extended kin relations in an industrial democratic society. In Shanas E, Streib G (eds): Social Structure and the Family: Generational Relations. Prentice-Hall, Englewood-Cliffs, NJ, 1965

4. Sussman MB: The family life of old people. In Binstock R, Shanas E (eds): Handbook of Aging and the Social Sciences. Van Nostrand Reinhold, New York, 1976

5. Women in the workplace. Working Age 3:1, 1988

6. Tabak HL: The role of the family. J Am Health Care Assoc 17:(3)293, 1979

7. Lebowitz BD: Old age and family functioning. J Gerontol Social Work 1:111, 1978

8. Mock S: A social worker's philosophy and treatment in rehabilitation. Ch. 17. In Kaplan PE (ed): The Practice of Physical Medicine. Charles C Thomas, Springfield, IL, 1984

9. Blenkner M: Social work and family relationships in later life with some thoughts on filial maturity. In Shanas E, Streib G (eds): Social Structure and the Family: Generational Relations. Prentice-Hall, Englewood Cliffs, NJ, 1965

10. Lewis MA, Binstock R, Cantor M, Schneewind E: The extent to which informal and formal supports interact to maintain the older people in the community. Presented at the Gerontological Society Annual Meeting, San Diego, 1980

11. Hawker M: Geriatrics for Physiotherapists and the Allied Professions. Queen Square, London, 1974

12. Purtilo R: Justice, liberty, compassion: analysis of and implications for "humane" health care and rehabilitation in the United States—some lessons from Sweden. Monograph 8. World Rehabilitation Fund, Inc., New York, 1979

13. McClusky HY: Education for aging: the scope of the field and perspectives for the future. In Gragowski SM, Mason D (eds): Education for the Aging. ERIC Clearinghouse on Adult Education, Syracuse, NY, 1974

14. Tibbitts C: Middle-aged and older people in American society. In Planning Welfare Services for Older People. Department of Health, Education and Welfare, Washington, DC, 1965

15. Hilliboe HE: A modern pattern for meeting the health needs of the aging. In Donahue W, Tibbitts C (eds): The New Frontiers of Aging. The University of Michigan Press, Ann Arbor, 1957

16. Tibbitts C: Can we invalidate negative stereotypes of aging? Gerontologist 19:1979

17. Tolliver L: Older Americans: our keys to the future. Aging 339:2, 1983

18. Grays on the go. Time 131(8):66, 1988

19. Williams TF: The Education of Health Professionals to Serve the Needs of a Growing Older Population. Association for Gerontology in Higher Education. Chicago, 1988

20. A Profile of Older Americans: 1987. American Association of Retired Persons, Washington, DC, 1987

21. U.S. Bureau of the Census, Washington, DC, 1986

22. Thompson WE, Streib G: Meaningful activity in a family context. In Kleemeier RW (ed): Aging and Leisure: A Research Perspective into the Meaningful Use of Time. Oxford University Press, New York, 1961

23. Hagestad G: Able elderly in the family context: changes, chances, and challenges. Gerontologist 27:417, 1987

24. Gutmann D: The parental imperative revisited: towards a developmental psychology of adulthood and later life. In J. Meacham (ed): Contributions To Human Development. Karger, Basel, 1985

25. Troll LE: The family of later life: a decade review. Marriage Family J May 33:263, 1971

26. Salber E: Don't Send Me Flowers When I'm Dead. Duke University Press, Durham University Press, Durham, NC, 1983

27. Anderson T: Rehabiliation management and the rehabilitation team. p. 375. In Basmajian J, Kirby R (eds): Medical Rehabilitation. Williams & Wilkins, Baltimore, 1984

28. Towle C: Common human needs. American Association of Social Workers, New York, 1952

29. Kramer C: Roundtable/family therapy: when the whole family needs your care. Patient Care, October, 1974

30. Cantor MH: Neighbors and friends; an overlooked resource in the informal support system. Presented at the Gerontological Society Meeting, San Francisco, 1977

31. Shanas E, Streib G (eds): Social Structure and the Family: Generational Relations. Prentice-Hall, Englewood Cliffs, NJ, 1965

32. Shanas E: Social myth as hypothesis: the case of the family relations of old people. Gerontologist 19:(1)7, 1979

33. Blenkner M: The normal dependencies of aging. In Kalish R (ed): The Dependencies of Old People. Institute of Gerontology, Ann Arbor, MI, 1969

34. Kreps J: The economics of intergenerational relationship. In Shanas E, Streib G (eds): Social Structure and the Family: Generational Relations. Prentice-Hall, Englewood Cliffs, NJ, 1965

35. Donahue W: Psychological changes with advancing age. In Planning Welfare Services for Older People. Washington, DC, 1965

36. Clark M: Is dependency in old age culture bound? Presented at the Gerontological Society Meeting, 1967

37. Cafferata G: Marital status, living arrangements, and the use of health services by elderly persons. Gerontology J 42:613, 1987

38. Sicker M: Some thoughts on a national policy for long-term care. Gerontological Social Work J 2:271, 1980

39. Finkelstein M: The impact on nursing homes of diagnosis-related groups. Long-Term Care Currents 10:15, 1987

40. Antonucci T, Akiayama H: Social networks in adult life and a preliminary examination of the convoy model. Gerontology J 42:519, 1987

41. Shanas E: The unmarried old person in the United States: living arrangements and care in illness, myth, and fact. Presented at the International Social Science Research Seminar in Gerontology, Markaryd, Sweden, 1963

42. Sussman MB, Burchinal L: Kin family network: unheralded structure in current conceptualizations of family functioning. Marriage Family Living 24:231, 1962

43. Blazer D; Working with the elderly patient's family. Geriatrics 33:117, 1978

44. Comptroller General of United States: The well-being of older people in Cleveland, Ohio. U.S. General Accounting Office, Washington, DC, April 19, 1977

45. U.S. Department of Health, Education and Welfare, National Center for Health Statistics: Home Health Care for Persons 55 Years and Over. Vital and Health Statistics Publication Series 10, No. 73, 1972

46. Califano JA Jr: The aging of America: questions for the four-generation society. Annals AAPSS 438:96, 1978

47. Adams BN: Interaction theory and the social network. Sociometry 30:64, 1967

48. Shanas E: A note on restriction of life space: Attitudes of age cohorts. Health Social Behav J 9:86, 1968

49. Stone R, Cafferata G, Sangl J: Caregivers of the frail elderly: a national profile. Gerontologist 27:616, 1987

50. Litwak E: Helping the Elderly: The Complementary Roles of Informal Networks and Formal Systems. Guilford Press, New York, 1985

51. Rosenmayer L: The family—a source of hope for the elderly. In Shanas F, Sussman M (eds): Family Bureaucracy and the Elderly. Duke University Press, Durham, NC, 1977

52. Horowitz A: Family caregiving to the frail elderly. In Eisendorfer C (ed): Annual Review of Gerontology and Geriatrics. Vol. 5. Springer, New York, 1985

53. Pearson J, Verma S, Nellet, C: Elderly psychiatric patient status and caregiver perceptions as predictors of caregiver burden. Gerontologist 28:9, 1988

54. Finley N, Roberts D, Banaham B: Motivators and inhibitors of attitudes of filial obligations toward aging parents. Gerontologist 28:73, 1988

55. Schmidt MG: Failing parents, aging children. Gerontol Social Work J 2:259, 1980

56. Brody EM, Spark GM: Institutionalization of the aged: a family crisis. Family Process 5:76, 1966

57. Hess B, Waring J: Parent and child in later life: rethinking the relationship. In Lernez R, Spanier B (eds): Child Influences on Marital and Family Interactions: A Lifespan Perspective. Academic Press, Orlando, FL 1978

58. Brahce CI, Silverman AG, Leon J: Altering a Service Delivery System to Improve Family Care of the Elderly: Final Report. Institute of Gerontology, Ann Arbor, MI, 1981

59. Silverman AG, Brahce CI: "As Parents Grow Older": an intervention model. Gerontol Social Work J 2:77, 1979

60. Butler RN, Lewis MI: Aging and Mental Health. 2nd Ed. CV Mosby, St. Louis, 1977

61. Milloy M: Casework with the older person and his family. Social Casework J p. 450, Oct 1964

62. Kirby H, Harper R: Team assessment of geriatric mental patients: the care of functional dementia produced by hysterical behavior. Gerontologist 27:573, 1987

63. Kapp M: Interprofessional relationships in geriatrics: ethical and legal considerations. Gerontologist 27:547, 1987

64. Campbell R, Chenoweth B, Kraus C: Peer supports for older adults, manual for replication. Turner Geriatric Clinic, University of Michigan Hospital, Ann Arbor, 1981

65. Crossman L, London C, Barry C: Older women caring for disabled spouses: a model for supportive services. Gerontologist 21:464, 1981

66. Hudis IE, Guchsbaum MD: Components of community based group programs for strengthening family supports to their aging relatives: implications for replication. Community Service Society of New York, Presented at the Gerontological Society Meeting, Dallas, 1978

67. Kahn BH, Silverman AG: Family service highlights. Family Serv Assoc Am 2(5):279, 1976

68. Adelman R, Marron K, Libow L, Neufeld R: A community-oriented geriatric rehabilitation unit in a nursing home. Gerontologist 27: 1987

69. Petchers M, Roy A, Brickner A: A post-hospital nursing home rehabilitation program. Gerontologist 27:752, 1987

70. Berman S, Delaney N, Gallagher D, et al: Respite care: a partnership between a Veterans Administration nursing home and families to care for frail elders at home. Gerontologist 27:581, 1987

71. Hanson S, Sauer W, Seelbach W: Racial and cohort variations in filial responsibility norms. Gerontologist 23:626, 1988

8 | Cardiac Considerations and Physical Training

Louis R. Amundsen
Corinne T. Ellingham

Before starting a physical therapy program for an elderly patient, it is necessary to determine that the patient needs exercise, that the cardiovascular effort is likely to be safe and beneficial, and that the patient is motivated and interested in physical training. In order to use effective and safe exercise intensity levels, it is necessary to evaluate the capacity for exercise of each individual who will participate in a physical therapy program. This is especially crucial with the elderly patient population because they have an increased susceptibility to the secondary complication of bed-rest deconditioning. For the physical therapy and rehabilitation program to be administered safely, it is necessary to determine the safe limits of exercise for every elderly patient. The assessment of exercise capacity needs to be sensitive enough to detect small changes and be specific to the goals of the treatment program.

Cardiovascular evaluation and training methods need to be convenient, inexpensive, and progressive in difficulty and intensity. These methods should also be easily adapted to the needs of the well, the frail, and the disabled elderly. There is also a need to be reasonably certain that a proposed training program will be effective.

The literature review and pilot study described in this chapter provide an overview of cardiopulmonary evaluation and training for elderly up to the age of 75 and extrapolate implications for evaluation and training approached for the very old (over 80 years of age).

NEED FOR EXERCISE FOR THE ELDERLY

Elderly persons need cardiovascular endurance training and instruction concerning appropriate activity levels because they tend to be inactive and to have an increased incidence of conditions that require supervised training, for example, heart and respiratory disease, obesity, chronic pain, arthritis, peripheral vascular problems, cerebrovascular accidents, and diabetes.[1-12]

Activity levels of the "healthy" elderly have been estimated.[4,10-12] The energy expenditures of older workers is the same as that of younger workers during the working day; however, a study of the male population of Tecumseh, Michigan, indicated that the frequency of participation in leisure activities decreased rapidly after age 40. Time spent swimming, bowling, fishing, dancing, and hunting decreased rapidly with increasing age. Walking and lawn-mowing with a power mower decreased after age 60. Gardening increased with age in the study sample (up to age 65).[11]

Sidney and Shephard[12] reported that a group of elderly university employees rarely reached or exceeded a heart rate of 120 beats per minute (bpm). A heart rate of 120 bpm is likely to represent the training intensity threshold for older employed persons. Other studies of representative groups of men and women over the age of 65 indicate that the drastic reduction of physical activity observed in middle-aged men continues in the population over age 65.[4,10]

For the frail and/or disabled elderly the ill effects of bed rest are well documented. Deficiencies in endurance and strength are a common consequence of prolonged bed rest, reduced mobility, and cardiopulmonary disease. Bed rest and inactivity will produce detrimental effects even when no other pathologic process is involved. Bed rest results in decreases in muscle strength, bone density, blood volume, and orthostatic tolerance.[13-17] Aerobic power will decrease dramatically after 3 weeks of bed rest for normal young healthy person.[13] Even 10 to 11 days of chair rest by healthy persons causes decreases in work capacity and orthostatic tolerance.[18] It is obvious that activity levels tend to decrease with advancing age and that inactivity will promote physiologic deterioration.[4,10-18]

FEASIBILITY OF TRAINING

If the premise is accepted that an optimal level of physical activity will minimize or eliminate the detrimental effects of inactivity in young normal persons and in cardiac patients,[19-25] then we still need to know if increasing the physical activity levels of the elderly will be beneficial. The specific effects of aging on skeletal muscle, on the cardiopulmonary system, and on the decline in bone mass have been studied[26-38] (see also Ch. 2). All these changes are similar to the physiologic deterioration caused by inactivity. However, aging per se does cause deterioration independent of the effects of inactivity. Even though the effects of aging will increase the risk and decrease the effectiveness of training, the feasibility of effective cardiopulmonary training for the elderly has been demonstrated.[38-46]

Logically, the key to effective training is the use of appropriate exercise intensity levels. These exercise intensities must be based on the exercise capacity of the individual being trained, on the use of exercises that are appropriate for these individuals, and on the functional analysis of the activity of the individual patient. A training program requires a pretraining evaluation, the use of exercises with known intensity levels, patient education to translate effort into implications for activities of daily living, and frequent assessment during training sessions.

ASSESSING EXERCISE CAPACITY

When assessing exercise capacity, it is necessary to know the normal and abnormal cardiovascular responses to physical exercise.[47-51] In the young the cardiovascular and pulmonary systems respond quickly to acute exercise by increasing heart rate, respiratory rate, stroke volume, tidal volume, and blood flow to active tissue. Advanced aging or progressive disease will lengthen the time required to reach steady state or homeostasis during exercise at a given intensity level.[30]

An equilibrium or steady-state condition will be reached if the functional reserve capacities of the cardiovascular and pulmonary systems have not been exceeded, however.[52] The exercise load that requires more oxygen and energy substrate, glucose, and free fatty acids than the cardiopulmonary systems are able to deliver can be identified when work loads are gradually increased. It is of course necessary to recognize the signs and symptoms of exercise intolerance early enough to prevent undue discomfort or risk to the patient. Before initiation of the exercise evaluation, the patient needs to demonstrate the ability to meet the demands of the resting state. The resting pulse rate should be between 60 and 100 bpm. If the heart rate is faster or slower than this range or is irregular, the resting electrocardiogram will need to be interpreted. Any unstable rhythm, ventricular arrhythmias, or ST segment shifts would contraindicate exercise testing or training.[47-50,53] Ideally, even for elderly persons the resting systolic blood pressure should be between 100 and 150 mm Hg. However, pressures greater than 150 mm Hg are common for the elderly and do not necessarily prevent safe exercise. If the resting pressure exceeds 225 mm Hg, however, it is not appropriate to initiate any exercise evaluation. At resting pressures approaching 225 mm Hg, greater caution and lower and smaller exercise levels and increments should be used.

A detailed description of the physical assessment and what to look for in a medical history concerning cardiovascular phenomena have been described previously in this series and elsewhere.[54,55]

The heart rate normally increases as the work rate increases, but in the elderly the rate of increase will be greater and/or the maximal heart rate observed will be lower (Figs. 8-1 and 8-2).[51-53] Normal active persons at any age will have a slower increase in heart rate than sedentary persons or cardiac patients.[48-50,53] Even at equivalent ages, cardiac patients will usually have lower maximal heart rates than persons with normal hearts. The maximal heart rate decreases as a function of age (Fig. 8-2).[48-53,56] The predicted maximal

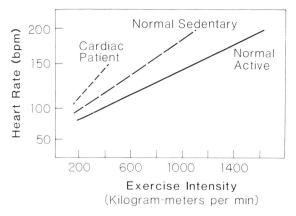

Fig. 8-1. Heart-rate responses during exercise. (From Amundsen,[101] with permission.)

heart rate (PMHR) plus or minus one standard deviation is equal to 220 minus the age in years.[57,58]

Blood pressure responses also can and should be used to assess responses to exercise (Fig. 8-3). Rhythmic isotonic exercise of the lower extremities normally cause large increases in systolic blood pressure but only minimal changes in diastolic pressure (Fig. 8-3).[48,56] An increase of 7.5 mm Hg per metabolic equivalent (MET) is considered normal for systolic pressure. If the systolic blood pressure (SBP) increases more than 12 mm Hg or less than 5 mm Hg per MET, the response is considered hypertensive or hypotensive, respectively.[57]

If the SBP fails to increase or falls when the exercise intensity is increased, the heart as a pump and/or the cardiovascular system as a shunt is failing, which of course requires stopping or decreasing the intensity of the exercise.

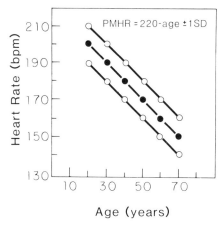

Fig. 8-2. Predicted maximal heart rate (PMHR). (From Amundsen,[101] with permission.)

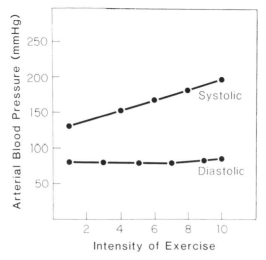

Fig. 8-3. Typical blood pressure response to progressively increasing work rates, METs (metabolic equivalents: 3.5 ml O_2/min/kg). (From Amundsen,[101] with permission.)

To minimize chances of overworking the heart or risking arterial rupture or aneurysm formation, the SBP should not exceed 225 mm Hg;[58] however, values up to 300 mm Hg have been observed during exercise without apparent untoward effects.[59]

In the young normal individual the diastolic blood pressure (DBP) changes very little as the intensity of ambulation, bicycling, or treadmill walking increases.[56] Elderly persons, even those classified as well elderly, are very likely to demonstrate increases in DBP in response to exercise. If the DBP exceeds 130 mm Hg, exercise should be stopped or the intensity should be decreased.[47,59–66] Decreasing the intensity of exercise is preferable to completely stopping it because continuing activity will promote the continued contribution of the auxiliary peripheral blood pumps, especially the gastrocnemius-soleus muscle group, and the respiratory system's contribution to venous return. If it is necessary to stop exercise completely, the elderly person should sit or lie in a head-up or Fowler's position. This position will prevent sudden overfilling of the heart and minimize the risk of promoting further heart failure due to excessive preload.

During physical exercise the therapist should estimate the adequacy of regional blood flow by observing skin color, changes in coordination, and levels of alertness. The cheeks, earlobes, and nose normally become pinker as the duration and intensity of exercise increases.[47] If these areas suddenly turn pale, the exercise intensity needs to be decreased. One can be relatively certain that the blood flow to the kidney and liver is being sacrificed in an attempt to maintain blood flow to the working muscles, the heart, and the brain when sudden pallor is accompanied by falling systolic blood pressure.

Pain and discomfort, such as angina pectoris, dyspnea, intermittent claudication, or joint pain, are also likely to be observed in the elderly and are reasons for decreasing/stopping a bout of exercise[47] or finding other evaluation procedures that do not cause lower extremity pain (e.g., upper extremity ergometry).

After exercise the heart rate, blood pressure, and respiration normally return rapidly to near-resting levels. The heart rate is expected to return to approximately 100 bpm within 6 minutes after exercise ceases. Blood pressure, cognition, equilibrium, and skin color need to be observed during the first 5 minutes of recovery after exercise in order to detect excessive pooling of blood in the lower extremities.[57,58]

These principles need to be applied in assessing tolerance for any exercise, especially when functional capacity is being determined before initiating an exercise training program for elderly persons.

Working capacity is usually expressed as maximal aerobic power and determined by submaximal or by symptom-limited progressive exercise tolerance testing.[57,60–64,66] It is possible to determine maximal aerobic power in elderly persons by conducting tests with the classic criteria developed on young normal persons for the establishment of maximal aerobic power.[65] Because progressive increase of work loads until an increase in work rate no longer causes an increase in oxygen uptake is perceived as extremely stressful and sometimes is impossible to achieve in young normal sedentary adults, this procedure is not reasonable for elderly persons, who are more likely to be sedentary and to possess hidden cardiosvascular disorders. In our opinion the test used must be safe and intense enough to allow an accurate estimate of maximal aerobic power and tolerance for the intensity levels to be used for physical therapy training.

We have used the exercise protocol given in Table 8-1 for evaluating well and frail elderly persons. Table 8-2 provides the conversions between metabolic equivalents and bicycle ergometer work loads.[63,66] Table 8-3 lists the metabolic equivalents for treadmill walking.[57] Tables 8-4 and 8-5 contain MET values for the step ergometer and for walking on a firm surface.[57,63,67] Any of these modes of exercise can and has been used for testing the elderly[39,41–43,46] with functional lower extremities. Although many functional evaluations have

Table 8-1. Submaximal Exercise Test Protocol for Elderly Persons

Exercise Stage	Duration (min)	Total Time (min)	METs[a]
1	3	3	2
2	3	6	3
3	3	9	4
4[b]	3	12	5
5	3	15	6
6	3	18	7

[a] Metabolic equivalents.
[b] Rarely achieved by subjects over age 75.

Table 8-2. Metabolic Equivalents (METs) of Bicycle Ergometer Work Loads

Work Load		MET According to Body Weight (kg)							
Watts	kpm/min[a]	50	60	70	80	90	100	110	120
10	60	2.1	2.0	1.9	1.9	1.8	1.8	1.8	1.8
25	150	3.0	2.8	2.6	2.5	2.4	2.3	2.2	2.1
50	300	4.6	4.1	3.7	3.4	3.2	3.0	2.9	2.8
75	450	6.1	5.4	4.8	4.4	4.1	3.8	3.6	3.4
100	600	7.7	6.6	5.9	5.4	4.9	4.6	4.3	4.1
125	750	9.2	7.9	7.0	6.3	5.8	5.4	5.0	4.7
150	900	10.8	9.2	8.1	7.3	6.6	6.1	5.7	5.4
175	1050	12.3	10.5	9.2	8.3	7.5	6.9	6.4	6.0
200	1200	13.8	11.8	10.3	9.2	8.4	7.7	7.1	6.6
250	1500	16.9	14.4	12.5	11.1	10.1	9.2	8.5	7.9
300	1800	20.0	16.9	14.7	13.1	11.8	10.8	9.9	9.2

The test protocol is given in Table 8-1.

[a] Kilopond meters per minute are equivalent to kilogram meters per minute.

Table 8-3. Submaximal Treadmill Exercise Test

Exercise Stage	Duration (min)	Total Time (min)	Treadmill Speed (mph)	Percent Grade (% incline)	METs
1	3	3	2.0	0.0	2
2	3	6	2.0	3.5	3
3	3	9	2.0	7.0	4
4[a]	3	12	2.0	10.5	5
5	3	15	2.0	14.0	6
6	3	18	2.0	17.5	7

[a] Rarely achieved by the elderly.

Table 8-4. Submaximal Progressive Step Test, 24 Ascents per Minute

Exercise Stage	Duration (min)	Total Time (min)	Step Height (cm)	METs
1	3	3	0	2.2
2	3	6	5	3.0
3	3	9	12	4.0
4	3	12	18	5.0
5	3	15	25	6.0
6	3	18	32	7.0

Table 8-5. Submaximal Walking Test

Exercise Stage	Duration (min)	Total Time (min)	Speed MPH	m/min^{-1}	METs
1	3	3	1.5	40.2	2.2
2	3	6	2.5	67.1	3.0
3	3	9	3.0	80.5	3.5
4	3	12	3.5	93.9	4.1
5[a]	3	15	4.0	107.3	4.8

[a] Rarely achieved by the elderly.

been used to assess activities of daily living and related functional ability, few standardized tests are based on physiologic phenomena.[68–78] The Kottke-Kubicek Five Stage Activity Test can be used to quantify physiologic responses to functional activities.[78] Our adaptation of this test is illustrated in Figures 8-4 and 8-5 and is described in detail later in this chapter.

TRAINING METHODS

Most studies of the effectiveness of training the elderly have demonstrated that subjects with an average age of 65 years can be trained by jogging and by riding bicycle ergometers.[39,40,45,79,80] Subjects of these studies and most persons 65 to 75 years of age are functioning independently in the community. Persons 75 to 85 years old often require some support or assistance from family members or community resources. Persons 85 years of age or older usually need considerable assistance and are most likely to require professional

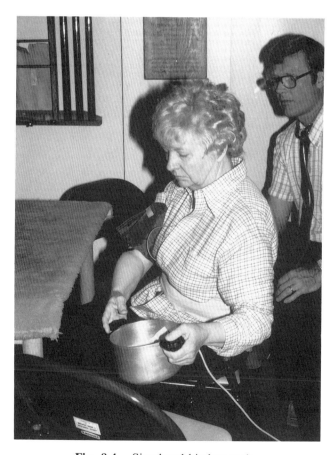

Fig. 8-4. Simulated kitchen task.

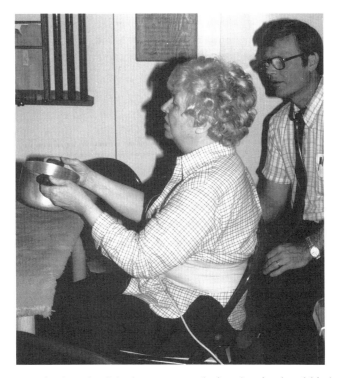

Fig. 8-5. Monitoring physiologic responses during the simulated kitchen task.

supportive services (nursing-home care or home care).[80] Obviously, arbitrary divisions based on chronologic age alone are not appropriate; however, these chronologic and functional divisions can be used to classify existing literature and to plan exercise testing and training regimens for elderly people.

Very little information is available that evaluates the effectiveness or safety of given exercise levels for persons over the age of 75.[29,42,80] However, it is likely that persons over the age of 75 and the frail elderly will benefit from training levels based on principles developed from research on normal young subjects, cardiac patients, the well elderly, and the young old.[20-25,39-46,80] It has been demonstrated that exercise intensities of 60 to 75 percent of maximal aerobic power will be sufficient to produce training effects in previously untrained subjects in these categories. Given that persons 65 to 75 years old can be expected to have maximal aerobic power of 5 to 7 METs and that ambulatory nursing home populations have demonstrated maximums of 2 to 4 METs,[80] it is possible to select and predict activities that will be effective for training persons older than 75 years. Walking, stationary bicycling, stationary stepping, light calisthenics, and various recreational activities, and activities of daily living (ADL) are likely to be appropriate (see Tables 8-6 and 8-7).[80-89] Calisthenic exercises of known low-intensity levels have been described previously in this series[63,86] and are discussed along with a model program later

Table 8-6. Approximate Energy
Requirements of Physical Activities

Activity	METs
Self-care activities and physical exercises in bed with back supported	
Feeding self	1–1.5
Washing hands and face	1–1.5
Washing body while sitting in a chair (excluding back and legs)	1.7
Brushing teeth	1–1.5
Care of fingernails	1–1.5
Shaving	1.6
Combing hair	1.6
Passive ROM[a] exercises to all extremities	1.0
Active ROM[a] exercises to all extremities	1.0–1.5
Active ROM[a] exercises with moderate resistance to all extremities	1.5–2.0
Calisthenics (by author)	
Greer[81]	2.0–4.5
Weise[82]	2.2–10.3
Fletcher[83]	1.4–4.2
Kellerman[84]	2.2–6.9
Amundsen[85]	1.7–5.9

Includes resting metabolic needs.
[a] ROM, range of motion.

in this chapter. MET levels have been determined for calisthenics by others,[81–84] but these values are meaningful only when determined at steady state or when the methods of the original literature report are duplicated. METs measured at steady state can be used for any time interval, usually 1 to 3 minutes per exercise, but MET values determined over short durations–for example, 30 seconds or 1 minute—can be applied only to exercise of the same duration.

When training heart rates are determined by the method first described by Karvonen,[20,90] the percentage of maximal heart rate will usually be achieved when exercising at the same percentage of maximal aerobic power. This is not true when the percentage of maximal heart rate is based on a starting point of zero. When a zero base is used, higher percentages of maximal heart rate are required to reach 60 to 75 percent of maximal aerobic power.[58]

SUMMARY OF THE RESULTS OF PILOT STUDIES

Our goal has been to identify practical exercise regimens effective for increasing the capacity of the elderly to perform activities of daily living. Effective training ideally decreases the physiologic effort required to perform

Table 8-7. Approximate Energy Requirements of Physical Activities

Category	Self Care or Home	Occupational	Recreational[b]	Physical Conditioning
Very light (<3 METs)	Washing, shaving, dressing Desk work, writing Washing dishes Driving auto	Sitting (clerical, assembling) Standing (store clerk, bartender) Driving truck[a] Crane operator[a]	Shuffleboard Horseshoes Bait casting Billiards Archery Gold (cart)	Walking (level at 2 mph) Stationary bicycle (very low resistance) Very light calisthenics
Light (3–5 METs)	Cleaning windows Raking leaves Weeding Power lawn mowing Waxing floors (slowly) Painting Carrying objects (15–30 lb)	Stocking shelves (light objects) Light welding Light carpentry[b] Machine assembly Auto repair Paper hanging	Dancing (social and square) Golf (walking) Sailing Horseback riding Volleyball (6 man) Tennis (doubles)	Walking (3–4 mph) Level bicycling (6–8 mph) Light calisthenics
Moderate (5–7 METs)	Easy digging in garden Level hand lawn mowing Climbing stairs (slowly) Carrying objects (30–60 lb)	Carpentry (exterior home building)[b] Shoveling dirt[b] Pneumatic tools[b]	Badminton (competitive) Tennis (singles) Snow skiing (downhill) Light backpacking Basketball Football Skating (ice and roller) Horseback riding (gallop)	Walking (4.5–5 mph) Bicycling (9–10 mph) Swimming (breast stroke)

Includes resting metabolic needs.

[a] May cause added psychological stress that will increase work load on the heart.
[b] May produce disproportionate myocardial demands because of use of arms or isometric exercise.
(Modified from Haskell,[102] with permission.)

any activity the patient is now able to complete, increase the number of activities the patient is able to perform, and delay the onset of dependent living. The immediate objective of this pilot study was to test and compare the effectiveness of the following exercise regimens: (1) aerobic calisthenics and (2) walking/stair climbing.

These exercise regimens were chosen because they provide very convenient and inexpensive exercise training methods that require little or no equipment and are especially applicable to group exercise. Calisthenics have the added advantage of requiring a minimum of space and of training all major muscle groups of the body. Because training is expected to decrease the cardiac effort of performing the specific movement being trained, a set of calisthenics that involves the movement of most parts of the body is likely to decrease the cardiac effort of a wide variety of activities needed for activities of daily living.

The effectiveness of these two regimens for increasing aerobic power and decreasing cardiac effort during a simulated kitchen task was tested and compared. The effects of training on body weight, spontaneous physical activity, and on selected psychological phenomena were also tested.

Twenty-three female residents of a high-rise apartment administered by the Minneapolis Housing Authority volunteered for the study. The Minneapolis Housing Authority administers 43 high-rise apartment complexes with approximately 6000 residents. Disabled persons or people over the age of 62 are eligible. The average age is 76.5 years (range 53 to 92); 8 percent of this population is under age 62 and disabled. The sample of 23 had an average age of 70.7 (range 57 to 80). All subjects signed an informed consent statement and completed a medical history form, which was reviewed by a physician. The subjects were medically stable but did not appear to be unusually healthy. The following medical conditions were present in one to eight subjects at the start of the study: blindness, rheumatoid arthritis, stable angina, peripheral vascular disorders, emphysema, asthma, orthopedic conditions, and hypertension.

All subjects were invited to attend a preliminary session designed to provide for practice pedaling of a bicycle ergometer. One week later during a single evaluation session subjects were weighed and measured, completed questionnaires concerning physical activity and state anxiety, and performed a bicycle ergometer test and the modified Kottke-Kubicek Five Stage Activity Test. A physical activity questionnaire was adapted from the form used by Cassel.[91] Anxiety levels were measured with the State and Trait Anxiety Inventory form STAI-1.[92]

The bicycle test protocol was given (see Tables 8-1 and 8-2). This test consisted of a series of 3-minute exercise bouts. The first bout or level was always performed at a 2-MET intensity. Exercise intensity was increased in 1-MET increments until the subject asked to stop, some sign of exercise intolerance occurred, or the heart rate exceeded 75 percent of the available heart rate range.

The Kottke-Kubicek Activity Test (simulated kitchen task) was modified to consist only of moving a weighted kettle from a 30-inch high table to a chair

on the right of the subject, returning it to the table, moving it to a chair on the left of the subject, and returning it to the table (see Figs. 8-4 and 8-5). This test was performed at a rate of 30 moves per minute. Each full cycle, from the table to the chair and back to the table, requires four moves. This test also consisted of a series of 3-minute bouts or levels. Level 1 was always performed with the kettle weighing 3.5 lb (1½ kg). After 1 minute of rest the subject was allowed to progress to 5.5 lb (2½ kg) if no signs or symptoms of exercise intolerance were observed or reported. Subjects progressed to 8.5 lb (4 kg) if the previous exercise levels were performed without exceeding the target heart rate or causing any indices of exercise intolerance.

Heart rate was recorded during the last 10 seconds of the third minute of each exercise level (see Fig. 8-6). Blood pressure was recorded immediately after each level of the kettle test and during the last 15 seconds of each level of the bicycle ergometer test.

The subjects who completed the pretraining evaluation were divided into high- and low-intensity groups and randomly assigned to the calisthenics or the walking group. The calisthenics are described in Figures 8-7 and 8-8, and the

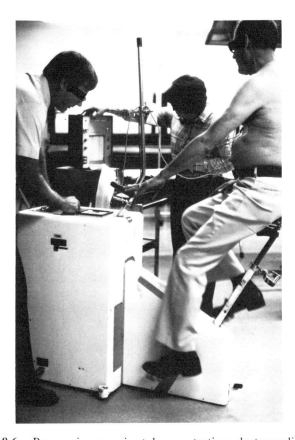

Fig. 8-6. Progressive exercise tolerance testing: electrocardiogram.

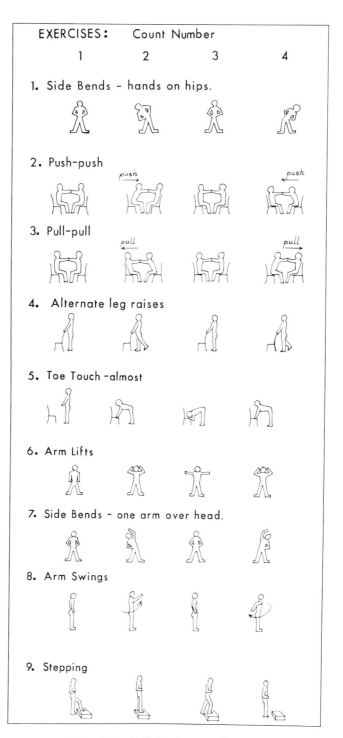

Fig. 8-7. Calisthenics exercises.

progression plan is given in Table 8-8. The calisthenics were performed at the following counts per minute (cpm):

Side bends	60
Push-push	120
Pull-pull	120
Alternate-leg raises	120
Toe touch—almost	60
Arm lifts	120
Side bends—one arm	60
Arm swings	120
Stepping	80, 100, and 120

The energy cost of stepping at 80, 100, and 120 cpm is 2, 2.4, and 2.8 METs, respectively.

The training regimen for walking/stair climbing is outlined in Table 8-10. The high-rise apartment selected for this study contains stairways at two ends of the building and balconies around two atria that provide a pleasant and convenient place to walk.

Target heart rates were set at 60 to 75 percent of the expected heart rate range. For a zero-based range this corresponds to 70 to 85 percent of the predicted maximal heart rate. However, target heart rates were never set higher than heart rates achieved during the bicycle ergometer test. Pulse rates were monitored at rest before each training session, during the last one third or immediately after each training session, and after 5 minutes of recovery. Subjects were taught to monitor their own radial pulse. The subjects were generally able to determine accurate pulse counts at rest but tended to report falsely low exercise counts. We believe that the subjects were able to count accurately, but were slow to locate the pulse after exercise, which would of course result in counts lower than those determined by the therapists.

Table 8-8. Exercise Program: Calisthenics

Week	Number of Exercises	Duration per Exercise (min)	Total Time (min)
1	1–9, 1	1	10
2	1–9, 1	1	10
3	1–9, 1	2	20
4	1–9, 1	2	20
5	1–9, 1	3	30
6	1–9, 1	3	30
7	1–9, 1	3	30
8	1–9, 1	3	30
9	1–9, 1	3	30
10	1–9, 1	3	30

An 8-oz (0.4 kg) weight (hand held) was added to exercises 6 to 8 for high-capacity subjects (done bilaterally).

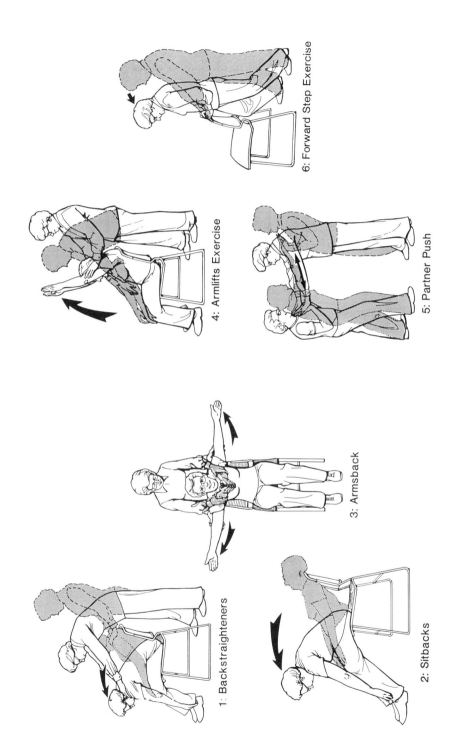

1: Backstraighteners

2: Sitbacks

3: Armsback

4: Armlifts Exercise

5: Partner Push

6: Forward Step Exercise

228

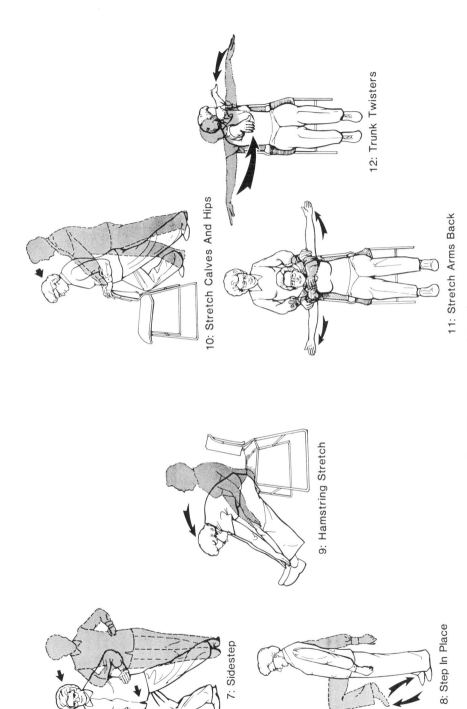

7: Sidestep

8: Step In Place

9: Hamstring Stretch

10: Stretch Calves And Hips

11: Stretch Arms Back

12: Trunk Twisters

Fig. 8-8. Partner calisthenics.

229

Table 8-9. Metabolic Equivalents (METs) of
Step Ergometer Work

8 inch bench		12 inch bench	
cpm[a]	METs	cpm	METs
40	3	44	4
60	4	72	6
80	5	104	8
104	6	136	10

[a] cpm = counts per min

Exercise sessions were supervised by physical and occupational therapy instructors and graduate students. Supervised sessions were provided on Monday and Thursday for 9 weeks. Subjects were encouraged to exercise one additional session each week.

Results of the Pilot Study

Maximal aerobic power was estimated by extrapolation from the results of the submaximal bicycle ergometer test. This estimate was based on the expected linear increase in heart rate as work load increased and on the predicted maximal heart rate.[63] The average maximal aerobic power of the eight subjects who completed training by the walking/stair climbing method increased from 4.5 to 6.0 METs after 9 weeks of training ($P < 0.01$). The eight subjects who completed the calisthenics regimen increased from a mean of 3.6 to 4.7 METs ($P < 0.05$). The gains of these two groups were not different ($P > 0.05$). Four subjects who did not train showed no significant change in maximal aerobic power (3.7 to 3.8 METs; $P > 0.05$). Physical activity scores increased from a mean of 9.6 to 11.5 ($P < 0.05$). State anxiety scores were generally in the low normal range for the subjects who completed the training program and did not appear to change after training. When only the low-capacity subjects are considered, the calisthenics regimen caused larger decreases in heart rate responses at a given work rate on the simulated kitchen

Table 8-10. Exercise Program: Walking/Stair Climbing

Week	Distance (miles)	Stairs[a] (loops)	Speed (mph)	Total Time (min)
1	0.3	0–2	2	10
2	0.50	0–4	2	14
3	0.70	0–6	2.5	16
4	0.80	0–6	2.5	20
5	1.00	0–8	2.5	25
6	1.20	0–8	2.5	30
7	1.30	0–10	2.6	30
8	1.40	0–10	2.8	30
9	1.50	0–12	3	30
10	1.60	0–12	3.2	30

[a] Each stair loop consisted of one to six flights of stairs followed by level walking.

task than did the walking/stair climbing regimen. The calisthenics regimen appears to provide more relevant changes in the cardiopulmonary capacity to perform upper-extremity-dominated ADL.

Pretraining aerobic power was higher than that reported for ambulatory nursing home populations. Posttraining values are comparable with values expected for the young old (5 to 7 METs).

This appears to be the only study that documents the effectiveness of calisthenics for increasing the aerobic capacity of the elderly. Kellerman et al.[84] reported that a training regimen consisting only of calisthenics did not increase the functional capacity of patients with angina pectoris.

Previous work by other investigators has demonstrated that jogging or riding stationary bicycles will improve the functional capacity of subjects with an average age of up to 65 years.[24,29,39,45] Reports concerning subjects older than an average of 65 years of age are rare. Smith et al.[93] have trained older female subjects ($\bar{x}$ 83 years of age) using low-intensity calisthenic-style activities. In the Smith study bone mineral loss was reversed in the trained group, but changes in functional capacity were not reported.

Further work by the authors has resulted in the development of a more practical yet reliable assessment tool for measuring aerobic power and a set of more effective calisthenics. The assessment tool is a graded exercise tolerance (GXT) test that uses a single height of 8 inches and cadences that are progressively increased.[94-96] The stepping rates and corresponding energy costs are given in Table 8-9. An audiotape that provides automatic control of durations and metronome-generated cadences is available (University of Minnesota, Media Distribution, Box 734 Mayo Building, 420 Delaware St. SE, Minneapolis MN). This GXT system has demonstrated good reliability when used on elderly persons.[97] Its feasibility has been amply demonstrated by successfully being used for approximately 300 tests. Almost all (about 99 percent) subjects living independently who volunteered for our testing and training programs were able to complete at least stage one of the step tests successfully, and more than 90 percent were able to complete two or more stages. Patients enrolled in day care were also usually able to complete at least two stages of the test. Day-care patients were most likely to experience difficulty with timing and coordination, whereas subjects living independently in a high-rise apartment for the elderly and handicapped who experienced difficulty with the test had orthopedic problems of the hip or knee.

Our newest calisthenics, as shown in Fig. 8-7,[96,98,99] have been proven to be feasible and have met with the approval of the approximately 200 subjects who have participated in our programs. We do need to emphasize that these calisthenics require good cooperation between participating partners. To achieve optimal results for the exercises designed primarily to improve local muscle endurance, strength, and flexibility (exercise numbers 1–5 and 11), the partner needs to be able to manually resist appropriately. Partners need to be reasonably well coordinated and appropriately matched according to strength and local muscle endurance. For day-care clientele or nursing-home residents we recommend using calisthenics that do not require cooperation between partners unless a skilled professional takes the role of the partner. Although variety is often recommended for exercise programs for healthy persons, we repeat these standard calisthenics for the 10-week sessions (refer to Table 8-11, for the recommended progression) and attempt to minimize changes in the program. Elderly persons or persons with traumatized joints need to be encouraged to adapt exercises in order to minimize muscle and joint discomfort. Almost all of our elderly subjects have appreciated the standardized routines. The intensities of exercise activity are regulated by adjusting resistances and rest breaks according to the capacity of the individual participant. The results of a study performed on 14 experimental and 5 control subjects showed a significant decrease in heart-rate responses to submaximal exercise by experimental but not by control group subjects.[98] This indicates that a training effect occurred for the heart and circulatory system and/or for the involved muscles as a result of this training program.

The circuit-training system described by Hagberg et al.[100] is theoretically similar to our calisthenics program. The effectiveness of these systems for improving strength and local muscle endurance is well established, but most authorities considered circuit training to be likely to worsen cardiovascular risk factors. Although we continue to recommend an emphasis on rhythmic lower extremity exercises (numbers 7 and 8), the evidence that exercise designed primarily to improve the local muscle endurance of all major muscle groups of the body caused improvement in cardiovascular risk factors indicates that our entire program will benefit the cardiovascular system.[100]

CONCLUSION

This review of the literature and pilot study description indicate that elderly persons are usually less than optimally active but are able to improve cardiopulmonary response to exercise through training. Pretraining evaluations capable of safely and specifically determining safe levels of physical therapy were recommended. Training regimens and training intensities appropriate for medically stable elderly persons were presented; these methods were especially effective for subjects with the following medical conditions: blindness, stable angina, peripheral vascular disorders, emphysema, and hypertension. The training regimens were readily adaptable to subjects with various orthopedic problems and for a subject with rheumatoid arthritis.

With the rapidly increasing population of elderly over the age of 75, and therefore the increasing frequency of lower-extremity dysfunction, research is needed to determine new evaluation and cardiopulmonary training regimens emphasizing upper extremity activities. The primary goal of evaluation of cardiopulmonary response to specific amounts of exercise is to avoid unnecessary secondary cardiac and pulmonary complications resulting from overexertion. In the very old it is common to find patients who require basic cardiac conditioning before other physical therapy procedures can be safely administered.

Table 8-11. Exercise Program: Partner–based Calisthenics

					Week Number			
	1	2	3	4	5	6	7	8–10
Warmup	3 min	3 min	3 min	3 min	3 min	3 min	3 min	3 min
Strength–Endurance (8–10 min)								
Ex. 1	5×	10×	15×	20×	25×	30×	30×	30×
Ex. 2	5×	10×	15×	20×	25×	30×	30×	30×
Ex. 3	5×	10×	15×	20×	25×	30×	30×	30×
Ex. 4	5×	10×	15×	20×	25×	30×	30×	30×
Ex. 5	5×	10×	15×	20×	25×	30×	30×	30×
Cardiopulmonary (5–30 min)								
Exs. 6–8	1 cycl	2 cycl	2 cycl	3 cycl	4 cycl	5 cycl	6 cycl	7 cycl
(1 min per side per exercise equals 1 cycle)								
Stretch–Cool-down (4–6 min)								
Ex. 9	5 sec × 1	10 sec × 1	10 sec × 2	10 sec × 3	10 sec × 3	10 sec × 3	10 sec × 3	10 sec × 3
Ex. 10	5 sec × 1	10 sec × 1	10 sec × 2	10 sec × 3	10 sec × 3	10 sec × 3	10 sec × 3	10 sec × 3
Ex. 11	5 sec × 1	10 sec × 1	10 sec × 2	10 sec × 3	10 sec × 3	10 sec × 3	10 sec × 3	10 sec × 3
Ex. 12	5 sec × 1	10 sec × 1	10 sec × 2	10 sec × 3	10 sec × 3	10 sec × 3	10 sec × 3	10 sec × 3
Approximate total time:	20 min	25 min	25 min	35 min	40 min	45 min	50 min	50 min

REFERENCES

1. Beall CH, Goldstein MC, Feldman ES: Social structure and intracohort variation in physical fitness among elderly males in a traditional Third World society. J Am Geriatr Soc 33:406, 1985
2. Borhani ND: Prevalence and prognostic significance of hypertension in the elderly. J Am Geriatr Soc 34:112, 1986
3. Hollenbeck CB, Haskell W, Rosenthal M, Reaven GM: Effect of habitual physical activity on regulation of insulin stimulated glucose disposal in older males. J Am Geriatr Soc 33:273, 1985
4. LaPorte RE, Black-Sandler R, Cauley JA, et al: The assessment of physical activity in older women: analysis of the interrelationship and reliability of activity monitoring, activity surveys, and caloric intake. J Gerontol 38:394, 1983
5. Payton OD, Poland JL: Aging process: implications for clinical practice. Phys Ther 63:41, 1983
6. Rosenthal MJ: Geriatrics. An updated bibliography. J Am Geriatr Soc 35:560, 1987
7. Vallbona C, Baker SB: Physical fitness prospects in the elderly. Arch Phys Med Rehabil 65:194, 1984
8. Zavaroni I, DallAnlio E, Bruschi R, et al: Effect of age and environmental factors on glucose tolerance and insulin secretion in a worker population. J Am Geriatr Soc 34:271, 1986
9. Bassey EJ: Age, inactivity and some physiological responses to exercise. Gerontology 24:66, 1978
10. Clarke HH: Exercise and aging. Phys Fitness Res Digest, Ser 7. No 2, April 1977
11. Shephard RJ: Activity patterns in the elderly. In Physical Activity and Aging. Year Book Medical Publishers, Chicago, 1978
12. Sidney KH, Shephard RJ: Activity patterns of elderly men and women. J Gerontol 32:25, 1977
13. Saltin B, Blomqvist B, Mitchel JH, et al: Response to submaximal and maximal exercise after bed rest and training. Circulation 38 (Suppl 7):1, 1968
14. Browse NL: The Physiology and Pathology of Bed Rest. Charles C Thomas, Sringfield, IL, 1965
15. Graf RS: Rehabilitation during the acute and convalescent stages following myocardial infarction. In Amundsen LR (ed): Cardiac Rehabilitation. Churchill Livingstone, New York, 1981
16. Brewer V, Meyer BM, Keele MS, et al: Role of exercise in prevention of involutional bone loss. Med Sci Sports Exerc 15:445, 1983
17. Robbins AE, Rubenstein LZ: Postural hypotension in the elderly (review). J Am Geriatr Soc 32:769, 1984
18. Serfass RC: What are the benefits and how do we get started? In Smith EL, Serfass RC (eds): Aging and Exercise. Enslow, Hillside, NJ, 1981
19. Michel TH: Physiological effects of endurance training. In Amundsen LR (ed): Cardiac Rehabilitation. Churchill Livingstone, New York, 1981
20. Karvonen MJ, Kentala E, Mustala O: The effects of training on heart rate. Ann Med Exp Biol Fenn 35:307, 1958
21. Amundsen LR: Establishing activity and training levels for patients with ischemic heart disease. Phys Ther 59:754, 1979
22. Carter CL: Cardiac rehabilitation of outpatients during the recovery phase following myocardial infarction. In Amundsen LR (ed): Cardiac Rehabilitation. Churchill Livingstone, New York, 1981

23. May GA, Nagle FJ: Changes in rate-pressure product with physical training of individuals with coronary artery disease. Phys Ther 64:1361, 1984

24. Adler JC, Mazzarella N, Puzsier L, Alpa A: Treadmill training for a bilateral below-knee amputee patient with cardiopulmonary disease. Arch Phys Med Rehabil 68:858, 1987

25. Hagberg JM, Ehsani AA, Holloszy JO: Effect of 12 months of intense exercise training on stroke volume in patients with coronary heart disease. Circulation 67:1194, 1983

26. Foster TA, Hale WE, Srinivasan SR, et al: Levels of selected cardiovascular risk factors in a sample of geriatric participants—the Dunedin Program. J Gerontol 42:241, 1987

27. Klausner SC, Schwartz AB: The aging heart. Clin Geriatr Med 1:119, 1985

28. Manvari DE, Patterson C, Johnson D, et al: Left ventricular diastolic function in a population of healthy elderly subjects. An echocardiographic study. J Am Geriatr Soc 33:758, 1985

29. Stamford BA: Exercise and the elderly. In Pandolf KB (ed): Exercise and Sports Reviews, Vol 16. Macmillan, New York, 1988

30. Shepard RJ: Gross changes in form and function. In Physical Activity and Aging. Year Book Medical Publishers, Chicago, 1978

31. Aniansson A, Sperling L, Rundgren A, Lehnberg E: Muscle function in 75-year-old men and women: a longitudinal study. Scand J Rehab Med (Suppl) 9:92, 1983

32. Aniansson A, Hedberg M, Henning G-B, Grimby G: Muscle morphology, enzymatic activity, and muscle strength in elderly men: a follow-up study. Muscle Nerve 9:585, 1986

33. Danneskiold-Samsoe B, Kofod V, Munter J, et al: Muscle strength and functional capacity in 78–81 year-old men and women. Eur J Appl Physiol 52:310, 1984

34. Murray MP, Duthie EH, Gambert SR, et al: Age-related differences in knee muscle strength in normal women. J Gerontol 40:275, 1985

35. Murray MP, Gardner GM, Mollinger LA, et al: Strength of isometric and isokinetic contractions. Knee muscles of men aged 20-86. Phys Ther. 60:412, 1980

36. Capuano-Pucci D, Rheault W, Rudman D: Relationship between plasma somatomedin C and muscle performance in a geriatric male population. Am J Phys Med 66:364, 1987

37. Gordan GS, Genant HK: The aging skeleton. Clin Geriatr Med 1:95, 1985

38. Stillman RJ, Lohman TG, Slaughter MH, Massey BH: Physical activity and bone mineral content in women aged 30 to 85 years. Med Sci Sports Exerc 18:576, 1986

39. Kriska AM, Bayles C, Cauley JA, et al: A randomized exercise trial in older women: increased activity over two years and the factors associated with compliance. Med Sci Sports Exerc 18:557, 1986

40. Boston AG, Bates E, Mazzarella N, et al: Ergometer modification for combined arm-leg use by lower extremity amputees in cardiovascular testing and training. Arch Phys Med Rehabil 68:244, 1987

41. Thompson RF, Crist DM, Marsh M, et al: Effects of physical exercise for elderly patients with physical impairments. J Am Geriatr Soc 36:130, 1988

42. Grimby G: Physical activity and muscle training in the elderly. Acta Med Scand (Suppl) 711:233, 1986

43. Mahler DA, Cunningham LN, Curfman GD: Aging and exercise performance. Clin Geriatr Med 2:433, 1986

44. Sager K: Exercises to activate seniors. Physician Sportsmed 12:144, 1984

45. Seals DR, Hagberg JM, Hurley BF, et al: Endurance training in older men and women. I. Cardiovascular responses to exercise. J Appl Physiol 57:1024, 1984

46. Seals DR, Hurley BF, Schultz J, Hagberg JM: Endurance training in older men and women. II. Blood lactate response to submaximal exercise. J Appl Physiol 57:1030, 1984

47. Amundsen LR: Assessing exercise tolerance: a review. Phys Ther 59:534, 1979

48. Amundsen LR, Nielsen DH: Normal and abnormal cardiovascular responses to acute physical exercise. In Amundsen LR (ed): Cardiac Rehabilitation. Churchill Livingstone, New York, 1981

49. Kispert CP, Nielsen DH: Normal cardiopulmonary responses to acute- and chronic-strengthening and endurance exercises. Phys Ther 65:1828, 1985

50. Irwin S: Abnormal exercise physiology. In Irwin S, Tecklin JS (eds): Cardiopulmonary Physical Therapy. CV Mosby, St Louis, 1985

51. Astrand I: Aerobic capacity in men and women with special reference to age. Acta Physiol Scand 49 (Suppl 169):1, 1960

52. Astrand P-O, Rodahl K: Textbook of Work Physiology. McGraw-Hill, New York, 1977

53. Irwin SC: Cardiac rehabilitation for the geriatric patient. Top Geriatr Rehabil 2:44, 1986

54. Schoneberger MB, Schoneberger B, Lundsford BR: Chart review and physical assessment prior to exercise. In Amundsen LR (ed): Cardiac Rehabilitation. Churchill Livingstone, New York, 1981

55. Hudson MF, Safeguard your elderly patient's health through accurate physical assessment. Nursing 13:58, 1983

56. Carlsten A, Grimby G: Effects of exercise on the central circulation. In The Circulatory Response to Muscular Exercise in Man. Charles C Thomas, Springfield, IL, 1966

57. Naughton J, Haider R: Methods of exercise testing. In Naughton J, Hellerstein H, Mohler IC (eds): Exercise Testing and Exercise Training in Coronary Heart Disease. Academic Press, Orlando, FL, 1973

58. Hellerstein HK, Hirsch EL, Adler R, et al: Principles of exercise prescription for normals and cardiac subjects. In Naughton J, Hellerstein H, Mohler IC (eds): Exercise Testing and Exercise Training in Coronary Heart Disease. Academic Press, Orlando, FL, 1973

59. Anderson KL, Shephard RJ, Denolin H, et al: Techniques for collection and evaluation of cardiovascular and respiratory data during exercise. In Fundamentals of Exercise Testing. World Health Organization, Geneva, 1971

60. American College of Sports Medicine: Guidelines for Graded Exercise Testing and Exercise Prescription. Lea & Febiger, Philadelphia, 1986

61. Serfass RC, Agre JC, Smith EL: Exercise testing for the elderly. Top Geriatr Rehabil 1:58, 1985

62. Roberts JM, Sullivan M, Froelicher VF, et al: Predicting oxygen uptake from treadmill testing in normal subjects and coronary artery disease patients. Am Heart J 108:1454, 1984

63. Nielsen DH, Amundsen LR: Exercise physiology: An overview with emphasis on aerobic capacity and energy cost. In Amundsen LR (ed): Cardiac Rehabilitation. Churchill Livingstone, New York, 1981

64. McAllister RG, Lowenthal SL: Progressive exercise tolerance testing. In Amundsen LR (eds): Cardiac Rehabilitation. Churchill Livingstone, New York, 1981

65. Sidney KH, Shephard RJ: Maximum and submaximum exercise tests in men and

women in the seventh, eighth, and ninth decades of life. J Appl Physiol 43:280, 1977

66. Physiological measurements and indices. In Larson: Fitness, Health, and Work Capacity: International Standards for Assessment. Macmillan, New York, 1973

67. Nielsen DH, Gerleman DG, Amundsen LR, et al: Clinical determination of energy cost and walking velocity via stopwatch or speedometer cane and conversion graphs. Phys Ther 62:591, 1982

68. Smith EL, Gilligan BA: Physical activity prescription for the older adult. Physician Sportsmed 11:91, 1983

69. George LK, Fillenbaum GG: OARS methodology. A decade of experience in geriatric assessment. J Am Geriatr Soc 33:607, 1985

70. Jette AM: Functional disability and rehabilitation of the aged. Top Geriatr Rehabil 1:1, 1986

71. Katz S: Assessing self-maintenance: activities of daily living, mobility, and instrumental activities of daily living. J Am Geriatr Soc 31:721, 1983

72. Kaufert JM: Functional ability indices: measurement problems in assessing their validity. Arch Phys Med Rehabil 64:260, 1983

73. Squires AJ: Physiotherapy assessment of the elderly patient. Physiotherapy 72:617, 1986

74. Kaufert JM: Functional ability indices: measurement problems in assessing their validity. Arch Phys Med Rehabil 64:260, 1983

75. Jackson O: Functional assessment of the aged. Allied Hlth Behav Sci 2:47, 1980

76. Lawton EB: Activities of daily living test: geriatric considerations. Phys Occup Ther Geriatr 1:11, 1980

77. Aniansson A, Rundgren A, Sperling L: Evaluation of functional capacity in activities of daily living in 70-year-old men and women. Scand J Rehabil Med 12:145, 1980

78. Kottke FJ, Kubicek WG, Olson ME, et al: Five stage test of cardiac performance during occupational activity. Arch Phys Med Rehabil 43:228, 1962

79. Fitzgerald PL: Exercise for the elderly. Med Clin N Am 69:189, 1985

80. Morse CE, Smith EL: Physical activity programming for the aged. In Smith EL, Serfass RC (eds): Aging and Exercise. Enslow, Hillside, NJ, 1981

81. Greer M, Weber T, Dimick S, et al: Physiological responses to low-intensity cardiac rehabilitation exercises. Phys Ther 60:1146, 1980

82. Weise RA, Karpovich PV: Energy cost of exercises for convalescents. Arch Phys Med Rehabil 28:447, 1947

83. Fletcher GF, Cantwell JD, Watt EW: Oxygen consumption and hemodynamic response of exercises used in training of patients with recent myocardial infarction. Circulation 60:140, 1979

84. Kellerman JJ, Ben-Ari E, Chayet M, et al: Cardiocirculatory response to different types of training in patients with angina pectoris. Cardiology 62:218, 1977

85. Amundsen LR, Takahashi M, Carter CA, Nielsen DH: Energy cost of rehabilitation calisthenics. Phys Ther 59:855, 1979

86. Fleischaker KF, Gower MA, Canafax LM, Holt LJ: Case study: Rehabilitation following a myocardial infarction, with a sample program. In Amundsen LR (ed): Cardiac Rehabilitation. Churchill Livingstone, New York, 1981

87. Lerman J, Bruce RA, Sivarajan, et al: Low level dynamic exercises for earlier cardiac rehabilitation. Aerobic and hemodynamic responses. Arch Phys Med Rehabil 57:355, 1976

88. Activities Which Require a MET Level in the Cardiac Rehabilitation Program.

Department of Physical Medicine, St. Joseph Mercy Hospital, Ann Arbor, MI, 1972

89. Stippig J, Berg A, Keul J: In Amundsen LR (ed): Cardiac Rehabilitation: Outpatient Physical Training Methods. Aspen, Publishers, Rockville, MD, 1988

90. David JA, Convertino VA: A comparison of heart rate methods for predicting endurance training intensity. Med Sci Sports 7:295, 1975

91. Cassel J, Heyden SH, Bartel AG, et al: Occupational and physical activity and coronary heart disease. Arch Intern Med 128:920, 1971

92. Spielberger CD, Gorsuch RL, Lushene RE: The State-Trait Anxiety Inventory (STAI), Test Manual for Form X. Consulting Psychologists Press, Palo Alto, CA, 1968

93. Smith EL, Reddan W, Smith PE: Physical activity and calcium modalities for bone mineral increase in aged women. Med Sci Sports 13:60, 1981

94. Patterson RP: Home computer based performance evaluation. Presented at the Twentieth Annual Rocky Mountain Bioengineering Symposium. Rochester, MN, 1983

95. Amundsen L, Ellingham C, Shore S: Cardiopulmonary fitness test. Cardiopul Rec 2:13, 1987

96. Amundsen L, Ellingham C: Safe and effective exercise for the elderly. Presented at the First World Congress of Allied Health Professions Elsinore, Denmark, 1988

97. Shore S: Stability of response by a geriatric population to submaximal step test. Plan B Paper. University of Minnesota, Physical Therapy Graduate Studies, Minneapolis, 1987

98. Amundsen LR, Ellingham CT, Pallasch JM: Physical training in the elderly. Phys Ther 64:724, 1984

99. Planning for Fitness: Part I. Cardiopulmonary fitness testing; Part II. Developing an exercise class. University of Minnesota, Media Distributions, Minneapolis, Videotape, Audiotape, and Instruction Booklet, Minneapolis, 1986

100. Hurley BF, Hagberg JM, Goldberg AP, et al: Resistive training can reduce coronary risk factors without altering VO_2 max or percent body fat. Med Sci Sports Exerc 20:150, 1988

9 | Comprehensive Functional Assessment of the Elderly

Osa L. Jackson
Rosalie H. Lang

Applied gerontology involves the process of taking didactic concepts and research findings out of the laboratory and using these to create a comprehensive functional assessment (CFA) that can be used as the starting point for effective rehabilitation intervention for the elderly. Comprehensive functional assessment is necessary for the elderly patient population because their medical histories are usually complicated by numerous related as well as unrelated conditions. The need for a multidisciplinary assessment with an emphasis on functional abilities is agreed on now as a basis for the practice of geriatric medicine.[1-7] The role of physical therapists and their contribution to the data collected for the CFA will vary, depending on where the CFA is performed. The important aspects for each geriatric rehabilitation team are to identify a format for patient assessment that will (1) reflect accurately the patient's abilities in the span of a 24-hour day; (2) be complete and assess the physical, emotional, social, cognitive, and environmental details of the patients unique situation; (3) assess the patient's maximum potential by avoiding unnecessary distortion of functional abilities arising from patient fear, tiredness, anger, and such; (4) provide data to periodic auditing of the effectiveness of intervention by all providers, including physical therapists; and (5) use the patient's values, life-style, goals, and sense of self-determination as a basis for

Ms. Lang's research supported by Administration on Aging grant 90-A-1618, a grant to The Assistance Group for Human Resources Development, Silver Spring, MD, a group she served as vice president in 1979–1980.

deciding the pace and process of intervention. The goal of all activity from the initial CFA to intervention and continued maintenance of maximum function at home (where possible) is to pace intervention so that the patient is empowered to choose to create a new life for himself or herself, whether after an acute illness or injury or in attempting to cope with chronic illnesses or disability.

A comprehensive data base will help the rehabilitation team be aware of the multitude of factors that can affect where a patient can live, whether on initial discharge from an acute-care hospital or in seeking to intervene to maintain a long-term patient at home. It is necessary to understand the multitude of factors that need to exist to enable independent living in the community in order to develop realistic plans for rehabilitation intervention for a patient with diminished function.

Policy issues abound from which the members of a geriatric rehabilitation team cannot isolate themselves. Repeated references are made throughout the discussion that follows to the gradual loss of functional ability in a growing aging and aged population. A geriatric patient could enter the circle of care at many points in the aging process, especially if the patient has a long-term disability. Yet, reimbursement policies of third-party payers make it most likely that rehabilitation will be available and affordable to the patient only after an acute medical problem resulting in hospitalization. But even for the postacute patient, reimbursement stops when therapeutic interventions reach the maximum level a patient can attain. For the elderly person striving to maintain independence at home, although rehabilitative services could effectively *maintain* functional status enabling independent living and sometimes prevent an acute medical crisis, payment is rarely available. The patient and his or her family must be both knowledgeable enough to seek help and sufficiently well off to pay for such care. Thus prevention and maintenance services are effectively unavailable.

Therefore, in discussing CFA and its role in ensuring effective care leading to maximum independence, we face major dilemmas. The demographic data point to a growing population, living to an ever older age, for whom preventive services to maintain function are not provided, largely because of financial constraints; yet we have increasing pressure on available resources that undergird postacute rehabilitation. This is so because the population to be served is larger and the number needing nursing-home care, which exerts the greatest drain on health resources along with hospitals and physicians, is both larger and more disabled because of lack of effective, timely intervention to maintain the functional independence of those with long-term disability.*

The data on need in the early sections of the chapter document these trends. The tools discussed in depth could result in systematic functional assessment and coordinated service delivery if incentives were in place to encourage such delivery. We urge health professionals seeking to benefit from this discussion both to consider the policy disincentives to the full exercise of their therapeutic skills as well as to address the narrower, though equally important, issues of comprehensive functional assessment within a service coordination system. As you consider how fully you can use these tools, assess also the policy changes necessary to enable you to enlarge your patient effectiveness through health policy changes, both systemic and financial, that are needed to support your therapeutic interventions in whatever setting they will be most effective.

(NOTE: An experimental project has been underway for the past 5 years in Hudiksvall, Sweden, that reflects many desirable health policy innovations. The project has thus far decreased the need for long-term care nursing-home beds and increased consumer satisfaction with health care delivery. In the town where the project is being carried out, there have been no other demographic or sociological changes that can account for the positive changes in the functional ability of elderly persons except the major modifications in health care policy to emphasize prevention, home care, and the nurturing of the ability and desire to care for oneself.) The overall result will be the creation of an organization, process, and philosophy of care that acknowledges the unique needs and functional capacities of the elderly as a group and of each individual.)

Evaluation/assessment of the aged patient requires a clear definition of the term rehabilitation and an understanding of the need for the primary emphasis to be placed on functional ability rather than on diagnostic labels. A discussion of the important interrelationship between activities of daily living (ADL) and mental health will be presented as the justification for the need for a circle of care for the elderly. As a physical therapist, how do you fit into the circle of care? How do the activities of the other providers of care in your community (hospital, short-term rehabilitation, long-term rehabilitation, nursing home, home care, adult day care, respite care, meals on wheels, homemaker and chore services) affect the potential effectiveness of your efforts? How can the organization and approach of institutional care affect the outcome of rehabilitation? Why is it that the majority of the elderly prefer and actually perform better in a home-based rehabilitation program? Are home-based rehabilitation programs realistic as an alternative to residential institutional rehabilitation? What are the major modifications needed? It is only with an understanding of the potential client and the total environment in which you are working that it is useful to examine the actual details of the process. If basic premises about the patient population are not accurate or if the environment in which you are working does not support the intended outcome of your efforts (improving self-care capacity and quality of life for the aged patient), the physical therapist cannot expect to see improvements in functional capacity in the elderly patient.

The elderly may come to rehabilitation after a stroke, cardiovascular problem, orthopedic problem, or a combination of problems or as a result of a disruption in self-care capacity stemming from chronic degenerative disabilities accumulating over time. The elderly cannot be squeezed into a rehabilitation model or program based on the evaluation/treatment approaches used for the middle-aged population. This chapter presents a discussion of a model rehabilitation program or system incorporating a record-keeping system designed for the multiple functional problems commonly seen in the elderly. A model for in-depth ADL evaluation and ongoing monitoring of progress as it relates to self-care capacity also is presented. The basic premise of this chapter is that the elderly are a special population requiring a special philosophy and process of rehabilitation and physical therapy if they are to achieve their full potential.

THE ELDERLY—A POPULATION WITH INTENSIVE REHABILITATION NEEDS

The 1975 report from the United States Federal Commission on Chronic Illness[8] estimated a rate of 4402 chronic diseases per 1000 people 65 years of age and older, compared to 407 chronic diseases per 1000 people under the age of 16. It has been noted that it is only when functioning in day-to-day activities is affected that chronic illness becomes a matter of both public and private concern.[9] For example, a household survey[10] of a Rhode Island population in 1975 noted that 66.7 percent of the respondents age 65 and older suffered a "longstanding condition" but that only 34.6 percent reported that it resulted in "some limitations in major activities." It is true that with advanced age there is increased incidence of chronic illness and disability, but it is a very small percentage of the elderly who require special, formal services.

In order to begin to examine the assessment process that helps to define the scope of the needed services, activities of daily living (ADL) will be defined as "all activities necessary during an ordinary day from waking up in the morning until going to sleep at night."[11] If it is possible to define the normal range of functional capabilities for the healthy and frail elderly, it will then be possible to begin to modify the assessment process to gain a better measure of the functional capacity of each elderly disabled patient. With realistic age norms, it is also possible to create increasingly appropriate restorative programs of care. The goal is to work to remove the age bias that now exists in evaluation of the aged as possible candidates for rehabilitation care, including the biases within the field of physical therapy. Increasingly targeted assessment procedures will facilitate independence and active lives for the aged, an outcome beneficial to society and the elderly individual. A more important by-product is that such procedures will make it possible to maintain independence among the healthy and better support frail elderly through environmental planning and modifications (e.g., housing design, kitchen organization).

The review of normative research findings in ADL capacity among the healthy and at-risk elderly will be divided as follows: basal ADL (upper extremity function, hygiene, and dressing); function in the kitchen (pronation, supination, and reach); mobility (standing from a seated position in a chair, maintaining a comfortable walking speed, climbing steps); gross mobility; common physical activities; and social disability (housekeeping, transportation, socialization, food preparation, and grocery shopping).

Basal ADL

The functional capacity of the upper extremities is closely tied to basal activities of daily living (upper extremity function, hygiene, and dressing). Because upper extremity strength and its functional use seems to be less affected by advanced aging than strength of the lower extremities, the basal ADL appears to change least with age.[12] Despite this fact, the Framingham Disability Study (FDS) found that the average healthy 75- to 84-year-old is likely to need more help to perform all basal ADLs except eating than persons 55 to 64. However, more than 90 percent of the 75- to 84-year-olds were still independent in all basal ADLs. Women in the study were also more likely to require help with basal ADLs than men.[13] The FDS examined a population that is slightly less disabled than the average older person in the United States because of a higher-than-average socioeconomic status and longstanding selective participation in the study (nearly 30 years) of the population studied. A comparison with Branch's 1976 Massachusetts Elders Survey of noninstitutionalized elderly confirms the finding that the Framingham group was slightly less disabled than the norm.[14]

The test for upper extremity mobility used four tasks (reach for opposite big toe, grasp earlobe on opposite side with arm in front of head, grasp earlobe on opposite side with arm behind head, and fit hand between buttock and seat). The only task that the average 70-year-old tested had any difficulty with was the reach for the opposite big toe.[15] In this study 7.3 percent of the men and 5.5 percent of the women were not able or were able only with difficulty to reach their opposite big toe. This movement involves the integrated function of the upper extremity with the pelvis and lower extremity. If the big toe reach cannot be performed, there will be functional problems with dressing and pedicure as well as ambulation. The need for assistive devices to compensate for the loss of integrated upper and lower extremity motion in the elderly is well documented.[16]

To facilitate improvement in basal ADL tasks, consider a review of the normative age-related changes in the component motions that has been made.[17] As compared to 20- to 30-year-olds, the average 70-year-old tested had no difference in strength of key grip or in endurance of the transversal volar grip. The lack of change in the key grip from young to old may be associated with the frequent use of this movement in ADL (e.g., handling keys, faucet handles). It was noted that there was a decrease in muscle coordination and strength of the transversal volar grip, visible in functional activities (e.g., handling an electric plug) for 70-year-old women, whose dexterity was found to be poorer than that of 70-year-old men at this task.[15] Researchers show a consensus in finding a decrease of hand strength in older men—35 to 43 percent between ages 25 and 74.[18,19] Asmussen[20] found a decrease in the strength of the transversal volar grip of 23 percent in men from age 25 to age 65. In women overall, the loss of strength noted was less than for men. It appears that as the elderly lose strength in the transversal volar grip there is an increase in the submaximal endurance of this movement. Functionally, this may mean that there is a normal compensation in endurance for the decrease in strength. The compensation is noted more in women than in men.

Functional Kitchen Activities

Carroll developed tests for pronation and supination as a part of a quantitative test of upper-extremity function.[21] Along with a reach test, these tests were used to examine the normative levels of function related to basic eating and food preparation activities. Pouring water from a jug to a glass was used to test forearm pronation in a power and precision activity. The jug contained 1 liter of water. Pronation and supination of the forearm were tested in a precision activity by having subjects pour water from one glass to another and back again. It was found that among elderly 2.3 percent of the men and 1.8 percent of the women had difficulty in carrying out one or more of the tasks involved in the water-pouring test. The subjects who experienced difficulty were noted to have some locomotor dysfunctions and could not be classified as healthy.[15]

Upper-extremity reach was tested by having subjects lift a glass and a 1-kg packet onto shelves 140 to 180 cm high. The shelves were mounted above a cupboard 60 cm deep and 90 cm high, simulating a kitchen counter. It was found that 1.1 percent of the men and 6.9 percent of the women were not able to lift the glass and the weight to the shelf 180 cm high. An equal number of participants could perform this task only with difficulty. With advanced age there is an associated decrease in height. It must be noted that even young women 158 cm tall or shorter have similar difficulty lifting a glass and a 1-kg packet to a shelf 180 cm high. Other causes that complicated the execution of the task were locomotor/neurologic problems or positional vertigo (head/neck extension). In the average elderly population living independently in the community, there appears to be enough difficulty with high reach to warrant systematic modifications of kitchen organization and design.

Mobility

The three components examined in this category are rising from a chair (seated position), walking speed (as it relates to pedestrian activity), and climbing steps (as it relates to use of public transportation). To rise from a seated position in a chair may require the assistance of the upper extremities. Sperling found no significant differences in strength of elbow extension between 70-year-old subjects and younger subjects.[17] This finding would imply that most elderly persons, if there is no pathologic problems involving the upper extremities, can assist themselves in coming to a standing position *if armrests are available*. Because lower extremity function for this task is often decreased, furniture design can directly compensate for the age-related losses in the ability to rise from a chair.

For the walking test, subjects were asked to walk 30 meters unassisted (the distance across an average urban street). The increased interest in examining walking speed in the elderly is the result of the increasing rate of traffic accidents involving the elderly as pedestrians. The elderly on average walk slower than the speed defined as safe for crossing at traffic signals (1.4 m/sec). In a study of Swedish pedestrians, the elderly averaged a speed of 0.9 m/sec for normal walking, 1.1 m/sec for "hurrying," and only 1.3 m/sec if they were trying to catch a bus.[22] These research findings concur with the work of Lautso,[23] who found that the average walking speed for the aged was 1.07 m/sec. The aged have been noted to have major gait changes,[24,25] and under stress elderly women particularly develop postural sway.[26] It was also noted that older men walk faster than older women; slower-walking men tended to be less physically active in leisure activities (no such correlation for women). The slowest-walking men and women were commonly dependent on a cane and often also had some upper-extremity problems or arthritis. It was found that walking speed correlated with height (taller persons tended to walk faster) but not with weight.[17]

As a person ages, ability to drive a car safely may decrease. The elderly become increasingly dependent on various means of public transportation, all involving some stepping into and out of the vehicle (bus, train). In the step test, all 70-year-old subjects could master steps of 10, 20, and 30 cm without handrails. All 70-year-old men and women tested could climb up and down a 40-cm step with a handrail. For a 40-cm step with no handrail, 4 of the men and 23 of women could not step up and 5 men and 10 women could not step down. At a 50-cm step nearly all men and women could manage, some with difficulty, with a rail, but without a handrail 10 men and 71 women could not get up and 9 men and 34 women could not get down. Women appeared to have more difficulties than men with the step test. Inverse correlations were found for 70-year-old women between step height and weight with no railing for both going up the step and coming down (no such correlation for men). For elderly women a correlation was also noted between maximum step height up/down without a railing and maximum dynamic muscle strength of the quadriceps muscle at the probable contractile velocity used when climbing up or down steps and isometric muscle strength at 60° and 90° knee angles. In both sexes a correlation was noted between maximum step height up/down and walking speed.[15]

The functional implication is that the average elderly person can manage to go up and down steps of up to 30 cm with no railing; 40 cm if a railing is available. A public transportation vehicle that has a step of 50 cm or higher, with or without a railing, represents a difficult obstacle, especially for elderly women. It has been found that older women (75+) seem to have less control stepping down than older men and younger women.[27] Given these basic data, it is crucial that we work to facilitate modifications in step height in all types of public transportation. The purchase of a poorly designed bus can result in 10 years of difficulty for the aged on that bus line until the bus wears out (for trains the life-span of a car may be up to 40 years). Yet moderate adaptation of step height and the use of handrails in public transportation can facilitate independence for the elderly by increasing their ability to be mobile.

Gross Mobility

The Rosow-Breslau test was used to examine the ability of the elderly, 55 to 84 years of age, to perform heavy housework, walk 0.5 miles (0.8 km), and climb stairs.[28] The results noted in the Framingham study demonstrate that a substantially smaller number of subjects are able to perform these activities than can perform all basal ADL. Only 50 percent of the oldest group (75 to 84 years old) were able to perform heavy household work as compared to 79 percent of the 55- to 64-year-old group; 77 percent of the oldest group were able to walk 0.5 miles, compared to 96 percent of the 55- to 64-year-old group; and 85 percent of the oldest group were able to climb stairs, compared to 97 percent of the younger group.

It is relevant that more than three-fourths of those 75 to 84 years old report that they are still able to climb stairs and walk at least 0.5 miles (but reporter reliability needs to be studied by actual task execution). Overall, women report performing more poorly than men, especially as age increases, but again this may not be realistic—actual task execution must be studied.[13]

These findings point up the need for supportive services to assist the elderly with heavy household work. As the maintenance of a home gradually deteriorates, the mental health of the high risk elderly may be affected, which could become a contributing cause of depression. A key to rehabilitation is that supportive intervention for heavy housework, if it is a task valued by the patient, may greatly improve the person's mental health and outlook.

Physical Activities Profile

In the FDS, 55- to 84-year-olds were asked to describe their ability to perform nine physical activities (extending arms below shoulders, extending arms above shoulders, lifting weight under 10 lb/4 kg, sitting for 1+ hours, standing for 15+ minutes, moving large objects, lifing weight over 10 lb/4 kg, stooping/crouching/kneeling). It was found that 80 percent of the total sample were able to extend their arms in both directions, lift weights under 10 lb/4 kg, sit for long periods, and hold small objects without difficulty. The proportion of elderly performing these five activities without difficulty decreased with advancing age (74 percent of the oldest members reported no difficulty). A notably smaller percentage of women than men stated that they could perform these five activities without difficulty. Among the group 75 to 84 years of age, only 67 percent of the women, compared to 90 percent of the men, reported no difficulty in lifting weights under 10 lb/kg (largest age-specific gender difference).

The remaining physical activities are highly significant for housekeeping, food preparation, use of public transportation, and grocery shopping, and they appear to be greatly affected by advanced age. Only 73 percent of the total sample reported that they experienced no difficulty standing longer than 15 minutes, and among the oldest group (75 to 84) only 58 percent of the women and 67 percent of the men reported no difficulty.* The loss or perceived loss of this physical ability increasingly limits the very old in their use of public transportation and in doing their own grocery shopping, because it becomes difficult to ensure a supportive environment (e.g., seats, benches, or chairs to rest on).

Some 66 percent of the total sample noted they could perform the task of moving large objects without difficulty. In the oldest group (75 to 85) only 48 percent of the women but 80 percent of the men felt that they could still perform this task without difficulty. Functionally, the loss or perceived loss of the ability to move large objects has direct impact on home maintenance and creates special problems for the older single or widowed woman.

Some 65 percent of the total sample ages 55 to 84 reported achieving the task of lifting weights over 10 lb without difficulty. For 55- to 64-year-olds, only 59 percent of the women could complete the task successfully, at 65 to 74 years of age only 55 percent, and for the oldest group (75 to 84) the success figure was 34 percent. The men reported less difficulty, with 87 percent of the 55- to 64-year-olds successful, 85 percent of the 65- to 74-year-olds, and 72 percent of the 75- to 84-year-olds.

Lastly, only 59 percent of the total sample reported completing the physical activity of stooping/crouching/kneeling without difficulty. The same trend was noted as was seen for lifting weights over 10 lb—the men reported greater success at all ages than the women, and a gradual decrease in ability noted for both sexes with advanced age. There are major functional implications for the finding that only 38 percent of the women and 59 percent of the men 75 to 84 years of age reported successful completion of this movement.[19]

Social Disability

The pivotal tasks affecting a person's ability to live independently are housekeeping, transportation, social interaction, food preparation, and grocery shopping. Studies of the capacity of elderly persons for physical activities such as standing for longer periods of time, lifting objects heavier than 10 lb/4 kg, and kneeling indicate that with advancing age there is increasing difficulty in performing the basic social tasks needed for independent living in the commu-

---

* It must again be noted that the subjects in the Framingham study tended to be healthier than the average older person in the United States. Shanas estimates that 12 of every 100 elderly (65 or older) have a major incapacity index, but the FDS only found 7 percent.[29] This discrepancy may be partly explained by the presence of persons over age 85 in the Shanas study; all subjects in the FDS were 84 years of age or younger.

nity. In the FDS only 6 percent of the total sample of 55- to 84-year-olds interviewed had unmet needs in one or more of the social tasks; however, one-fourth of the elderly were *at risk* of developing unmet needs in one or more of the social tasks.

Housekeeping and transportation were the two social tasks with the highest prevalence of unmet need or risk of unmet need. It was found that three times as many 75- to 84-year-olds as 55- to 64-year-olds had unmet needs (but this was still only 12 percent of the oldest group). Housekeeping tasks involved the greatest reported difficulty; 15 percent of 55- to 64-year-olds and 25 percent of the oldest group experienced difficulty with housekeeping. Women were found to have more unmet needs for housekeeping and transportation than the men. Housekeeping—the ability to keep the home orderly, neat, and clean by one's personal standards—and transportation to carry out basic tasks for independence and meaningful survival in the community are pivotal to the mental as well as physical well-being of the elderly. The loss of the ability to perform these social tasks can contribute to depression and related physical dysfunction due to stress.

It is estimated that in the year 2000 20 percent of the United States population will be age 65 or older and half of this group will be 75 years of age or older.[30] Physical capacity to perform tasks involving mobility and the basic survival activities for independent living in the community decrease with increasing age. The research documenting the functional abilities of the elderly as a group, particularly the very old (85+), is only in the beginning stages. The data that already exist (FDS, Shanas, Aniansson, etc.) point to the increasing need to modify the environment to facilitate independent living for the elderly, especially the very old. Should not the hospital, clinic, and nursing home provide the basic environmental and organizational modifications to support maximum function for elderly with rehabilitation potential? What is the role of health-care providers (rehabilitation team) in facilitating the postfacility adjustment of the disabled elderly in the community in light of their special needs (e.g., housekeeping, transportation) during the early weeks of home care? The special functional needs of some elderly mandate examination of the evaluation procedures used for rehabilitation and discharge planning to ensure that they incorporate the potential areas of high risk unique to the very old.

REHABILITATION FOR THE ELDERLY— A SPECIAL APPROACH

To assure an effective outcome, it is important at the outset to define the desired goal clearly. The entire rehabilitation team, including the physical therapist, interacts with the patient to promote above all else the patient's urge to use his or her full potential (physical, emotional, cognitive, and spiritual). To assure that the process of interaction supports the patient's sense of self-determination (motivation), the assessment demands placed on the patient need to be paced to avoid the patient feeling overwhelmed, anxious, angry, or extremely tired. At the outset it is important to agree that in the rehabilitation process the mind-set is different from the emergency room or intensive care unit, where the patient is necessarily dependent and gives up some or all of his or her sense of control to receive life-sustaining help. In the rehabilitation process the mind-set of all staff is to teach and support the patient in learning how to use his or her body more effectively. It is also important to acknowledge that learning how to use your body more effectively is an interaction between physical, emotional, cognitive, and spiritual aspects of oneself. If the assessment is not paced to the emotional/cognitive needs of the patient, the result can be that the patient withdraws, refuses to cooperate, or becomes clinically depressed. Modification in the total health-care delivery system to incorporate the special functional characteristics of the elderly population will allow a greater number of elderly to reach a higher level of self-care capacity (with the self-determination that is necessary to function independently in the community after discharge).

Barry indicates that there is potential for better mental and physical health among older people if their independence can be supported.[31] The ability to perform ADL affects mental health, and the description or diagnosis generally does not predict the functional capacity of the patient mentally or physically. A discussion of interrelationship of function, diagnosis, and mental health is used here as the basis for the development of the concept of total care or a circle of care for the elderly. The need for a comprehensive approach to care of the disabled elderly forces us to examine the components of care, their interrelationship, the organization and the role of home-based care, and its unique contribution to the social and emotional well-being of the aged.

Independent Living Rehabilitation

The elderly are an increasingly visible group who are conscious of the positive potential of rehabilitation. Yet the disabled elderly have been unserved or underserved by all members of the rehabilitation team.[32,33] This lack is largely related to the original definition of rehabilitation, which was based on the potential for return to employment, as the majority of persons needing rehabilitation were of employable age. The demographics are changing, and the elderly population will increase in percentage of the total population for many years. The advent of independent-living rehabilitation (ILR) can be seen as a beginning toward promoting self-help, consumer involvement, and prevention of premature institutional care for the disabled elderly. A contemporary definition of ILR is as follows:[34]

> [ILR requires] control over one's life based on the choice of acceptable options that minimize reliance on others in making decisions and in performing everyday activities. This includes managing one's own affairs; participating in day-to-day life in the community; fulfilling a range of social roles; and making decisions that lead to self determination and

the minimization of psychological or physical dependence on others. Independence is a relative concept, which may be defined personally by each individual.

Statistics show that independent living is an issue of grave concern as a part of advanced aging:

- 17 percent of the elderly were "unable to carry on their major activities;"[35]
- The baseline average is one disabled in 10 Americans, but for those age 65 it is one in three;[36]
- 20 percent of older people 65 to 74 years of age and almost 42.5 percent of those over 75 have "substantial and severe limitations in physical and emotional performance;"[37]
- 11.5 percent of disabled 65 to 74 years of age need mobility or personal care assistance for independent living, and the percentage increases to 25.8 percent for those over 75 years of age.[37]

The elderly are underrepresented as rehabilitation clients, particularly in light of their proportion in the population of persons with disabilities.[38]

ILR is an approach that can work for the elderly disabled because older disabled persons require the same basic services as other disabled, although they may require them for a longer period of time. Among the services that are crucial (owing to the unique physical, emotional, and functional abilities among the elderly) are the following:

1. Group counseling, with special emphasis on motivation, reality, and support groups;
2. Mobility assistance—e.g., shopping help, transportation, and adaptive training for those with failing sight;
3. Homemaker services—e.g., attendant care, meals on wheels, "Friendly Visitor"
4. Information, referral, and advocacy;
5. Coordination among the various agencies, programs, and services; service system management on behalf of individual elderly to assure care and support appropriate to their functional status.

In 1978 the Rehabilitation Services Administration (RSA) funded five ILR demonstration projects in the United States, but only one of the projects included the aged as part of the target population.[34] The emphasis needs to change—the Urban Institute estimates that in 1974 there were 10 million noninstitutionalized severely disabled persons in the United States, and 4 million of them (40 percent) were 65 years old or older.[36]

ILR should emphasize restoration of independent living skills during short- or long-term-facility care for acute illness. Driscoll and co-workers noted that if the elderly can avoid taking on the role of the "good patient," they then avoid the need to lose this dependency and the lack of self-directed behavior at the moment of discharge to the community.[39] This may be an unrealistic expectation, however, in view of the dependency-creating characteristics of institutional care.

ADL—Functional Versus Diagnostic Emphasis

In the presence of unlimited fiscal resources, health care for the elderly can be built on a crisis intervention, diagnostic model. Even with unlimited resources, given the chronic nature of most disabilities, crisis care could never provide the most effective model of improved function as the goal. The reality of health care today is that there are limited fiscal and manpower resources available, in light of which it is crucial that any intervention beyond the life-or-death or emergency situation be focused on facilitating the elderly clients' independence and overall well-being. For the disabled elderly, it is crucial to build from two concepts that have been shown to affect their adjustment in any new situation: (1) what the person desires or values, and (2) the extent to which it is obtainable.

The joint interaction of these two factors is referred to by Reid and Ziegler[40] as a person's "locus of desired control;" their research has shown substantial and reliable correlations between locus of desired control and psychological adjustment. The physical ability of the elderly to carry out the ADLs described in the previous section decreases gradually over time. The functional losses in the ability to perform ADLs related to normal aging is itself minimal. At this point other factors, such as physical fitness, emotional overload (too many life changes in a short period of time), or ongoing social/family relationships that are not supportive, need to be evaluated. It is recognized that a person who is in a stressful interpersonal relationship will present with limbic symptoms such as tight muscles, particularly in the flexors, adductors, and internal rotators.[41] It is crucial to note that there is great variability among the elderly; the majority even in the oldest groups studied (75 to 84 years of age) were able to carry out the ADLs needed for independent living in the community.

When an elderly person has a stroke or a hip fracture, there are no predictable functional changes. A stroke patient does not always lose the ability to perform an ADL task. The loss of functional ability to perform an ADL task requires the identification of deficits concomitant with assessed visual/motor impairment. The significance of an organic or pathologic diagnostic label must be interpreted individually with each elderly person in order to identify the behavioral implications. That is, the "organic difficulties should be interpreted in terms of the patient's observable function."[42] Only if assessment is done with a functional emphasis is it possible to help the client think in concrete *self-help* terms, such as, "I've had a stroke and I want to learn to get on and off the toilet—that is important to me." The alternative is to evaluate the aged as we do with the young, examining range of motion, strength, spasticity, and so on as the primary emphasis, which can only lead to a reinforcement of loss rather than self-help. The young tend to have more psychological stamina and broader support networks, thus the lack of functional emphasis does not impact as severely as for the aged. The process of care, not just the intended outcome, must support psychological adjustment as part of rehabilitation of the functional losses. (NOTE: Use of range of motion, strength evaluation, etc. can and should be used once functional goals are identified to evaluate details of loss and to help design a treatment program, but such factors should never be used as the primary approach.)

There are psychologic implications of the ability to perform ADLs, and a loss of such ability will result in a direct loss of self-esteem and perceived control.[43] *If the rehabilitation team and therefore the elderly disabled client can focus on self-care capacity as a starting point, the patient will begin to understand that the component skills of basal self-care are also the foundation skills of the ability for independent living.*

It has been noted that physical impairment, age, depression, and disorientation have a strong interrelationship.[44] Therefore with any loss in the ability to perform basal ADLs (temporary or permanent), the psychological reaction must also be examined. If depression develops in response to a temporary or permanent loss, an evaluation of the extent of emotional reaction must be examined if realistic evaluation and plan of care are to be developed.

A person needs some mental clarity to relearn ADL;[45] however, with use of assessment tools with a functional emphasis (i.e., tools that give insight into how the individual learns and communicates), it is possible to improve functional status of elderly persons with major distortion of emotional and cognitive abilities.[46] Ultimately, the goal of independent living is achieved only by working with the whole person—physical and mental dysfunctions and the emotional and functional implications of those dysfunctions.

Accuracy of Clinical Judgment Versus CFA

Pinholt and associates[47] compared the use of clinical judgment with comprehensive functional assessment to determine clinical effectiveness in noting moderate as well as severe functional problems in elderly patients. The elderly patients studied were 79 inpatients over the age of 70. It was found that clinicians recognized severe impairments in cognitive status, nutrition, vision, gait, and continence. It was found that the sensitivity for noting moderate impairments was poor, especially as it relates to vision, cognitive status, nutrition, and continence. The physical therapist, as a member of the rehabilitation team, needs to be aware that without a CFA process he or she will need to screen the patient to rule out the possibility that the functional losses that are present may be related to moderate losses of vision, disturbances in nutrition, cognitive problems, or incontinence. With early detection, the moderate impairments can respond more easily to intervention and avoid secondary functional losses. In treating the elderly patient, it is an advantage to the patient to have the data base (medical, cognitive, social, emotional, environmental) developed by a multidisciplinary team to assure a real understanding of all variables that are contributing to the problem and that need to be taken into account when choosing the pace and types of intervention.

Circle of Care for the Disabled Elderly

The circle of care for the elderly consists of the full range of medical, social, and environmental services, including meals on wheels, chore services, housekeeping, home health (including in-home rehabilitation specialists), senior centers, adult day care, telephone reassurance, respite care, homes for the aged, nursing homes, rehabilitation centers, and hospitals. For the disabled elderly who have had a major medical problem, the point of entry into the circle is usually the hospital. For the disabled elderly who have severe chronic degenerative disease, the point of entry may lie with any provider in the circle. The intent of a circle of care is to assure that once identified, the elderly client receives care, over time, appropriate to need and functional status and becomes a part of a preventive health maintenance effort. The fact that one-fourth of the independent elderly over age 75 in the Framingham Disability Study were found to be at risk for problems related to social survival in the community should sensitize us to the precarious independence of the disabled elderly.

Interrelationship and intercommunication among components of the basic health and social service network are crucial for support of the maximum level of independent living among the elderly. Owing to the differences between young and old in psychological and sociological status and functional skills, the high-risk/frail elderly need the support of the entire network to remain in *their* preferred living environment, which is usually their own home. Implicit in the need for intercommunication among the network of providers who track and provide services to maintain health and independence is the need for longitudinal record-keeping with a problem-oriented focus. Such need is especially acute if the elderly client has any form of mental status decline.

Organization and management of care of the elderly disabled client must include respect for confidentiality and the client's own needs and desires concerning plans of care. One way of dealing with the decrease of physical capacity or mental status of the client is to have an independent evaluation process that will assist and enable implementation of flexible, dynamically changing plans of care for the frail or high-risk aged who because of their physical and/or mental status are unable to coordinate effectively the network of care they require to remain independent in the community (see the discussion of Model Approach—Rehabilitation for the Elderly).

If the elderly disabled do require hospital care, the quality of the experience can affect every other component within the circle of care. The hospital environment and program of care should support maximum independence and self-directed behavior in patients beyond life-or-death crisis, which should involve individual plans of care allowing for self-care in all areas where the patient is able to perform.

The philosophy of care within the hospital must clearly be defined from the emergency room and the recovery room to the patient's room. For the elderly, as for other age groups, the emergency room and the recovery room are situations in which staff are in charge and are doing things *for* the patient. Once the elderly patient is back in his or her own room, the hospital staff must reorient themselves and the patient to support a philosophy of independent and self-directed behavior. The work load of the nursing staff is affected by the intent of the care plan in effect for the patient. Basal ADLs must be the concern of nursing care both to reduce the work overload caused by an increasingly aged hospital population and to assure care that supports the dignity and choices of patients regardless of illness and disability. For example, incontinence is not a factor that contributes to staff work load if an adequate toileting policy is implemented; however, if there is inadequate staff and concomitantly a poor toileting policy, the nursing work load will increase, patient morale will decrease, and the overall rehabilitation outcome will be negatively affected.

It is probably true that to facilitate rehabilitation, especially in the acute-care hospital, staff levels must be above those required for acute care, because the partially mobile patient requires more and different types of care than a bedridden patient.[48] If this challenge can be met, the 80-year-old stroke patient, for example, may need a longer rehabilitation effort but will do as well as the younger stroke patient.[49]

If the level of functional disability but not age[49] relates to future placement, is a geriatric rehabilitation unit a positive step after acute hospital care? In a time of limited resources, the key to the effectiveness of a geriatric rehabilitation unit is the ability to pick patients who need the special benefits of such a unit. Hall[50] noted that patients with a favorable diagnosis can make progress in any hospital setting as long as the basic medical and rehabilitation components are present, but patients with unfavorable diagnoses need total environmental and organizational support in order to improve to desired levels of independence. Available research data indicate that bowel and bladder function, ability to walk, and mental status are the major predictors of rehabilitation outcome.[51] In a study of 76-year-old patients admitted to a geriatric rehabilitation unit, 20 percent went home, 28 percent to a home for the aged, and 52 percent to a nursing home; it is significant that age was not a predictor of rehabilitation outcome.[49]

The plan of care within an institutionally based geriatric rehabilitation program must take account of experience demonstrating that patients can be out of their own environment no more than 3 months and still be likely to reintegrate at the completion of rehabilitation.[52] It is essential not to distort or displace the informal support network available to the elderly patient if that informal network is to be available on discharge. In fact, in rehabilitation of the elderly special efforts must be made to evaluate, orient, and train those within the informal network so that they can accept and support the patient at discharge, another reason for identifying clearly the intended outcome of rehabilitation (independent living) and helping all within the circle of care (patient, family, friends, rehabilitation team) to focus on functional ability.

As a part of the evaluation procedures for a rehabilitation unit, the Barthel Index (or the modified Barthel Index) has received a lot of attention. The Barthel Index measures the degree of physical handicap regardless of the particular diagnostic designations. It is an accurate measure of the degree of physical impairment as it relates to basic ADL function. It is thus a screening tool that can describe overall functional capacity, physical function, decision making, and ability to fulfill usual or customary roles. The screening of a patient with the Barthel Index can lead to a referral for in-depth ADL evaluation by physical or occupational therapists.[36]

Home care or home-based rehabilitation programs (using visiting physical therapists, occupational therapists or nurses, adult day care, etc.) is the part of the circle of care most sought by the majority of the elderly.[53] This fact may be related to how our needs for belonging, love, and esteem can better be met in the community than within the structure and process of institutional care.[54]

The current emphasis of reimbursement for care in institutions is based on the visible, tangible physical intervention and the ease for providers of facility-based intervention, but home-based rehabilitation programs offer special support by the very structure of care for the patient (own environment, familiarity) and by involvement of the informal network.

The home-care setting allows rehabilitation with an emphasis on the needs of the patient and an acceptance of the patient's preferred environment. For the rehabilitation team, home care allows the clinician to examine the interrelation and complexity of management of multiple problems (diagnostic and functional) involved in the care of the aged. It is not unusual to have a case history based on an isolated systems review that results in a problem list like the following:[55]

List 1—Medical
   1. Hearing impairment
         Unable to hear normal speech tones
   2. Vision impairment
         Difficulty seeing small print
         Difficulty seeing distant objects
   3. Speech and language impairment
         Relies on spouse to answer
   4. Respiration impairment
         Shortness of breath with exertion
   5. Neuromuscular/skeletal function impairment
         Limited range of motion
         Inability to manage some ADL
         Poor coordination

6. Circulation impairment
      Edema in lower extremities
      Occasional irregular heart beat
7. Digestive function impairment
      Anorexia
      Some weight loss
8. Dentition impairment
      Ill-fitting dentures
9. Bowel function impairment
      Incontinence
      Constipation
10. Urinary function impairment
      Incontinent
      Inability to empty bladder
11. Nutrition impairment
      Lacks proper caloric intake
      Improper feeding schedule
      Lacks essential vitamins, minerals, and food groups
12. Physical activity impairment
      Sedentary life-style; lacks regular exercise
13. Therapeutic regimen noncompliance
      Failed to return to ophthalmologist for postcataract lenses
14. Income—possible deficit
      Noncompliance due to worry about bills

A problem-oriented approach coordinated with a home-care process facilitates the examination of the interrelation of function and diagnostic problems. Such an approach enables clinicians to direct limited time and resources to the cluster of services that can improve or facilitate maximum independence within a rehabilitation framework.

For example, in the sample case above, when the problems were studied and reorganized based on a functional approach, targets of intervention changed drastically:[55]

List 2—Functional Problems in Light of Medical and/or Social Problems
1. Social isolation
      Overdependence on wife, who speaks for patient
2. Related medical
      Bowel function impairment: incontinency, constipation
      Urinary function impairment: incontinence, inability to fully empty bladder
      Hearing impairment
      Vision impairment
3. Nutrition/digestive
      Anorexia
      Lacks proper calorie and nutrient intake

Dentition (poorly fitting dentures)
Constipation—see problem
4. Mobility/ADL limitation
Related medical
Respiration—shortness of breath
Circulation—edema, irregular heart beat
Neuromusculoskeletal—limited range of motion, balance/coordination
See problem 2—vision impairment
5. Income
Vision impairment—failure to return for glasses after cataract surgery
Dentition—ill-fitting dentures

List 1 resulted in a plan of care that relied primarily on the nursing care of the home health agency, with physician oversight. List 2 includes all the medical problems identified in list 1, but it relates those problems to *loss of function*. Therefore a high priority was placed on the following:

Congregate meals program
Male companionship for the husband
Respite for the wife, who was giving total care
Financial counseling to facilitate purchase of glasses and attention to dentures
Attention to balance, coordination, breathing difficulties, and effective therapeutic exercise program

The medical problems required continuing physician oversight and collaboration with the home health agency, which worked on bowel and bladder control, diet control, and monitoring of respiration and circulation. However, the medical regimen took on goals for mobility and social interaction implicit in a rehabilitative framework.

Home care intervention must be focused on functional needs in order to preserve the precarious independent living situation of the disabled elderly; this focus *can* be cost effective.[56] The reality today is that the cost of all institutional care is increasing. The organization and process of care must be reexamined and modified—the care provided in many hospitals and nursing homes is not therapeutic and diminishes the independence of the disabled elderly. Yet in the wake of rising costs the U.S. Federal Health Care Policy strongly supports institutional based care. In 1977 the budget for facility care was $12.6 billion, compared to $575 million for Medicare and Medicaid ambulatory and home care services. It is necessary to modify national health policy if the physiologic, psychological, and social needs of the aged are to be supported to enable independent living into very old age for as many as possible.[57]

Current policies and related systems of care do not acknowledge the increasing *risk* of functional changes with advanced age (e.g., ability to stand for 15+ minutes, lift 10 lb/4 kg or heavier, kneel) and the risk of social disability (loss of ability to shop for groceries, prepare meals, and use public transportation). Identification of the risk is the first step in appropriate management of the range of problems. More research will be valuable to gain more precise understanding of this population and their needs, but the effectiveness of rehabilitation coupled with attention to environmental and organizational modification to support independence of the high-risk elderly through all components of the circle of care has been amply demonstrated.

MODEL APPROACH— REHABILITATION FOR THE ELDERLY

The elderly as a group sustain many physiologic, psychological, and social losses as a part of the normal aging process. Despite this, the majority of the elderly continue to maintain the basic functional skills needed for independent living in the community. Through research, patterns of functional loss (ADL and social) have been identified as common in the healthy elderly, and there are distinctive patterns defining elderly as being *at risk* of loss of basic functional skills necessary for independent living. When the elderly become disabled owing to acute or chronic degenerative illness, it is necessary that rehabilitation and patient assessment incorporate not only the current illness or disability but also any previous functional losses, temporary functional losses due to the current illness, and the risk of future ADL and social functional losses.

The Service Coordination System (SCS) provides a system of assessment that can enable continuity of care through information sharing among hospital, home care, and community providers, patient, and family. The SCS is a way to organize service delivery for the aged from the community (preliminary problems), hospital (crisis), home care (short-term restorative care), nursing home (long-term restorative care), and then back to the community. The structure of SCS provides a tracking and coordination capacity in support of high-risk elderly as they move through a complicated and fast-paced health-care delivery system. As health and service systems become increasingly accommodated to the elderly, SCS will be needed only in the nonhospital environment; until that time, the elderly will require a coordination program such as SCS to integrate their service needs at each level of medical/social intervention.

The Client Screen

The potential client's first contact with SCS is through a screening process designed to target care intensively to those at risk of functional losses. The screen has various formats, depending on whether patients are self-referred, are referred by others, or are referred during hospital stay. It can be adapted to multiple settings.

The screening interview (by phone or in person) is standardized and can be carried out by relatively unskilled interviewers. The interviewer gathers information on all ADLs that affect survival in the community: communication/cognition—can patients communicate, can they remember (especially short-term memory); mobility/transfer, feeding; toileting—both volitional control and self-care; emotional state; and home situation—level of assistance available, level of social support.

It is significant that the emphasis of the screening process is self-care tasks and identification of task limitations. It seeks to determine what persons can or cannot do for themselves. It is a function screen.

The screen probes for short-term memory loss in a functional way. Patients are asked to describe the primary problem(s) and how the problem(s) affect their life and their ability to do what is important to them. At the end of the screening interview, patients are asked to review their primary problem(s) for the interviewer to assure accuracy. A person with significant and functional memory loss is likely not to be able to remember what was described the first time, even a few minutes earlier.

Because the organic brain syndromes (including senile dementia of the Alzheimer type) and depression mimicking senility are among the most significant predictors of institutionalization, *early* identification of short-term memory loss is crucial to a successful screening and intervention program. Equally important is the fact that for the person for whom memory loss is not a problem, the request to review the primary problem(s) to ensure that the interviewer understands them accurately will not be offensive. The screen is designed to assess the patient's capacity to function at home, either alone or with assistance.

For situations where the client is not self-referring, the screen elicits information that is especially important if the caller is the primary caretaker. The need may exist for assistance to the primary caretaker to enable the caretaker to continue in that role. The screen can identify supporter stress that unless relieved can lead to an institutional placement undesired by client and family.

If the client is referred by a hospital, other institution, or social agency, the screen is adapted to integrate standardized isolated medical data with functional data related to self-care, community networking, and client goals. Throughout SCS, an effort is made to facilitate self-directed behavior in the client by the format and process of care. It is only in this way that it is possible to motivate patients to work with commitment toward realizing their potential.

Client Orientation and Confidentiality

If the interview or referral indicates that the patient is experiencing functional problems and an assessment in depth is required, the client is given a brochure and letter describing the SCS. A consent form for basic information-sharing among practitioners is also included. In this way the patient and family or significant others have time to review the documents and prepare questions or voice concerns. When the members of the assessment team (a rehabilitation nurse or physical or occupational therapist *and* a social worker) arrive, they can answer any questions about the SCS.

Rules governing staff conduct relative to confidentiality and disclosure of records must be prepared as part of the implementation of SCS. Staff training includes emphasis on informed consent and the importance of confidentiality.

A questionnaire (patient history—self-report) is also sent to the patient as part of the introductory packet. The assumption is made that most people, given a chance, want to take responsibility for their own lives and will do so if they can. The self-report gathers information from the patient about past and present illnesses, bed days in home and in hospital, and significant losses and includes a full checklist of symptoms (Fig. 9-1). The self-report form is presented in nonmedical language and large print to facilitate elderly client participation. It communicates to the patient and family that "you are a participating partner in your care; you and your family have the best information about how you feel and what you are experiencing."

SCS by its format of information collection attempts to strengthen the independence of the client. Clients fill out the form at their own pace and have time to reflect on the questions asked. The self-report provides a valuable tool for cross-validation of client responses during the actual assessment and with the physician summary. The fact that a given client cannot or chooses not to complete the self-report is also a valuable datum. The goal of the patient self-history is to build a "locus of control," which is known to facilitate psychological well-being.[40]

Do you experience any of the following:	Check No	Yes	When did it start?	What tasks does this keep you from doing?
Tired				
Unwell				
Weak				
Gain in weight				
Loss in weight				
Hoarseness				
Sore tongue				
Difficulty swallowing				
Headache				
Dizziness				
Noises in ears				
Belching				
Heartburn				

Fig. 9-1.   Excerpt from patient self-history chart.

Assessment

The goal of the assessment procedure is to produce sufficient information to allow valid and reliable judgments about service needs. Potential services can be formal or informal, free or paid for, but they should match the needs of the patient/client at any given time. Decisions about service needs based solely on medical and social data or the inability to purchase a service in isolation from the other variables have at least some probability of being wrong. To be patient-effective and cost-effective, services must be appropriate to needs. An unneeded service, no matter how fine, may sap independence in the client and is always wasteful.

The core assessment has nine basic categories of data collection:

Socioeconomic Data

This category contains basic descriptive data to enable determination of financial eligibility for services, primary language, education, employment history, and source of referral.

History

The history consists of three parts:

1. Directory of services/providers—A descriptive list of all services/providers used by the client, the date that client was last seen or services were last used, the types of services received, and the goal or purpose of those services (this directory allows SCS to build on the system already in place).
2. Family history—Family illness history and a brief examination of family interaction, identifying primary source of information during the assessment.
3. Self-history—A review of the self-report form to assure that the client understood the questions and to discuss the answers.

Risk Factors

Nutrition, obesity, dentition, substance abuse (including smoking and alcohol), are all risk factors.

Medications

A special emphasis is given to this segment (Fig. 9-2). A review is made of the 18 basic categories of medications, the client's use of over-the-counter and

Problem No.	Category	Specific Medication	Dose	Freq.	Route	Length/ Time	Half- Life
	Analgesics/ narcotics						
	Antacids						
	Antibiotics/ antiinfectives						
	Anticoagulants						
	Anticonvulsants						
	Antihypertensives						
	Bowel regulators						
	Bronchodilators						
	Cardiac regulators						
	Diuretics/ electrolytes						
	Insulin/ hypoglycemics						
	Sedatives barbiturates						

Fig. 9-2. Excerpt from medication review. Specify each medication by category. Include dose; frequency; route of administration; length of time on medication; and half-life. Data also requested: Does patient understand purpose and side effects of medication? Who gave the medication instructions? Medication No.? Date of original Rx? Date last filled? MD ordering? Pharmacy (see service directory)? Date terminated?

prescription drugs, the patient's understanding of the medications and their use, and patient compliance (including review of patient education about medication use). At the completion of the assessment, a review is made of medication–medication and medication–food interactions, which are significant problems for the elderly.

Sensation, Balance and Proprioception

A review of the patient's sensation, balance, and proprioception is made to examine his or her status—functional with compensation (if so, what type?, partial loss of function with compensation, full loss, date of onset, and whether gradual or sudden.

Musculoskeletal

A full review of the patient's functional range of motion (amount of joint motion needed for basic self-care tasks) is made. If the patient's motion is limited, a comparison of active and passive movements of affected joints is made, and functional tasks affected are noted.

[NOTE: The core assessment team is composed of a rehabilitation nurse or a physical therapist/occupational therapist to ensure the ability to provide a functional emphasis to the initial evaluation. The assessment is not meant to replace the in-depth physical therapist/occupational therapist evaluation that is ordered as more details are required (after the core team has reviewed the assessment, physician summary, and the patient's self-history).]

Activities of Daily Living

A systematic review is made of the client's ability to do each of the following tasks, along with the amount and type of help needed (as applicable) and related health care status and mobility status as they relate to each ADL task:

1. Personal care (bathing, grooming, dressing, eating/feeding);
2. Communication (spoken and instrumental—telephone, writing, electronic);
3. Excretory functions (bowel and bladder);
4. Mobility skills (transfers and ambulation).

Mental Status

Assessments of subjective mental status (how the patient feels and relates to others) and objective mental status (competence to direct one's own life, to remember, to comprehend, to follow instructions, to calculate, to understand basic spatial relationships, and to behave within acceptable norms) are made. The mental status assessment has a functional orientation and emphasizes all the primary component skills used in communication and teaching. It is designed to facilitate identification of any special therapeutic support necessary to increase the client's potential to participate in the plan of care. (For example, if a client were unable to copy a simple design, such as a pair of interlocking pentagons, how would you modify the process of teaching this patient to use a walker?)

Environment

A review of support resources as well as constraints to independence, including a detailed survey of the physical environment and economic status, is made. The family and significant others within the social network are asked about specific assistance and support they are willing and able to provide (Fig. 9-3) as well as the degree of training they seem willing and able to accept.

All of the above information should be assessed in the person's home, if possible. Barriers to independent living are often obvious in the home and are not considered within a facility setting. Examples abound:

Activities of Daily Living	Needed		If Needed			Recommendations (Cross-check to Plan of Care)
	No	Yes	Willing but Needs Training	Willing if There Is Respite	Not Able (Reason)	
Mobility						
Transferring						
Walking (ambulation)						
Wheeling						
Personal care						
Bathing						
Dressing						

Fig. 9-3. Excerpt from care assessment record involving the assistance/support the family or significant other is willing and able to provide. The provider should cross-check to ADLs and include as part of the plan of care.

1. The multiple sclerosis or stroke victim who faithfully undergoes rehabilitation in the hospital until able to walk 40 steps with a walker, on a tile floor—only to become immobilized at the first step on the carpeting at home.

2. The patient with Parkinson's disease and related severe muscle weakness who can get out of a hospital bed alone but cannot transfer at home because the bed is too low and lacks a side rail to grasp for leverage.

3. The patient with heart disease recovering from a broken hip at home whose neighbors bring hot meals daily with high salt content.

4. The patient who is ordered to have six small meals a day but receives meals on wheels twice daily and has no way to divide them into appropriate portions.

5. The patient who sleeps most of the day as well as at night, gradually weakening because medications are not adjusted downward to mitigate soporific side effects and bed-rest deconditioning secondary to steadily decreasing activity.

6. The grieving patient who displays severe memory loss presenting as senile dementia when what is needed is therapy to deal with loss plus social interaction and systematic memory help.

All the information needed does not have to be gathered at the face-to-face interview. The assessment process is augmented by the physician summary, a brief description by the primary physician of conditions under medical management, management regimen, residual problems, relevant laboratory data, precautions, and short- and long-term goals. Just as delivery of medical care is incomplete without knowledge of the social and environmental needs of the patient, so it is irresponsible to the person with chronic disabilities to make judgments about service needs without knowledge of medical conditions and their current management.

In addition, if the assessment team finds cause, an in-depth psychological evaluation can be requested. The underlying questions always exist—How is this problem(s) affecting the patient's life? What are the functional implications?

All this information plus the client's self-report complete the basic data base, providing the raw material on which a plan of care can be built *in cooperation* with the patient, the family network, friends, and the full spectrum of care providers.

(NOTE: The terms patient and client have been used interchangeably throughout the SCS. We must focus on the person who is seeking help and not allow ourselves to be trapped or confused by the labels that we or others place on the person.)

Data Integration—The Problem-Oriented Record

The assessment provides information. It is important information—but by itself it is not useful. It must be integrated across functional, medical psychosocial, and environmental aspects of the person's life to identify problems and potential solutions.

The assessment instrument is cross-referenced to support easy correlation of data. Where two areas are particularly related, each is cross-referenced. However, once all data are assembled, the difficult job must be done of analyzing the material and recording it in an easily understood and manageable form. The problem-oriented record (POR) facilitates the analytic process by which data—discrete pieces of information—are reorganized into defined problems requiring solution. Once the problem(s) is identified, a plan of care complete with action steps to reach specific goals can be developed and monitored.

In a good record, problems are clearly described, the information supporting the problem definition is clear and identifiable, the actions to be taken to deal with the problem are also clear, and those actions are related to goals set within a time frame to facilitate follow-up and monitoring. Such a record can be audited, and another caregiver can pick it up and assure continuity of care. It also becomes a useful teaching tool because it can be reviewed objectively for successes and problems.

The working parts of the SCS are modeled on the basic components of the POR, problem list, planning flow sheets, process notes, objective data (listed separately for easy review), and medication directory. This system standardizes *how* data are integrated in order to arrive at decisions about needed care. As new providers replace old (staff turnover, vacations, etc.) there is a logical record of how decisions were arrived at, a record that can then be built on. In the care of the elderly, because of the multiple chronic degenerative problems and their ever-changing functional impact, it is often difficult to determine with a standard descriptive record-keeping system the rationale for care or services provided earlier. With SCS the record becomes a tool that can be used quickly by any provider or caregiver to identify the current problems under management by a SCS. If needed, a detailed rationale for particular services can be discerned by systematic tracking of a problem number through the chart.[58]

Problem List

The problem list is the first page of the record. It serves as the index to the record. Each problem is given a name and a number, which are reserved for that problem only and never reused. All entries relative to each problem carry that name and number, so that a review of all actions in relation to each problem is simple. The problem list enables computerization of the record and cross-referencing of related problems by problem number, facilitating quality review and utilization review and thus creating an easily audited and checked record.

Planning Flow Sheets

The entries on this sheet are the action steps, dated relative to each problem. They are numbered and named as on the problem list. The flow sheets facilitate a quick review of action relative to the goals, by problem, with a date for initial action and one for review.

The more dynamic a case, the more useful this part of the record is because the care coordinator/manager does not have to wade through lengthy notes or complex analysis to find out what happened. Problem, goal, action, and dates are easy to follow. The index number allows easy reference to the analysis in the process notes if one needs to understand the reasons for any action or set of actions.

Process Notes

This part of the record is done first because it provides the analytic framework that leads to definition of the problem. Each problem definition is tentative until the care manager (any designated member of the rehabilitation team) has analyzed the supporting information across all relevant aspects of function and is fairly confident as to what the problem is.

It is important to recall that the focus of service management is to maximize function. Therefore the object in defining a functional problem is to ask what difference it makes in the person's life. The question is—So what? If it makes no difference, it probably needs no action.

A simple example makes this focus clear. If a person cannot see well and the medical problem is the specific vision impairment (e.g., cataracts or myopia), the functional problems could be, say, inability to read, or restricted mobility, or restricted socialization; once this person has glasses that correct the vision impairment, a great many problems are resolved. But if the person had an uncorrected vision problem because of an inability (real or perceived) to afford the glasses, the physician's prescription will remain unfilled until the financial problem is resolved. Solving the functional problems that are secondary to the medical problems depends on resolving the financial problem.

Such an example is deceptively simple. Teasing out the functional problem and relating it appropriately to medical, psychosocial, and environmental factors is usually a complex process.

The process is further complicated by the styles of each profession. Nurses (and physicians) tend to review a patient by body system. Such review pinpoints medical problems but makes it hard (though not impossible) to see how the person's life is affected. A review of the same problem list first by body system and then by function shows how a functional list that considers medical problems as they relate to function can refocus a plan of care (see lists 1 and 2, Circle of Care).

Analysis

SOAP—the analytic process used to organize the data and the analysis of data—begins with the client's view of the situation.

S stands for *subjective*—the patient's description. Patients are the ultimate experts on how they feel and what is being experienced. The use of subjective does not imply that the client's feelings are not real, only that what the client experiences is being discussed.

O stands for *objective*—verified findings from clinical or laboratory tests (listed separately for easy retrieval).

A stands for *assessment meaning analysis*. Given all the information that has been gathered, where does it lead? *What is the problem?* At this point the problem has a name and can be numbered and entered in the problem list.

P stands for the *plan of care*. The actions for long-term patients always fall into two categories. First, what does the person and/or the family have to know to take maximum responsibility for care? This involves client education, family education, and possibly training if there are identified services that patient and family are willing and able to carry out. Second and complementary to client and family education and service mobilization are the formal services required. These may need to include regular respite for caretakers who bear the lion's share of responsibility for care. It sometimes means providing actual services to the caretaker along with the client services, such as meals on wheels, financial counseling, therapy, or counseling to deal with stress or to help the caretaker understand the plight of a loved one (especially for spouses of clients with Alzheimer's disease, where memory, personality and cognition diminish).

Fundamentally, the plan of care must be responsive to the needs of the client. The client is viewed holistically, with function as the prime focus and predictor of services. The client also must be viewed within the context of a system—the family and community that share informally and formally in service and care.

The initial assessment and SOAP process are time-consuming, but they provide the service manager with a firm foundation from which to define problems, monitor progress, change services as conditions change, and termi-nate services no longer needed. Further, the chart with its integrated problem list and plan, when shared appropriately with physician or other caretakers, educates the community of providers to the need for a shared enterprise on behalf of impaired clients. Everyone can come to realize that they cannot and need not operate alone if chronic problems are to be managed.

Medications

The medications record is virtually a chart within a chart. It is pulled out of the assessment and made a part of the client's ongoing chart. It allows an examination of the interactions between medications as well as interactions with food. (For example, eating licorice when taking digitalis is contraindicated.) Gathering the complete medications record and sharing it with the physician, with the client's consent, can lead to dealing with overmedication and even some underlying problems, often for the first time.

Service Coordination Action Log

Because the SCS was a demonstration project and the first step to eventual statewide implementation, the SCS plan of care goes several steps beyond normal charting. The service management team was asked to develop an ideal plan of care, then to enter in the chart what actually could be delivered. The providers were then asked for an analysis of the reasons for the difference between actual and ideal plans. The reasons that needed services cannot be delivered are information relevant to policy and rarely available to decision-makers.

To faciliate easy notations of barriers encountered when implementing the plan, we developed the action log for the service manager's use as a record of barriers by problem. This log functions as a vital part of regular chart review because it fosters mutual help among staff in dealing with and overcoming barriers to appropriate care.

The POR as a Teaching Tool

A chart review should be held regularly for all staff involved in the evaluation process. At that time new cases are reviewed, assessment data are summarized, problems are listed by function in light of medical and social problems, and actions in the plan of care are reviewed. The training by consultants established a model for constructive critique of the record. Shared experience about real problems to which innovative solutions must be sought creates an environment conducive to self-assessment, staff development, and growth. It also creates an environment in which diverse viewpoints across professional differences can be appreciated.

The record becomes the source of data that can be tracked by individual client, cross-tabulated to develop profiles of client characteristics with service need, and collected for planning purposes. It keeps the system accountable to clients, because services must be arranged acceptable to and, at least in part, implemented by them; to providers, who share in the care of each client; and to public and private payers, whose fiscal support enables care.

Training and Implementation

To implement the SCS, initial training for the assessment team, composed of the rehabilitation nurse or physical therapist/occupational therapist and social worker, can be done in approximately 48 hours. The initial 24 hours (3 days) provides a theoretical foundation plus experience with the assessment and charting process. After the staff have gained actual field experience in assessment and service management, follow-up training for 8 to 16 hours is provided. Additional problem-solving sessions of 8 to 16 hours should be offered as part of a staff development process. The SCS coordinator builds from this training through weekly or bimonthly chart reviews and problem-solving sessions as a means of ongoing in-service training.

The instruments discussed earlier were used as basic curriculum materials in the original program. Each staff person received two notebooks. Volume 1 included the screening and assessment instruments and the POR format with detailed instructions for its proper use.

Two case studies were used to introduce the processes of assessment and of integration and analysis of data, leading to a plan of care. An assessment was demonstrated on film, and the staff analyzed what they had heard and attempted to formulate a functional problem list. A second case study presented assessment data in an organized form, and the staff formulated the functional problem list and plan of care.

Volume 2 was a service manual. It included a description of the system; a section on reimbursement, with special emphasis on Titles XVIII, XIX, and XX of the Social Security Act, and on OAA funds; and descriptions of three simple conceptual tools that helped communicate the meaning of the service delivery system: the circle of care, the health team and its composition, and a chart of the continuum of care/services for the elderly.

The chart illustrating the continuum of care was divided into 10 columns: it functioned as the index for the service manual. A survey was made of all the providers in the five-county area of the demonstration project. Each section of the notebook, correlated to a column of the chart, contained descriptions of the service providers that fit the particular category. Thus there was a concrete way to talk about the range of services and types of providers. It supported discussion of the essential interaction among medical, social, and environmental services (income, housing, transportation) and the role of client, family, social supports, and the service management team in building an appropriate minisystem of care for each client.

MODEL APPROACH FOR PHYSICAL THERAPY
EVALUATION OF THE DISABLED ELDERLY

When the CFA by the rehabilitation team results in a referral to physical therapy, the goal of the physical therapy evaluation is to develop a detailed description of the functional losses. Given a description of the ADL tasks affected, the amount of physical and mechanical assistance needed, and the time needed to perform the complete task, it is then possible to study the component factors of the impaired functional skills (range of motion, coordination, strength, proprioception, sensation, balance, posture, etc.). The final treatment plan will use physical therapy procedures chosen to achieve improvement in the total function of the patient.

The ADL assessment developed by Edith Buchwald-Lawton[59] is ideally suited for the initial review of ADL losses or dysfunction because of its precision in evaluation, its reproducibility and reliability as a testing tool, and the low cost of its implementation and utilization. The Lawton ADL evaluation is ideally suited to the evaluation required for the aged because it can measure very small increments of progress. The Lawton assessment has evolved from years of testing and is a precision tool for the evaluation of ADL. The form is divided into an initial summary, 47 indoor ADL tasks, 44 ADL tasks related to mobility in the home and the community, equipment inventory, discharge summary, and a home situation checklist for barriers to independence.

The initial summary provides a description of the basic demographics about the patient with a functional emphasis (time in bed or wheelchair per day, ADL-related equipment owned, patient goals, means of communication, etc.). The initial summary provides an overview, but the core of the assessment is the systematic review of the 91 ADL tasks (fewer as ability allows), with the description of the grade of physical help required to perform a task, the time needed, and, as called for, the distance or number of steps and the height of stairs or curbs. The 91 tasks are each broken down, and it is presumed that the client will perform the task in both directions as it applies (e.g., into bed from wheelchair and out of bed to wheelchair).

The grades of physical assistance are lifting (L), performing for patient (P), assistance (A), supervision (S), independent (I), not pertinent (X), not feasible at present (O), and not tested or patient refused (N). The grading of physical assistance has been defined on the same model as traditional muscle testing (Fig. 9-4). For a specific grade it is clear to the therapist what quantity of help must be required (100 percent, 75 percent, etc.).

In addition to the grade for physical assistance, the time required to perform the ADL task is also measured. The time to complete a task requires the inclusion of all activities done by the patient and the helper/assistant. The sequence of motions for a particular task are identified, so that it is clear when to start timing, when to finish, and what to include (Fig. 9-5). Time is the only measure of minor improvement currently available, as it measures the patient's coordination/organization of the performance of the ADL task. For the aging patient, use of both grade (physical assistance) and time allows documentation

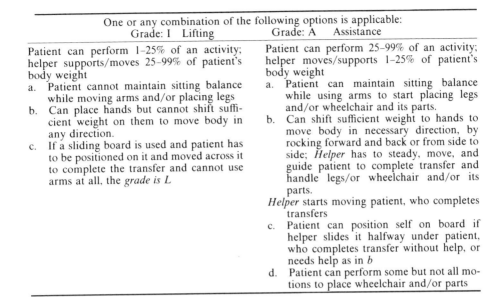

One or any combination of the following options is applicable:

Grade: I Lifting	Grade: A Assistance
Patient can perform 1–25% of an activity; helper supports/moves 25–99% of patient's body weight	Patient can perform 25–99% of an activity; helper moves/supports 1–25% of patient's body weight
a. Patient cannot maintain sitting balance while moving arms and/or placing legs	a. Patient can maintain sitting balance while using arms to start placing legs and/or wheelchair and its parts.
b. Can place hands but cannot shift sufficient weight on them to move body in any direction.	b. Can shift sufficient weight to hands to move body in necessary direction, by rocking forward and back or from side to side; *Helper* has to steady, move, and guide patient to complete transfer and handle legs/or wheelchair and/or its parts.
c. If a sliding board is used and patient has to be positioned on it and moved across it to complete the transfer and cannot use arms at all, the *grade is L*	*Helper* starts moving patient, who completes transfers
	c. Patient can position self on board if helper slides it halfway under patient, who completes transfer without help, or needs help as in *b*
	d. Patient can perform some but not all motions to place wheelchair and/or parts

Fig. 9-4.   Excerpt from Part I of the Lawton ADL evaluation. G, grade; T, time. L indicates an activity involving lifting. (Courtesy of Dr. Edith Lawton.)

of small increments of progress and can also function as positive feedback to the patient when visible progress is slow.

The Lawton assessment also lists any equipment that the patient uses to achieve maximal independence in each ADL task. The description of how the patient achieves maximum independence (physical assistance, time, equipment) can be of great help to nursing staff and the family to ensure follow-through of the training conditions required for independence (e.g., patient requires supervision to transfer wheelchair to toilet but can accomplish it only in a wheelchair with swing away leg rests, with a grab bar to the left of the toilet, wearing glasses, and with Velcro adaptation for trousers). The charting format allows multiple assessments to be recorded on one page, thereby

Bed to wheelchair	Start	Sitting in bed
	Time	Placing wheelchair, removing parts, locking brakes, placing necessary equipment, replacing wheelchair parts
	Finish	Sit in wheelchair, all parts replaced, feet on footrests
	NOTE:	*If helper has to place wheelchair, include in time and grade*
Wheelchair to bed	Start	Sitting in wheelchair near bed, feet on footrests
	Time	Placing wheelchair, removing parts, locking brakes; transfer, placing legs, replacing wheelchair parts
	Finish	Sit on bed

Fig. 9-5.   An example of timing in the Lawton ADL evaluation. (Courtesy of Dr. Edith Lawton.)

facilitating its use by aides and family for daily care as well as noting progress (Fig. 9-6). From the flowchart of ADL tasks an inventory is generated of equipment currently in use, any equipment that will be needed on discharge, what has been ordered, and what has been received. The rehabilitation team can use this form to assure accurate acquisition of assistive devices needed at discharge; at all times it is possible in 1 or 2 minutes to identify any outstanding or missing pieces of equipment essential for independent action.

The validity and relevance of any assessment tool is determined in the day-to-day use with patients. The Lawton form has been found to be realistic in design, layout, and length of time needed to maintain it. Its development was facilitated by practitioner criticism. The effectiveness of the Lawton ADL instrument was tested formally in a study by Willard. The goal was to examine reproducibility and reliability—agreement between the grades given by different therapists who evaluated the same patients for physical assistance, time, and equipment. The instrument was found to have high reliability in this regard. For example, for different therapists using the "wheelchair mobility" segment of the form there was 94 percent agreement in evaluation. The high percentage of agreement means that evaluation should consistently show high reproducibility from tester to tester, ensuring effective communication among practitioners.

The Lawton ADL Test is ideal for functional testing and as a base for generating a physical therapy treatment plan. The tester needs 6 to 8 hours of orientation to the form. The Lawton ADL test allows organization of large quantities of data, and several assessments can be recorded on a single page.

| | | Date: | | | Date | | |
| | | Sign: | | | Sign: | | |
Patient:		G	T	Equipment	G	T	Equipment
1	*BED:* Rolling over (L)						
2	Sitting up and reverse (L)						
3	Using signal bell						
4	Using telephone						
5	Bladder care (L)						
6	Bowel care (L)						
7	To commode chair (L)						
8	Reverse (L)						
9	*WHEELCHAIR TO:* Bed (L)						
10	Reverse						
11	Sink (wash and dry hands)						
12	Toilet (L)						
13	Shower (L)						
14	Tub (L)						
15	Car–taxi (L)						
16	Reverse						
17 (L)	Placing wheelchair into car						
18	Reverse (L)						

Fig. 9-6. Examples of grading activities involving gross body motions. This excerpt involves transfer from bed to wheelchair. (Courtesy of Dr. Edith Lawton.)

The form is concise, and the flowchart format allows quick scanning of previous and current status. The strongest argument for the use of this form, as opposed to individual practitioners attempting to design their own forms, is that it has been tested for reliability and validity. The Lawton instrument, used as a starting point for planning physical therapy care of the aged, promotes humane care for a fragile population because it can measure small increments of improvement. It thus increases the motivation of the patient to work hard to increasing function. Evaluation must consider patient age, disabilities, and cause of those disabilities as well as emotional needs. The Lawton ADL test is designed to provide a testing environment and approach that considers the unique abilities and needs of the elderly. It is constructed to allow the amount of detail necessary to effectively evaluate and monitor the *slow* but *possible* progress as the elderly go through a process of rehabilitation.

THE PROCESS OF ASSESSMENT

Specific considerations that the physical therapist can implement in order to allow an elderly patient to perform as effectively as possible on the CFA could include preassessment planning and assessment considerations.

Preassessment Planning

1. The patient is oriented by oral and written input to the purpose of the assessment (e.g., the physician/nurse leaves a pamphlet describing activities as they generally relate to this patient).
2. The patient is given the maximum amount of control in scheduling the appointment (e.g., Do you prefer early morning or afternoon appointments?).
3. The patient is oriented as to requirements for clothes, shoes, and such needed during assessment.
4. If the patient is not independently mobile (walking or in a wheelchair), the initial assessment will begin in the patient's room if the patient is comfortable in the room and will focus on all aspects needed to teach mobility skill, as soon as possible.
5. The patient is helped as is needed to groom and dress to his or her habitual standard.
6. The patient is offered assistance as needed to go to the restroom before the assessment starts.
7. The patient is offered a glass of water as needed.
8. If the assessment is not in the patient's room, the patient self-propels to the site of assessment (walking or in a wheelchair) accompanied by an aide. (If the patient is unable to self-propel, the first assessment is in the patient's room.)
9. The patient is oriented to the environment (where the restroom and water fountain are, how to call for assistance, etc.,) and if possible has

companionship of an aide until the assessment can start (this allows the patient to pose questions and become familiar with the environment). One primary task the aide attends to is the patient's level of preferred visual and auditory privacy and needed level of lighting.

Assessment Considerations

- Practitioner bias will affect patient outcomes. Yearly attendance at continuing education courses will increase self-awareness of personal attitudes and value system. The attitude of therapeutic interaction involves unconditional acceptance of the patient and avoids value judging (e.g., age bias).
- The patient self-description of the situation is the starting point for the assessment and is focused in the present with historical data recorded as it is significant.
- The patient is encouraged to take responsibility for participation in the assessment. Periodically, check with the patient to be sure that he or she is comfortable.
- The patient sets the pace.
- The patient's interest in the assessment is a direct process.
- The patient's ease (emotional and physical) is a controlling factor that influences the progress of the assessment.
- All assessment data are reported to the patient in statements about what is functioning (regardless of how data are recorded for clinicians use).
- Questions are posed to the patient, and the patient is given time to interpret them.

As assessment proceeds, all questions are posed to promote the urge to do for oneself and to increase self-awareness. For example,

- How does this feel to you—better, worse, or about the same?
- Does this feel natural to you? If not, how would you prefer to do it?

At the end of the assessment:

- Ask the patient if there are any questions.
- Ask the patient to describe what he or she has experienced.
- If a home program has been given, as a last review session, ask the patient to demonstrate how he or she is going to carry out the program.
- Set the time for the next appointment by posing options for the patient.

Assessment is an interpersonal interaction. If it is carried out with respect for the patient's physical/cognitive/emotional needs, it is likely that it will set a tone for all the rehabilitation intervention, so that the patient will choose to participate (be motivated).

REFERENCES

1. Besdine R: The educational utility of comprehensive functional assessment in the elderly. J Am Geriatr Soc 31:651–656, 1983
2. Rubenstein L: The clinical effectiveness of multidimensional geriatric assessment. J Am Geriatr Soc 31:758-762, 1983
3. Rowe J: Health care of the elderly. N Engl J Med 312:827–835, 1985
4. Linn R, Linn B: The rapid disability rating scale. J Am Geriatr Soc 30:378–381, 1982
5. Rubenstein L: Specialized geriatric assessment units and their clinical implications. West J Med 135:497–502, 1981
6. Kane RA, Kane RL: Assessing the Elderly: A Practical Guide to Measurement. Lexington Books, Lexington, MA, 1981
7. Warshaw GA, Moore JT, Friedman W: Functional disability in the hospitalized elderly. JAMA 248:847–850, 1982
8. Commission on Chronic Illness: Chronic Illness in the United States, Vol 4, Chronic Illness in a Large City, The Baltimore Study. Harvard University Press, Cambridge, MA, 1975
9. Sherwood S: Long term care issues, perspectives and directions. p. 3. In Sherwood S (ed): Long Term Care: A Handbook for Researchers, Planners and Providers. Spectrum, New York, 1975
10. Rhode Island Health Services Research, Inc. (SEARCH): Profiles from the Health Statistics Center, Series 4, No. 1, Results of the 1972 and 1975 Health Interview Surveys, 1977
11. Lawton EB: ADL: Activities of Daily Living Test, A New Form. Rehabilitation Monograph No. 57, Institute of Rehabilitation Medicine, New York University Medical Center, New York, 1979
12. Aniansson A: Muscle function in old age with special reference to muscle morphology, effect of training and capacity in daily living. Thesis, Departments of Rehabilitation Medicine and Geriatric and Long-Term Care Medicine, University of Goteborg, Sweden, 1980
13. Jette AM, Branch LG: The Framingham Disability Study: II. Physical Disability among the Aging. Am J Public Health 71:No. 11, 1981
14. Branch LG: Understanding the Health and Social Service Needs of People over Age 65. Center for Survey Research of the University of Massachusetts and the Joint Center for Urban Studies of MIT and Harvard University, Cambridge, MA, 1977
15. Aniansson A, Rundgren A, Sperling L: Evaluation of functional capacity in activities of daily living in 70-year-old men and women. Scand J Rehabil Med 12(4):145–154, 1980
16. Hook O, Nordquist D, Magnussen K, Sjovall E: Teknik for aldringar. Styrelsen for teknisk utveckling. Utredning 27, Stockholm, 1975
17. Sperling L: Evaluation of upper extremity function in 70 year old men and women. Scand J Rehabil Med 12(4):139–144, 1980
18. Donnelly RJ: A study of the dynamometer strength of adult males ages 30 to 79. Doctoral dissertation, University of Michigan, Ann Arbor, University of Michigan Microfilm, 1664, 1953
19. Burke WE, Tuttle WW, Thompson CW, et al: The relation of grip strength and grip strength endurance to age. J Appl Physiol 5:628, 1953
20. Asmussen E, Heeboll-Nielsen K: Isometric strength of adult men and women. Communications from the Testing and Observation Institute of the Danish National Association for Infantile Paralysis, vol. 11, 1961

21. Carroll D: A quantitative test of upper extremity function. J Chronic Dis 18:479, 1965

22. Petrofsky JS, Lind AR: Isometric strength, endurance and the blood pressure and heart rate responses during isometric exercise in healthy men and women with special reference to age and body fat content. Pfluegers Arch 360:49, 1975

23. Lautso K: Jalankulkuliikennie, ominaisuuksia ja teoriaa. Liikennetekniikka OY, Helsinki, 1971

24. Ayalon A, von Gheluwe B: A comparison study of some mechanical variables from daily life activities in elderly and young people. In Physical Exercise and Activities for the Ageing. Proceedings of an International Seminar. Wingate Institute of Physical Education and Sport, 1975

25. Peszcynski M: Senile Gait. Restorative Medicine in Geriatrics. Charles C Thomas, Springfield IL, 1963

26. Hasselkus BR, Shambes GM: Aging and postural sway in women. J Gerontol 30:661, 1975

27. Azar GJ, Lawton AH: Gait and stepping as factors in the frequent falls of elderly women. Gerontologist 4:83, 1964

28. Rosow I, Breslau H: A Guttman health scale for the aged. Gerontologist 21:556, 1966

29. Shanas E: Self-assessment of physical function: White and black elderly of the United States. In Haynes SG, et al. (eds): Second Conference on the Epidemiology of Aging. U.S. Department of Health and Human Services, NIH Pub. No. 80-969, Bethseda, MD, 1980

30. Uhlenberg P: Changing structure of the older population of the United States of America during the twentieth century. Gerontologist 17:197, 1977

31. Barry J: Pro/con: Rehabilitation of the aging. J Rehabil 46:3, 1980(b)

32. Benedict RC, Ganikos ML: Coming to terms with ageism in rehabilitation. J Rehabil 47:4, 1981

33. Blake R: Disabled older persons: A demographic analysis. J Rehabil 47:4, 1981

34. Independent Living Research Utilization Project: Source Book. Texas Institute for Rehabilitation and Research, 1978

35. United States Department of Health Education and Welfare: New Facts About Older Americans. Administration on Aging. U.S. Government Printing Office, Washington, DC, 1973

36. The Urban Institute: Report of the Comprehensive Service Needs Study. Department of Health, Education and Welfare, Office of Human Development, Rehabilitation Services Administration, Washington, DC,1975

37. Nagi S: An Epidemiology of Adult Disability in the U.S. Mershon Center, Ohio State University, Columbus 1975

38. Rehabilitation Brief, Independent Living Rehabilitation: Results of Five Demonstration Projects. National Institute of Handicapped Research, Washington, DC, 1979

39. Driscoll J, Marquis B, Corcoran P, Fay F: Second generation: New England. Am Rehabil 3:6, 1978

40. Reid DW, Ziegler M: A desired control measure for studying the psychological adjustment of the elderly. Paper presented at the symposium on Goal-Specific Locus of Control Scale—A New Step in I-E Research held at the meeting of the American Psychology Association, Toronto, Sept 1978

41. Umphred D: Neurological Rehabilitation. 2nd Ed. CV Mosby, St. Louis, 1989

42. Boll TJ: A rationale for neuropsychological evaluation. Prof Psychol 8:64, 1977

43. Center for the Study of Aging and Human Development: Multidimensional Functional Assessment: The OARS Methodology. 2nd ed. Duke University Medical Center. Durham, NC, 1978

44. Fortinsky RH, Granger CV, Seltzer GB: The use of functional assessment in understanding home care needs. Med Care 19:5, 1981

45. Stewart CPU: A prediction score for geriatric rehabilitation prospects. Rheumatol Rehabil 19:239, 1980

46. Kahn RL, Goldberg AI: The relationship of mental and physical status in institutionalized aged persons. Am J Psychol 117:120, 1960

47. Pinholt EM, Kroenke K, Hanley JF, et al: Functional assessment of the elderly—a comparison of standard instruments with clinical judgment. Arch Intern Med 147(3):484–488, 1987

48. Magid S, Hearn CR: Characteristics of geriatric patients as related to nursing needs. J Nurs Studies 18:2, 1981

49. Adler MK, Brown CC, Acton P: Stroke rehabilitation—Is age a determinant? J Am Geriatr Soc 28:11, 1980

50. Hall MRP: The assessment of disability in the geriatric patient. Rheumatol Rehabil 15, 1976

51. Carroll D: In Nichols PJR (ed): Proceedings of a Symposium on the Motivation of the Physically Disabled. 1968

52. Report by the Comptroller General to the Congress: Entering a Nursing Home—Costly Implications for Medicaid and the Elderly. U.S. Government Printing Office. Washington, DC, PAD-80-12, Nov 29, 1979

53. Currie CT, Moore JT, Friedmen SW, Warshaw GA: Assessment of elderly patients at home: report of 50 cases. J Am Geriatr Soc 29:9, 1981

54. Tickle LS, Yerxa EJ: Need satisfaction of older persons living in the community and in institutions. Part 2, Role of activity. Am J Occup Ther 35:10, 1981

55. Developing Comprehensive and Coordinated Service Systems for Older People: Lessons from the Nebraska Demonstration. Project funded by the Administration of Aging, Office of Human Development, Department of Health and Human Services. Grant No. 90-A-1968

56. Hicks BC, Segal J, Quinn JL, Raisz H: Triage: Coordinated Services to the Elderly. Final Report. National Technical Information Service, Springfield, VA, Pub. Order PB-135-824

57. Future Directions for Aging Policy: A Human Service Model. A Report of the Select Committee on Aging, U.S. House of Representatives, Ninety-sixth Congress. Comm. Publ. No. 96-226, U.S. Government Printing Office, Washington, DC, May 1980

58. Weed LL: Medical Records, Medical Evaluation and Patient Care. Case Western Reserve University Press, Cleveland, 1971

59. Buchwald-Lawton E: ADL—Activities of Daily Living: A New Form. New York University Medical Center, Institute of Rehabilitation Medicine, New York, 1979

Index

Page numbers followed by f indicate figures; page numbers followed by t indicate tables